LESS-TOXIC ALTERNATIVES

~ Revised Edition ~

By Carolyn Gorman
with Marie Hyde

PUBLISHED BY
OPTIMUM PUBLISHING
TEXARKANA, TEXAS

Dedication

The increased incidence of environmental sensitivity and allergies is in direct proportion to the increased usage of chemicals in our daily lives. This book is dedicated to the awareness of the toxicity of specific and excessive chemical exposure and to the provision of Less-Toxic Alternatives.

We want to thank all who have had a part in the development of this work, and we pledge my continued research of *Less-Toxic Alternatives* for the development of a healthy lifestyle.

Sincerely,
Carolyn Gorman & Marie Hyde

LESS-TOXIC ALTERNATIVES
~ Revised Edition ~

Replaces *Less-Toxic Alternatives* – First Edition
Which replaced *Less-Toxic Living* – Sixth Edition
Second Printing – May 2002

See 2002 Updates on pages 252-253

Cover photo by Bill Gorman *(used by permission)*
Treasure Falls (West of Wolf Creek Ski Area), Colorado

ISBN #1-57397-015-8
Printed in the United States of America

PUBLISHED BY

OPTIMUM PUBLISHING

P.O. BOX 7435 ~ TEXARKANA, TX 75505
www.optimumpublishing.com   e-mail: gorman@optimumpublishing.com

Bobby A. Mohler
965 Seabrook
Waldport, OR

Contents

> > < <

Introduction

The future of the world depends on you. You are the answer to the health of your family and your world. To make intelligent decisions, you must have correct information. We hope to provide you with the knowledge that enables you to make health-wise decisions. We have provided information about possible problems and submitted Less-Toxic Alternatives for your selection.

The items mentioned for *"Avoidance"* are known or suggested to contain volatile organic compounds, aldehydes, pesticides, herbicides, dyes, scents and/or inks. Those interested in the stewardship of our world or a healthy lifestyle should avoid their use. Likewise, those with sensitivities, neurological or breathing problems, older adults and the very young should avoid or minimize the use of known toxins that can adversely affect health. Alternatives should be selected which offer reduced risk to you and your world.

We have found the items offered as *"Less-Toxic Alternatives"* to be tolerated by the majority of people. We believe these items contain fewer undesirable substances; however, not everyone tolerates all products. We can thus make no guarantees that all these items will be safe and effective for you. Individuals must make their own selections in regard to their individual sensitivities. Everyone is encouraged to test all products before making decisions regarding their safe usage.

The information provided covers several areas, all of which are related to daily living: food, personal needs, household cleaning agents, building or home maintenance, natural insect control, office needs, and air and water purification.

> < <

KNOWLEDGE ENABLES YOU TO MAKE HEALTHY CHOICES

RECOGNIZE EXPOSURE SOURCES
Chemicals ~ Pesticides ~ Climate Control Systems,
Building & Maintenance ~ Diet ~ Allergen Control
RECOGNIZE YOUR RESPONSE
RECOGNIZE MEDICAL OPTIONS
& REACH OPTIMAL HEALTH

> < <

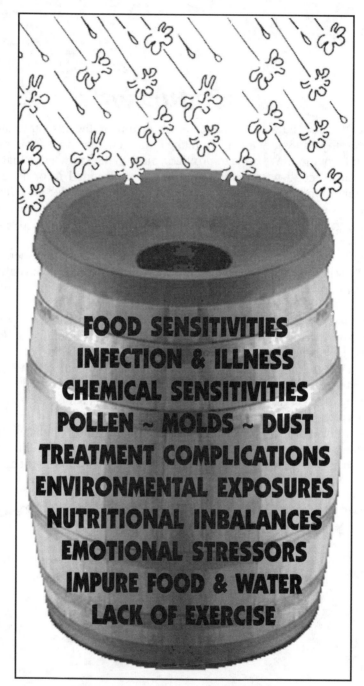

FOOD SENSITIVITIES
INFECTION & ILLNESS
CHEMICAL SENSITIVITIES
POLLEN ~ MOLDS ~ DUST
TREATMENT COMPLICATIONS
ENVIRONMENTAL EXPOSURES
NUTRITIONAL INBALANCES
EMOTIONAL STRESSORS
IMPURE FOOD & WATER
LACK OF EXERCISE

Illustration 1: The Rainbarrel Effect
Your total body stressors can be compared to a rainbarrel. When your rain barrel overflows, your immune system is compromised, and illness may result.

Less-Toxic Alternatives

Part I: Understanding Environmental Sensitivity

The twentieth century will be remembered as a century of phenomenal achievements for mankind. Advances in engineering, chemistry, and other sciences enabled mankind to soar to outer space. Satellites orbiting our shrinking earth now link communications, once limited by wires. Electricity has progressed from kite string to atomic fission. Advanced computer technology has revolutionized the marketplace and opened the windows of the world to school children and adults alike. Agriculture, once bound to horse and plow and earth, now encompasses sophisticated mechanized equipment, hybrids, grafts, chemicals, and irrigation. Medicine, once challenged by the bubonic plague and smallpox, now encompasses laser surgery, computerized body imaging, and transplanted organs.

The wonders of our victories are amazing, and the human race seems limited only by its imagination. However, the discoveries and miracles of progress may be proceeding too rapidly. Rapid change has stressed the social, economic, and cultural fibers of our society; and the resources of our earth. Over-population, the irresponsible use of the earth's resources, and total disregard for the eco-system's delicate balance have created problems that require the genius of mankind for solution.

For many, these advances make life in today's world exciting, rewarding, bountiful, and fulfilling. However, for an increasing number of individuals, daily life on our shrinking planet is a continual struggle to remain healthy. These people are victims of the rapid changes that have taken place since the early 1900's. Their struggle is with their environment; their condition is called environmental illness.

Environmental Sensitivity is a relatively new term that better identifies what has, for many years, been called an allergy heightened sensitivity acquired through exposure to a particular allergenic substance with re-exposure causing an altered capacity to react.

> > < <

Causes of Environmental Illness

This new illness is a result of the body's overactive immune response to seemingly innocuous substances which are perceived by the body as a threat to continued good health. These may be inhalants (pollen, dust, or mold), food, water or chemicals; and the symptoms are a result of the interplay of the body's reaction to the many forms of physical and psychological stress affecting it. The condition reflects the unique metabolic characteristics and nutritional status of the body, the biological individuality and genetic background, and the integrity of the body's immune and enzyme systems. This concept of multiplicity of factors contributing to the body's total stress load is illustrated by the rain barrel effect on page 8.

Equally as important as the immune reaction is the uniqueness of each person's biological makeup. Differences that exist in the number and action of bodily enzymes can create considerable variations in the ability to metabolize and utilize nutrients, to detoxify chemicals, and to respond to offending inhalants. Inadequate blood levels and disordered cellular balance of necessary nutrients are important factors affecting multiple sensitivities and perhaps auto-immune reactions.

Forty million Americans have pollen sensitivities, and an additional twenty million have adverse food reactions. Many more may have either food or pollen sensitivities, but are not aware of them because of the "masking" effect. For example: if a person eats beef occasionally, he or she may notice a runny nose or coughing after ingestion of the beef. However, if the food is eaten daily, symptoms may not be noticeable, illness may develop, and the person may be totally unaware of any systemic response to the offending food. Sneezing, runny nose, watery eyes, sinus pain and pressure, and asthma are common symptoms of the inhalant sensitive. Indigestion, joint pain, headaches, diarrhea, nausea, depression, and even asthma can often be linked to food sensitivity.

These varied symptoms may occur as a vigorous response to naturally occurring substances encountered every day. Food, pollen, dust, and mold existed for ages and are not unique to the world today; however, there is another aspect of environmental illness that enhances the body's response to food, air and water. This is the body's reaction to innumerable chemicals that increasingly permeate our world. The presence of man-made chemicals in air, food, water, and soil is an unnatural addition to the natural environment and is a major factor in the development of a complex pattern of illnesses.

Dr. Theron Randolph, a Chicago physician, first identified Environmental Illness (EI) in the late 1950s. Its presence and recognition have paralleled the industrial, technological, and chemical revolutions that began in America in the early 1940s.

Environmental Illness does not discriminate regarding age, sex, or ethnic origin; but those with pre-existing sensitivities to pollen, dust, mold and food are certainly at risk. Like traditional allergies, this type of reactivity to environmental triggers is sometimes an inherited familial tendency. Because of their continuing immune response, sensitive patients may lack the reserve to deal effectively with the growing list of environmental chemicals to which they are exposed.

Individuals who have inadequate nutritional status may be susceptible to illness of an unexpected magnitude. Persons who have difficulty absorbing

Less-Toxic Alternatives

nutrients and are unable to maintain the proper balance of minerals (storing some and excreting others) may develop serious health problems. This imbalance of vitamins and minerals frequently stresses the immune and enzyme systems of the body. This can then contribute to an individual's developing multiple sensitivities and progressing to other symptoms of environmental illness.

Occupational exposures to synthetic chemicals can also make some individuals more susceptible to environmental illness. People who are acutely or chronically exposed to hydrocarbons found in paints, plastics, solvents, degreasers and glues are prime candidates for developing sensitivities to these and other chemicals. Aldehydes, alcohols, acetones, ketones, pesticides, fungicides and herbicides are examples of other chemicals that can precipitate environmental illness.

Life in today's world can be very stressful. These stresses originate from many sources, and can produce various problems. There are the mental stresses of everyday living such as the pressures of job, traffic, money, child rearing and marriage. There are also the emotional stresses that emerge from such events as the death of a loved one or the death of a marriage. Diseases such as infections and environmental reactions also stress our vigilant immunoglobulins that are an essential component of our immune response.

An unparalleled stress is that of insidious and undetected chemical exposure. The effort required by the enzyme detoxification system as it tries to metabolize environmental toxins, protect cells and tissue from attack, and maintain healthy organ function is indeed stressful. Sometimes individuals who are limited by their own biological uniqueness and weakened by the stresses of today's world cannot maintain the delicate balance. They become victims of environmental illness.

> > < <

Symptoms of Environmental Illness

Unfortunately, individuals suffering from this condition do not always have symptoms characteristic of a specific disease process. Symptoms are as varied as the incitants. Sometimes, because of the phenomenon known as masking, an individual may be adapted to the presence of some stressor, but be unaware of the effect it produces. In this way, many people fail to perceive the cause and effect relationship between the substance and symptom. It has been estimated that as much as sixty percent of all illness may be linked to or influenced by these environmental triggers.

The organ targeted by the illness is not necessarily specified by definition. It may be the lungs or the heart, the brain or the liver, or any combination of organs. The condition may affect the bone marrow, blood vessels, colon, or the joints and muscles. In some instances, symptoms of environmental illness may not be limited to organ response alone, but may become a condition involving the entire body.

Headache, arthritis, joint pain, muscle spasms or pain, indigestion, difficulty breathing, runny nose, itchy eyes and skin, sinus pain and pressure, asthma, hay fever, gastrointestinal upset, arrhythmias, central nervous system distress, hyperactivity, learning problems, depression, vasculitis and anemia may all be symptoms of environmental sensitivities. It is no wonder that overwhelming fatigue of mind, body, and the immune, enzyme, and detoxification systems is the chief characteristic of environmental illness.

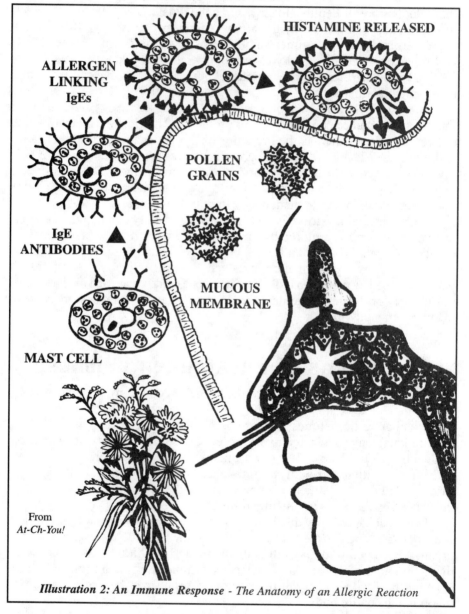

Illustration 2: An Immune Response - The Anatomy of an Allergic Reaction

Allergens & Contaminants

Illustration 2 *(previous page)* shows the dynamics of an IgE mediated immune response. However, an allergy can also be T-cell directed, with mediation through IgG and the complement cascade; or through the circulation of immune complexes, a combination of antigen and antibody.

Allergens can be any of the following:

Pollens: weed, tree, or grass and must be light, buoyant, numerous, and possess a special chemical or allergenic nature.

Molds: A mold is a Thallophyte or the lowest member of the plant kingdom. Molds have no chlorophyll, no stem, leaves, or flowers. They do not make their own food. Molds are everywhere.

Dust and Dust Mites: Household dust contains many allergens including feces of microscopic dust mites.

Foods: The most common food offenders are eggs, corn, cow's milk, baker's and brewer's yeast, wheat, and cow's milk.

Chemicals: Hydrocarbons, aldehydes, and chlorine are common chemical allergens. These and many others are found in cleaning products, paints/varnishes, pesticides/herbicides and even in clothing, furnishings, food and water.

Smuts: mold-like substance on grass and grains

Terpenes: organic aromatic hydrocarbon with the chemical formulation $C_{10}H_{16}$ – smell of pine, sage, cedar, etc.

Fabrics: cotton, linen, wool, silk or synthetics

> > < <

Pollens

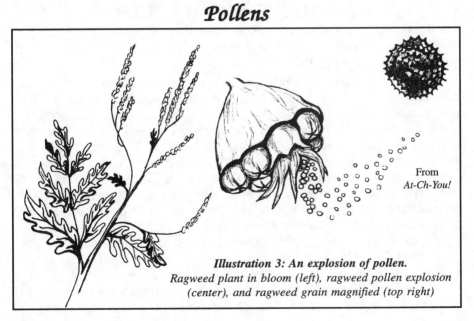

From
At-Ch-You!

Illustration 3: An explosion of pollen.
Ragweed plant in bloom (left), ragweed pollen explosion
(center), and ragweed grain magnified (top right)

Revised Edition

13

Pollen is the male reproductive cells or microspores of flowering plants, which is produced by and discharged from the plant. Many airborne pollens are proteins capable of sensitizing persons and producing allergic type symptoms. Pollen can be large or small, heavy or light, and is carried by the wind or by bees and other insects from anthers to stigma for fertilization and reproduction. Plants that depend on insects for pollination are less apt to cause allergic reactions than those that are wind pollinated.

Forty million Americans suffer from some form of allergy that usually includes pollens. These can be diagnosed through skin and blood tests. Pollen allergies depend on the chemical composition, the buoyancy and abundance of pollen. One-quarter of a million plants use the wind as a vehicle for cross-pollination and produce pollen dust clouds of generally small, dry, smooth, uniform, light and buoyant grains. The wind can carry them for miles to their destination. Airborne weed, tree, and grass pollens in spring, summer and fall are most closely associated with pollinosis.

Pollen is the miracle of life for plants and a hoped-for miracle for man. It is used in archeology to reveal vegetation, climate and customs of ancient man; in oil exploration to pinpoint drilling accuracy; and pollen grains representative of plants in a certain area have aided in crime solving. Pollen is important in genetic engineering of plants and was used by American Indians and other cultures in special ceremonies. Pollen supplements are sold to improve a runner's competitive edge and an immune system's vitality. Additional pollen is harvested for use in immuno-therapeutic allergy extracts to treat allergies. Even though pollen is a blessing to many, it can also be a curse to those who respond to it with

A WHEEZE OR A SNEEZE!

Blood and skin testing can determine pollen allergies. The history of symptom occurrence can also be a guide to defining pollen allergies.

TREATMENT OPTIONS

Individuals need to be knowledgeable about various treatment options and, with their doctor's help, choose those options that are best suited for them. Immunotherapy often provides the most effective, long-term relief for the allergic patient. Medications for the allergic patient include Nasalcrom (Cromolyn Sodium), Seldane, Hismanal, Sudafed and Benadryl. Alternative and homeopathic treatments are also available. Vitamins, minerals and herbs can often promote health and reduce symptoms (see Supplements on page 64).

Environmental Controls that help fight pollen allergies include HEPA (High Efficiency Particulate Arresting) or electrostatic air filtration and portable air purifiers. A filtration mask made with cotton or silk material and containing a charcoal filter can be helpful with pollen exposure whenever it becomes necessary to go outside on a high pollen count day. A 3-M high efficiency mask is most efficient, removing 99.97% at .3 microns.

You should be aware of local daily pollen count (the number of grains per cubic yard of air), and be alert to days when your particular allergens are most prominent. Carefully plan your outdoor activities for low pollen days to minimize exposure to high pollen counts. Known allergens should be removed from your yard.

Certain foods are concomitant or interactive with pollen sensitivities. For example: during ragweed and elm pollinating seasons, milk consumption may produce allergic symptoms; likewise, an allergy to cedar can enhance an allergic reaction to beef and brewer's or baker's yeast; while sage may enhance a reaction to potatoes. *(Also see list of Concomitant Foods on page 19)*

> >< <

Mold

Mold is a simple plant of the fungus group with no leaves, stems, or flowers, and no chlorophyll or green coloring matter. Molds can appear as blue, black, green or white and can be microscopic or grow to be over two feet in diameter.

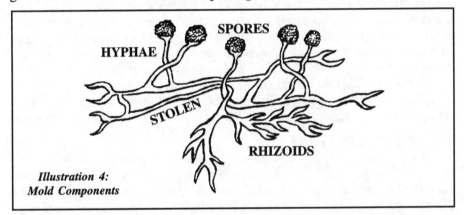

Illustration 4:
Mold Components

Molds can live anywhere (in water, soil or the air, on plants, and in man and animals). Molds especially like to live in cool, damp, dark places such as the refrigerator drip pan, garbage pails, bathrooms, humidifiers, and central air ducts. They also choose gardens, houseplants, compost piles and sewage sludge; and find fruits, breads and cheeses a friendly host.

Any organic material that remains wet for 24 hours (drywall, carpet, or fabrics, for example) is likely to result in fungal growth.

Molds cannot produce their own food, so they are parasitic in nature. Molds get food by absorbing minerals, sugars and water from the plants, soil, animals or decaying matter upon which they live.

Molds are important in medicine, fermentation, fertilization of soil, and in the production of some foods. Mold is everywhere!

Mold can also cause allergy and illness. Some molds cause fungal diseases of the skin, nails, ears and lungs. Other molds cause allergy symptoms that can include sneezing, wheezing, joint pain, muscle ache, headache, fatigue, depression, itching, hives and rashes and digestive distress. Mold symptoms can be flu-like in nature.

Molds far outnumber pollens as part of the total airborne allergy count. There are many different mold offenders, but the most common molds are Alternaria, Aspergillus, Cladosporium and Sporobolomyes. These peak at various times in various regions; i.e. Alternaria generally peaks in the fall, but is a problem from June through November in the Midwest. Thus different molds may be causing you problems during different seasons of the year, much like pollen's seasonal cycles.

Studies have shown a relationship between dampness and mold and nausea, blocked nose, breathlessness, high blood pressure and nervousness. According to one study, children living in moldy dwellings have a greater prevalence of wheeze, sore throat, runny nose, cough, headache, and fever. Recent outbreaks of unexplained infant respiratory problems and skin reactions have been traced by health care investigators to mold growing in basements or other water damaged areas of their homes. Stachybotrys atra (found on water-damaged ceiling tiles and sheetrock/wallboard) can be deadly to infants and young children. In a study conducted at Georgia Tech University, molds were found to emit volatile organic compounds that are known to cause disease and health problems upon repeated inhalation. Mold contamination is serious contamination.

A mold-related problem can be discovered through blood and skin testing, symptom response, and environmental history. Mold testing plates and air quality tests can identify and enumerate types of molds present in indoor air.

TREATMENT OPTIONS

Individuals need to be knowledgeable about various treatment options and, with their doctor's help, choose those options that are best suited for them. Immunotherapy often provides the most effective, long-term relief for the allergic patient. Medications for the allergic patient include Nasalcrom (Cromolyn Sodium), Seldane, Hismanal, Sudafed, and Benadryl. Alternative and homeopathic treatments are also available. Vitamins, minerals and herbs can often promote health and reduce symptoms *(see Supplements on page 64)*.

Environmental Controls are very important to individuals who are sensitive to molds. Exhaust fans, air filtration and purification, dehumidification, and the cleaning of air conditioner coils and ducts are vital factors in the control of mold growth. Maintaining proper humidity levels (50% or less) and the use of light and ventilation help prevent mold growth.

It is important to keep kitchens, bathroom and closets mold free and clean. Because the dirt in houseplants is a breeding ground for mold, they should be kept to a minimum or completely eliminated from the inside environment. Yards should be kept clean and mold free. Care should be taken in the use of fungicides and mold retardants because some contain toxic chemicals. Vinegar should not be used as a cleaning agent by those allergic to molds.

A Low-Mold Diet includes avoidance of mushrooms, dried fruits and products containing vinegar (such as mustard, ketchup and salad dressings). Cook and peel all root vegetables, roast all nuts, and minimize contact with yeast. **A Four-Day Rotation Diet**, where foods are eaten only once every four days and food families every two days, minimizes allergen contact.

Care must be taken when storing baker's yeast, vegetables, fruits, cheeses, nuts and grains. Fruits and vegetables can be washed in hydrogen peroxide and grapefruit seed extract to remove mold spores.

> > < <

Dust Mites

Illustration 5 – Dust Mites
European Mite (left), D. farinae (center), and Predatory Mite (right)

Dust mites are microscopic members of the Arachnid family and are second cousins to ticks and chiggers. The most common dust mites in homes and offices of North America are D. farinae and D. pteronyssinus.

They live in our homes and offices, and are found primarily in our carpets, draperies, bedding, mattresses, pillows, upholstered furniture, books and dust. They thrive in an environment that includes high humidity and warm temperatures.

Dust mites eat microscopic fungi and are especially fond of human and animal skin scales that they find in abundance in upholstery, carpet and bedding.

Their secret weapon is their abundant population and alarming reproductive rate. Although they live only three weeks, during that time each produce 25-50 babies, and each mite produces 10-20 fecal particles per day.

Dust mites and their waste particles can produce severe allergic reactions in individuals. Symptoms can include ear infections, runny noses, itchy eyes, wheezing, sneezing, etc. If you experience these symptoms, blood and skin testing can determine the cause.

TREATMENT OPTIONS

Individuals need to be knowledgeable about various treatment options and, with their doctor's help, choose those options that are best suited for them. Immunotherapy often provides the most effective, long-term relief for the allergic patient. Medications for the allergic patient include Nasalcrom (Cromolyn Sodium), Seldane, Hismanal, Sudafed and Benadryl. Alternative and homeopathic treatments are also available. Vitamins, minerals and herbs can often promote health and reduce symptoms (see Supplements on page 64).

Environmental Controls. Create a healthy inside environment for yourself and an unhealthy environment for dust mites by keeping the humidity in your office or home below 50% with a temperature around 65 to 70 degrees. They can be killed if the humidity is below 35%.

Use HEPA and electrostatic air filters, and portable air purifiers. A regularly cleaned vacuum, with a water and/or HEPA filtration system, removes dust mites and particulates from floor, air and furnishings. Several good systems are available *(see Air Handling on page 107)*.

The bedroom is an area where dust mites proliferate. To destroy the mite's happy home, clean thoroughly with Tannic Acid or Eucalyptus oil. Clean the closets regularly and keep them uncluttered. Use washable barrier cloth covers for mattresses and pillows, and wash regularly. Dust mites can be destroyed in bedding by washing at temperatures over 140 degrees for 20 minutes. Use mini blinds instead of draperies, and either steam clean carpets regularly or replace with wood, tile or safe vinyl flooring. Dust catchers, books, and clutter should be banned from the bedroom.

> > < <

Food Reactivity

There are three different ways in which individuals react to foods – allergies, sensitivities and intolerances. Food allergies can also be affected by mold, pollen or dust sensitivities.

These allergic reactions are mediated by immune globulin E (IgE), the white blood cells most generally associated with allergic responses. This type of reaction is immediate and can lead to anaphylaxis.

Sensitivities are related to white blood cells, IgG and IgM antibodies with complement activation or to the formation of immune complexes (antigen and antibody mediate these reactions) with platelet and complement activation. These sensitivities sometimes lead to delayed food reactions.

Intolerances are caused by the lack of a specific enzyme that is necessary for digestion of a particular food. Examples of this are lactose or milk intolerance, and gluten or grain intolerance.

The symptoms of food reactions are individual in nature and include nausea, diarrhea, headache, muscle and joint pain, hyperactivity, skin irritations, respiratory problems, depression, sinus and nose irritation and throat swelling. Some reactions can be quite severe, and acute cases can lead to anaphylaxis.

Food reactivity may be indicated if you have a history of symptoms when exposed to certain foods. This may be confirmed through allergy skin testing (scratch or intradermal) for specific food reactivity. Nutritional analysis and vitamin/mineral assessment or a rotary elimination diet may provide useful information. Other diagnostic tools may include blood testing to determine lack of specific enzymes; RAST testing for IgE, IgG levels of sensitivity response; or ELISA/ACT testing for delayed food sensitivity reactions.

Food reactions may be caused or increased by untreated food and inhalant allergies, or past chemical exposures. They may also be related to dyes, preservatives, pesticides, or improper food preparation. Enzyme depletion, parasite or bacterial infestations, extensive and/or prolonged antibiotic usage, GI or abdominal surgery, or bowel disease may also complicate food reactions.

CONCOMITANT FOODS

Sensitivity to a mold, pollen, dust or chemical can make food allergy worse or create a food allergy when none existed. Eating the food during exposure to the concomitant item can increase allergic reactions.

Cedar	Beef, Baker's & Brewer's Yeast
Cottonwood	Wheat, Tea
Dust	Nuts
Elm	Chocolate, Lettuce
Goosefoot	Egg
Grass	Legumes
Latex (rubber)*	Banana, Kiwi, Avocado
Marsh Elder	Wheat
Oak	Egg, Apple
Pecan	Corn, Banana
Pigweed	Pork
Ragweed	Milk
Sage	Potatoes

Used extensively around medical facilities

TREATMENT OPTIONS

Individuals with food reactions usually suffer from specific nutritional deficiencies. After a proper nutritional analysis, a hypoallergenic regimen of vitamins and minerals can be beneficial in restoring a proper balance.

Food antigens can sometimes be utilized for the treatment of specific food reactions as established through blood or skin testing.

You should reduce exposure to dyes, preservatives, pesticides and other chemicals in foods by eating only organically grown food. Use only filtered or glass bottled spring water for drinking and cooking.

Since most individuals who experience food reactions usually suffer from other environmental sensitivities, it is recommended that individuals who are health wise and conscious of multiple health risks choose only stainless steel, enamel, iron, ceramic and/or glass cookware for cooking. Glass or cellophane is recommended for freezing and storing foods. It is best to prepare foods by boiling, steaming, baking or frying in their own or a non-allergenic oil.

It is important to eliminate from your diet foods that have proven to cause serious reactions. The most common reactions are usually caused by cow's milk, eggs, sugar, corn, wheat, and baker's and brewer's yeast.

After avoiding problem foods for a period of time, the body often develops a tolerance for them, and they can be individually reintroduced into the diet over a period of time. Reintroduction of foods should always follow a rotational diet plan. Your physician should be consulted before any attempt is made to reintroduce foods that produced severe reactions.

Plan your meals according to a rotational diet plan where the same food item is not eaten more often than once every four days. This helps in the management of food reactions in two ways:

1. A rotational diet helps you determine to which foods you react. It allows you to compare good and bad days with the foods you have eaten on those days. In this manner you can more easily determine the culprit food(s). In extreme cases, food families must also be rotated.

2. A rotational diet helps prevent the development of new food allergies caused by patients regularly substituting a new food for a problem food (i.e.: substituting orange juice daily for milk often leads to sensitivity to orange juice). This can often be eliminated by the rotational diet because no food is used more than once every four days. Two excellent rotational diets books are:

If It's Tuesday, It Must be Chicken by N. Golos & F. G. Golbitz. New Canaan, CT: Keats Publ., Inc., 1983. *(Available at health food and bookstores).*

Rotational Bon Appetit by Stephanie Bauer and Barbara Maynard. Dallas: Environmental Health Center, 1986. *(Available from AEHF)*

PARTIAL SAMPLE ROTATION DIET						
SUN	MON	TUES	WED	THURS	FRI	SAT
		1 LIST 1	2 LIST 2	3 LIST 3	4 LIST 4	5 LIST 1
6 LIST 2	7 LIST 3	8 LIST 4	9 LIST 1	10 LIST 2	11 LIST 3	12 LIST 4
13 LIST 1	14 LIST 2	15 LIST 3	16 LIST 4	17 LIST 1	18 LIST 2	19 LIST 3
20 LIST 4	21 LIST 1	22 LIST 2	23 LIST 3	24 LIST 4	25 LIST 1	26 LIST 2
27 LIST 3	28 LIST 4	29 LIST 1	30 LIST 2	31 LIST 3		

LIST 1
Protein: venison, pork, duck, catfish, tuna or halibut
Vegetables: broccoli, cabbage, yellow squash or pumpkin
Fruits: cantaloupe, grapefruit, grapes, raisins or limes
Flours/Cereals: wheat, bran, rice, millet, milo or spelt
Nuts: pumpkin or sunflower seeds, cashews or coconut
Fats/Oils: sunflower, canola, grapeseed or coconut
Sweeteners: sorghum, rice syrup or date sugars
Beverages: rice, coconut or cashew milk; chamomile tea; or juices from fruits/
    vegetables lists

LIST 2
Protein: chicken, pheasant, lamb, salmon, shark or shrimp
Vegetables: onion, asparagus, sweet potatoes, lentils, beets, carrots, eggplant,
    green beans or soybeans
Fruits: banana, apricot, plum, prune, pears or cherries
Flours/Cereals: amaranth, soy or arrowroot

Nuts: pecans, filberts, almonds or peanuts
Fats/Oils: almond, soybean, avocado, peanut or pecan oil
Sweeteners: honey or beet sugar
Beverages: soy or goat milk or juices from fruits/vegetables lists

LIST 3

Protein: turkey, rabbit, goose, sole, haddock or whiting
Vegetables: lettuce, zucchini, artichokes, corn, cauliflower or cucumber
Fruits: blueberries, orange, lemon, figs or mangos
Flours/Cereals: corn, rye, barley, oats, wild rice or teff
Nuts: Brazil, macadamia or pistachios
Fats/Oils: corn, olive or safflower
Sweeteners: molasses, corn syrup, cane sugar or brown sugar
Beverages: tea or juices from fruits/vegetables lists

LIST 4

Protein: beef, eggs, veal, trout, lobster or cottage cheese
Vegetables: potatoes, tomatoes, peppers, spinach, pinto beans, green peas, celery or okra
Fruits: apples, pineapple, strawberries or peaches
Flours/Cereals: potato, buckwheat, tapioca or quinoa
Nuts: walnuts, sesame seeds, pinenuts or chestnuts
Fats/Oils: sesame, walnut, cottonseed, butter or flaxseed
Sweeteners: pure maple syrup
Beverages: cow's milk, mint tea or juices from fruits/vegetables lists

> > < <

 Chemicals

Chemical sensitivity is an adverse reaction to ambient levels of chemicals found in food (preservatives), air (cigarette smoke, perfume, natural gas, gasoline, and formaldehyde) or water (chlorine). The nature of the reaction depends on the substance's chemical composition, the length of exposure, the type of immune response, the person's biological uniqueness, the tissue involved, and the total body burden.

Symptoms of chemical sensitivity are individual in nature but can include: anaphylaxis, anemia, cancer, depression, disorientation, dizziness, fatigue, headache, heart irregularities, irritated eyes, joint pain, kidney/bladder/prostate infections, multiple sensitivities, muscle weakness, numbness, poor memory, runny nose, seizures, shortness of breath, skin rashes and sneezing.

Chemical sensitivity can result in allergies, auto-immune disease, blood count irregularities, or lung and respiratory disease. They can also cause problems with the central nervous system problems, heart, kidney, or liver.

Chemical sensitivity can be determined by a history of symptoms when exposed to chemicals, allergy skin testing (patch or intradermal) for specific chemicals, booth testing (controlled chemical exposure), Spirometry and brain SPECT Scans. Blood testing can be used to determine the levels of chemical contaminants or their metabolites, level of antibodies to specific chemicals, levels of depollution enzymes and liver-kidney functioning.

Chemical sensitivity can be complicated by several different factors including inhalant sensitivities such as dust mites, pollen, molds, smuts and terpenes. It can also be related to past chemical exposures, untreated food sensitivities, immune system dysfunction, nutritional deficiency due to malabsorption or malnutrition, or enzyme depletion.

It is important to discover the source of your chemical exposure. Some forms of chemical exposure include air pollution (cars, industry and ozone), food contamination (pesticides, parasites and mercury), water contamination (TCE), formaldehyde or radon gas contamination, pesticide/herbicide application, and cleaning chemicals. Chemical exposure can also occur from "sick buildings" (home, school or workplace). Poor ventilation or improper air exchange, HVAC problems (location/type), construction or renovation can create sick buildings. They may also be a result of a gas or oil leak in the heating system or lines, or sewer/septic system that leaks methane gas (hydrogen sulfide and carbon monoxide). Some chemical exposures may be a result of occupation or hobby exposure. Chemical dangers in the workplace include paint, plastic, fiberglass, toxic metals, nitrates and solvents (degreasers).

When chemicals enter the body, body functioning quickly eliminates some. Others circulate in the blood until metabolized or stored in fatty tissue, liver and/or brain. Repeated exposures can deplete the chemical enzyme detoxification system, allowing chemicals to circulate in the blood, to become stored in the body, and sometimes to cause the spreading phenomenon of sensitivity to many substances. Medically supervised detoxification techniques (sauna or intravenous therapy) can help remove harmful chemicals from the body.

TREATMENT OPTIONS

Since those who are chemically sensitive are in an overload situation, it is important that they reduce demands on the immune system and reduce their total body burden. Stress and environmental exposures should be minimized whenever possible. Also treat and control food and inhalant allergies.

Chemically sensitive individuals usually suffer from specific nutritional deficiencies that can be evaluated by blood and urine tests. Problems may be improved by a rotary/diversified balanced diet and by supplementation with vitamins, minerals and antioxidants. They should reduce exposure to pesticides and other chemicals in foods by eating only less chemically contaminated meat and produce. They should also use only bottled or filtered water for drinking, cooking and bathing.

Avoidance of harmful chemicals is vital to the control of chemical sensitivities. Personal products should be chosen carefully, and exposure to chemicals that can be present in bedding, clothes, cosmetics, deodorants, soaps, shampoos, toothpaste, sunscreens and body lotions should be minimized and carefully monitored. Less-toxic building products, heating and air conditioning systems, appliances, cleaning products, and pest control should be used.

Create a healthy environment for yourself by using HEPA (High Efficiency Particulate Arresting) filtration, electrostatic air filters, charcoal filters, and formaldehyde-free portable air purifiers in your home and workplace.

CHEMICALS IN OUR AIR

OUTSIDE AIR QUALITY

Air pollution is an international problem. In 1986 radioactive material from the Chernobyl nuclear explosion in Russia fell around the globe. Sulfur dioxides and nitrous oxides forming clouds in one part of our country can travel thousands of miles to deposit acid rain in other areas. Man-made air pollutants compose from 45 to 55 percent of outdoor air pollution.

According to EPA studies, there has been no fresh air in the United States in over 20 years. A 1989 EPA study of toxic air chemicals released by industry showed over 2.45 billion pounds per year, with the chemical industry releasing the most at 886.6 million pounds per year (primary metals 21.5 million and paper 207 million). The five most toxic states were Texas (229.9 million), Louisiana (134.5 million), Tennessee (132.5 million), Virginia (131.4 million), and Ohio (122.5 million). The least toxic was Hawaii with just under a million).

Major sources of chemical pollution are transportation, stationary fuel combustion, industrial processes, forest fires and solid waste disposal. The most common inorganic chemical pollutants known to adversely affect health are sulfur dioxide, carbon monoxide, nitrous oxides, carbon dioxide, ozone, lead and ammonia; and their percentages in outside air composition steadily increase. (As one moves inland from the sea to the desert, the composite air pollution gradient can increase 10 fold. On the best days in cities of 100,000 or more, the average pollution gradients may be 1000 times that of sea air.)

A Harvard School of Public Health Study of 6 cities for 11 to 16 years was released in 1994 and documented a direct correlation between pollution and mortality. It showed that the higher the air pollution rate, the higher the mortality rate. Another study of 7 large U.S. cities, released in 1995, showed a 10-parts-per-million increase in outdoor carbon monoxide concentrations resulting in a 10 (New York) to 36% (Los Angeles) increase in Medicare admissions for congestive heart failure.

Outside air contains natural allergens, pollens, molds, terpenes, and synthetically created chemicals. To coordinate outside activity with your health needs and to afford cellular protection you should know the ozone level, mold count, pollen count and pollination times for your area. It is advisable to use a pollen mast or a charcoal mask for chemical pollutants. You should also keep your car properly maintained, and use recycled air or an in-car air purifier. Restrict outside chemical usage for lawn care and pest control to less-toxic products. It is also important to maintain good nutritional status through proper supplementation *(see Pesticides and Lawn Care on page 187)*.

> > < <

INSIDE AIR QUALITY

Indoor air quality is paramount to health and has been a problem since Ben Franklin's day. He stated, "no common air from without is so unwholesome as the air within a closed room that has been breathed and not changed."

Most of us spend 90% of our time indoors; therefore, the quality of the indoor air we breathe is vitally important. Indoor air is not an exact reflection of outdoor air because it can have higher concentrations of chemicals, and there are some indoor contaminants that pose little or no problem when found outside. Indoor air quality is affected by ventilation, filtration, heat source, humidity, building products, furniture and equipment, and personal products used indoors. Over the past several decades our exposure to indoor pollutants has increased due to insulated/sealed buildings, reduced ventilation rates, synthetic building materials and furnishings, and the use of pesticides, disinfectants, deodorizers and chemically based detergents.

One of the most common indoor air contaminants in home and office is cigarette smoke, which can contain formaldehyde, cadmium, acrolein, benzo-a-pyrene, ammonia and pesticides. In 1985, *Newsweek* reported that British researchers had discovered that eighty-five percent of the non-smokers they tested had measurable levels of tobacco substances in their urine, even though only half felt they had been exposed to cigarette smoke. Cigarette smoke is a widely proven health hazard to those who smoke, but it is also a hazard to those who do not smoke but have to breathe it as a part of their air. It is especially troublesome to those with respiratory ailments and tobacco/smoke sensitivity. Research findings during the mid-1990s have caused most medical facilities to adopt smoke-free environments, and increased public pressure is placed on businesses and industries to become smoke-free.

The Environmental Protection Agency tells us that indoor air is two to five times more polluted than outside air. Why? One major reason is the use of chemical products indoors. There are over eight million distinct registered chemical compounds, and 6000 new ones are added each year. Of these, as many as 70,000 are in current production, and human life is both directly and indirectly affected by them. We come in contact with these chemicals both at home and at work, in the air we inhale, the things that touch us or we touch, and the food and water we consume.

According to D. W. Schnare, et. al, in "Evaluation of a Detox Regimen for Fat Stored Xenobiotics" (*Medical Hygiene* 9, 1982, pp. 265-282), "Over 400 have been identified in human tissue, 48 in adipose tissue, 73 in liver tissue and 250 in blood plasma." This presents a major health issue.

Indoor air particles are measured in microns. One micron (or micrometer) is one-millionth of a meter. The human eye can see particles of 10 microns or more, but a microscope must be used to see particles of 0.2 to 10 microns. In order to see smaller particles of .001 to 0.2 microns, an electron microscope must be used.

Some of the most common air contaminants and their usual sizes are: bacteria (0.35 to 10 microns), molds (2 to 20 microns), pollens (20 to 50

24   *Less-Toxic Alternatives*

microns), plant spores (20 to 40 microns), human hair (70 to 100 microns), and lung-damaging particles (0.50 to 9 microns). By comparison, a postage stamp is approximately 25,400 microns and about 400 microns would dot the "i" in the word micron.

The Occupational Safety and Health Administration (OSHA) has done extensive testing of indoor air, particularly in the workplace, in an effort to define Sick Building Syndrome (SBS). In 1983 the World Health Organization listed eight non-inclusive symptoms that characterize SBS:
1. Irritation of the eyes, nose or throat
2. Dry mucous membranes and skin
3. Erythema
4. Mental fatigue or headache
5. Respiratory infections and cough
6. Hoarseness or wheezing
7. Hypersensitivity reactions
8. Nausea or dizziness

In SBS, these reactions are not generally traceable to specific substances, but are attributed to some unidentified contaminant or combination of contaminants. A 1987 telephone survey of randomly selected office workers indicated 20% perceived their performance hampered by poor indoor air quality. OSHA assumes, however, that in actuality 30 percent of American office buildings have indoor air quality problems which translates to 1.4 million buildings and approximately 21 million employees exposed to poor indoor air quality.

The climate control system is vitally important in protecting indoor air quality. Heating systems that burn natural gas, kerosene, oil, and wood emit varying quantities of respirable particles along with carbon, sulfur, and nitrogen oxides, and trace organic chemicals. Other indoor air contaminants include asbestos, pesticides, formaldehyde, and volatile aromatic, aliphatic and chlorinated hydrocarbons. Fungi, dust, bacteria and other disease-causing organisms add to the indoor air contaminants that make breathing hazardous to one's health.

Chemicals, dust and dust mites, mold, pesticides, toxic furnishings and synthetic building materials adversely affect indoor air quality. Restricted ventilation rates, insulation, improper heat sources and contaminated ductwork also contribute to sick buildings.

Care must be taken in the type system, its location and the location of fresh air intakes. Ventilation and airflow should be at least 20 cfm per person. HEPA or HEPA-quality filter media, granular activated carbon, and UV lighting in the climate control system can remove over 99 percent of all airborne contaminants and chemicals found indoors. The use of a combination of these two filters with sufficient airflow can effectively clean most indoor environments *(see Air Handling on page 107)*.

Indoor air quality can be improved and protected when you know your enemies (allergens) and neutralize them, and use good judgement in selecting less-toxic products. Any discoloration on walls or ceiling may be a sign of mold or chemical contamination and should be corrected immediately. Be aware of odors as they can be a clue to existing problems.

When there is an appropriate balance between natural materials and less toxic household products, coordinated with a proper climate control system, the air and its occupants experience less risk of disease. When these factors are not considered, indoor air can become humid, contain allergens and chemical toxins, and health problems can arise.

> > < <

CHEMICALS IN THE HOME

There are many opportunities for chemical exposure in the home. Toxic fumes may be released by:

- Air fresheners and odor absorbers
- Bedding (synthetic fabrics, vinyl pads, foam rubber mattresses, foam or feather pillows, chemical treatment of mattresses and pillows)
- Books (new), magazines and "junk" mail often outgas chemicals used in the printing process
- Building and remodeling materials including particleboard
- Carpets and rugs may be synthetic, chemically treated with formaldehyde, and cleaned with toxic chemicals
- Chemicals generated by appliances and home computers
- Cleaning products, disinfectants, furniture polishes, floor waxes, etc.
- Cosmetics, perfumes and other personal care products
- Dry cleaned clothing in closets
- Dyes in clothing. Absorbed dyes from clothing can affect skin, brain, or respiratory system; cause abnormal cell growth; and decrease blood oxygen
- EMF exposure (high voltage lines, computers, printers, fuse boxes, etc.)
- Energy source for heating / air handling system (type/location)
- Laundry detergents, bleaches, pre-washes, fabric softeners, etc.
- Particleboard, plastics, and stain-resistant materials in furnishings
- Pest management in the home and lawn *(see below)*
- Pet care products
- Plastic or vinyl coverings over clothing
- Polyester and other synthetic fabrics in clothing
- Poor circulation and tight buildings that restrict movement of fresh air and removal of chemical contaminants
- Synthetic draperies and curtains that may be chemically treated and cleaned
- Synthetic upholstery fabrics, padding and chemical treatments of furnishings
- Volatile organic chemicals in paints, sealers, glues, polishes, and flooring

Most people spend eight to ten hours in the bedroom, so it is important to eliminate indoor air contamination problems in that part of the house. If you feel worse upon arising, you need to carefully consider your bedroom, its furnishings, and your closets in the light of the above list. You should also evaluate your cleaning schedule for dust mite control, and consider EMF exposure from TVs, radios, clocks, electric blankets, etc.

> > < <

CHEMICALS WE ARE EXPOSED TO DAILY

Many products used inside can contain harmful chemicals. It is important to use less-toxic products throughout the home and workplace. These may include less-toxic goods and furnishings ; alternative building and remodeling materials; heating and air filtration products; less-toxic laundry, cleaning and dishwashing products, and safer pest management *(see less-toxic, alternative products in Part III - page 107).*

COMMON AIRBORNE CHEMICALS & THEIR DANGERS

The following common chemicals are found in most homes and offices, and their dangers are often overlooked.

Alcohols: CNS and mucous membrane irritant

Aldehydes: Carcinogenic and mucous membrane irritant

Aliphatic hydrocarbons: CNS depressant and respiratory irritant

Aromatic hydrocarbons: CNS depressant, liver and kidney irritant, immune and vascular system irritant

Chlorinated hydrocarbons: CNS depressant, liver, kidney and mucous membrane irritant

Fungicides: CNS depressant, skin, respiratory and GI irritant

Organochlorides: CNS depressant, liver, kidney and mucous membrane irritant

Organophosphates: Nerve toxin

Petroleum distillates: Affects liver, lung, heart and blood

Acetone (art supplies, paint, and nail polish remover): Headache, fatigue, and bronchial irritant

Ammonia (household cleaners): Respiratory irritant

Asbestos: Carcinogen

Benzene: Carcinogenic and mucous membrane irritant

Butyl Alcohol: Irritant

Butyl Cellosolve (lacquers, solvent): CNS depressant, poisonous

Carbon monoxide (auto exhaust): Affects brain, blood and heart, causes bone damage and low birth weight in fetus

Carbon tetrachloride (grain fumigant, solvent and cleaners): Poisonous, CNS depressant, causes nausea, liver and kidney irritant

Chlordane (termiticide): Headache, dizziness, nausea, CNS depressant, carcinogenic, poisonous, kidney irritant

Chlorine (sodium hypochloride): Lung and respiratory irritant

Chloroform / Trichloromethane (solvent): Fatigue, carcinogenic and CNS depressant

Chlorpyrifos/Dursban (pesticide): CNS depressant, kidney, liver, eye and skin irritant

Cyclohexane (solvent): CNS depressant, skin irritant

DDT – Dichloro diphenyl trichloroethane (pesticide with biotransformation to DDE and dechlorination to DDD): CNS depressant, decreased respiration, birth defects/reproductive problems, myocardia irritability and indefinite half-life

Dieldrin (pesticide): CNS depressant, headache and malaise

Endrin (pesticide): More toxic than chlorpyrifos

Ethanol / denatured alcohol: Mucous-membrane irritant

Ethylene Dichloride (grain/soil fumigant, and degreaser): Conjunctivitis, CNS depressant and respiratory irritant

Glycol Ethers (paints, adhesives, glues, caulking): Affects reproductive system, liver, red blood cells, bone marrow

Heptachlor/Heptachlor Epoxide (pesticide-termites): Poisonous, carcinogenic, liver necrosis and blood dyscrasias

Isopropanol/isopropyl alcohol: Headache, dizziness, nausea, and CNS depressant

Lead (paint, solder, and insecticidal sprays): Affects brain and blood, causes hyperactivity and low birth weight in fetus

Mercury (paint, dentistry, tatoos, fungicide): Affects brain

Methanol: Poisonous, headache and fatigue

Methylene Chloride - Dichloromethane (paint thinners and removers): Heart, cancer, and asthma

Methyl Bromide (grain and soil fumigant): Nausea, vomiting and headaches, CNS depressant and kidney irritant

Nitrogen oxide (auto exhaust): Affects immune system

N-Butyl acetate: Irritant, conjunctivitis

N-Hexane: CNS depressant, peripheral neuropathy

Ozone and sulfur dioxide (auto exhaust): Lungs/respiratory irritant

Pine oil: GI irritant

Toluene: CNS depressant, affects liver and heart

1,1,1 Trichloroethane: CNS depressant, affects liver and heart

Xylene: CNS depressant, affects liver and heart

NEUROTOXICITY TESTING	*not tested	**not adequate
Pesticides	67%	100%
Cosmetics	100%	-
Drugs	47%	88%
Food Additives	73%	100%
Chemicals in Commerce >1,000,000 lbs	100%	-
<1,000,000 lbs	90%	100%

*Percentage of products not subjected to neurotoxicity testing.
**Percentage of products which were tested that were judged to be inadequate.
Source: National Academy of Science – 1980

> > < <

CHEMICALS IN CLEANING PRODUCTS

Cleaning agents are frequently used at home, school and in the workplace including: personal care products and cleaners for clothes, dishes, silverware, cookware, bathrooms, kitchens, floors, furniture, ovens, drains, etc.

Cleaning agents should be less toxic and contain the least amounts of formaldehyde, phosphate, chlorine, petrochemicals and other irritating compounds. Natural cleansers and less-toxic compounds like baking soda, washing soda, zepheran chloride, borax, tri-sodium phosphate and oxygenated bleaches are helpful for maintaining the integrity of indoor air.

The health-conscious individual will proceed with caution in the use of or exposure to any cleaning agent, will read all labels, and test all products before use. It is also important to realize that no product is safe for everyone. Whenever possible, household cleaning should be done when the allergic individual is away from home. However, since the after-effects of any cleaning remains for hours or even days, it is advisable to use less-toxic alternatives to achieve a cleaner, safer indoor environment *(see Part III - page 107)*.

In choosing cleaning agents it is important to clean without contaminating the air. Removal of dirt and destruction of bacteria and germs is very important, but we do not want to victimize our lungs, skin and other living cells.

HARMFUL CLEANING CHEMICALS

Several chemicals commonly occur in cleaners, pesticides, etc. that can be harmful to children and adults alike. Some of the most common and where they are found are listed below. This list is not intended to be all-inclusive, but only designed to give you an idea of the most common occurrences of these dangerous chemicals. Their dangers are listed on the previous two pages.

Aldehydes: Laundry and dishwashing detergents, cosmetics and shampoos, plywood, paints, building products, mold inhibitors, fabrics, bedding, clothing, and shoes

Alcohol: Cosmetics and personal care products, air fresheners, paints and building products

Aliphatic hydrocarbons: Carpet cleaning solutions, paint and solvents

Aromatic hydrocarbons: Floor wax, paint, disinfectants

Chlorine: Tap water, household cleaners, disinfectants, laundry bleach and detergents

Chloroform: Household cleaners

Chlorinated hydrocarbons: Carpet cleaning solutions, room deodorizers, carpeting

Fungicides: Furnishings, wallpaper, mold inhibitors

Glycol Ethers: Antifreeze, paints, glues, sealants, caulks

Lead: Paints, building products, dishes, crayons, water pipes and faucets

Methylene chloride: Degreasers, waxes, lubricants, pesticides, paint, thinners

N-Hexane: Glues, paints, varnishes, printing inks

Organochlorines: Pesticides/insecticides

Organophosphates: Pesticides/insecticides

Petroleum distillates: Pesticides, paints, thinners, adhesives, furniture polish, spot removers, caulks

Pine Oil: Household cleaners

Toluene: Gasoline, glues, paints, thinners, nail polish

1,1,1-Tricholoroethane: Drain cleaners, spot removers, shoe polish, insecticides, printing inks, degreasers

> > < <

CHEMICALS IN PERSONAL CARE PRODUCTS

We all want to look our best and present a pleasant natural aroma. But many of the products we choose to nourish our skin and hair are actually drying and irritating. Some can even cause cellular damage. It is therefore important to investigate your product choices, understand the ingredients and your sensitivities, and arrive at the correct formula for yourself.

Soaps with a moisture retention base can be allergenic. They often contain glycerin or coconut oil. Since we do absorb some of the ingredients, it is important to choose a base to which you are not sensitive. What touches your skin is as important as what enters your body. You may get more than you expect with chemical additives in soaps, shampoos, suntan lotions, etc. Personal products may contain:

ALLERGENS

1-4 Dioxane (an emulsifier) – contained in ingredients identifiable by prefix "peg," "eth" or "oxynol"

Cellulose

Detergents

Glycerin

Gums

Imidazolidinyl urea (a preservative which causes dermatitis)

Oils

Orris root

Parabens (allergenic)

Paraffins

Quaternium 15 (an emulsifier which can release formaldehyde, is very allergenic and can cause dermatitis)

Synthetic fibers

Thimerosol (contains mercury)

CHEMICALS

Alcohols

Ammonia

Boric acid

Dyes

Hexachlorophene

Mercury

Perfumes

PEG – Polyethylene Glycol (degenerates into formaldehyde)

Phenyl mercuric acetate

COAL TAR DYES – DRUG & COSMETIC (D&C)
Blue 1 (allergenic)
Green 5
Orange 17
Red 4, 5, 8, 9, 19, 36 and 37
Yellow 10 (carcinogenic)

DRYING AGENTS
Alcohol, camphor, menthol
Propylene Glycol (a vegetable glycerin mixed with grain alcohol, has been know to cause allergic and toxic reactions)

IRRITANTS
EDTA (Ethylenediamine Tetraacetic Acid)
Esters to delay moisture escape: Butyl Stearate, Isopropyl Myristate and Octyl Palmitate
Laureth-4 (detergent)
Sodium lauryl sulfate (detergent) causes eye irritations, skin rashes, hair loss, scalp scurf and allergic reactions

MICROBIAL GROWTH INHIBITORS
Methyl, propyl and butyl paraben (can cause skin rashes and allergic reactions)

PRESERVATIVES
2-bromo-2-nitropropane-1,3-diol (decomposes to formaldehyde and nitrosating agent, may cause cancer)
Formaldehyde (heart, mucous membrane and eye irritant)
Imidazolidinyl urea and diazolidinyl urea (causes contact dermatitis – can release formaldehyde)
Phenylmercuric acetate (phenol, mercury)
Thimerosol (may contain mercury)
Tri- and di-ethanolamine (nitrosating agent)

CHECK ALL LABELS
Carefully read all labels to see if they contain any harmful chemicals or allergens. Self-administered skin patch tests can also assist in your selection. If uncertain about a product, rub a very small amount on the inside of your wrist and wait 10-15 minutes, check for skin irritation or systemic reaction. Your sensitivities will determine your product choices.

> > < <

PESTICIDES USED INSIDE
It has been estimated that 85 percent of the private households in the United States have pesticide products on their premises. Many people think of them simply as routine cleaning products because they are unaware or unconcerned about the harm they cause.

An EPA study of selected homes in Florida and Massachusetts released in 1990 revealed the following:

- The most common compounds were chlorpyrifos, propoxur, diazinon, o-phenylphenol and chlordane^.; also found were heptachlor^, lindane, dieldrin^, aldrin^, dichlorvos, alpha BHC^, bendiocarb, malathion, and hexachlorobenzene. (^ = banned)
- Indoor concentrations were 5 to 100 times higher than outdoor.
- Air in older homes contained more banned substances than new.
- Pesticides were found in house dust samples
- Occupants often could not remember when termite treatment was done, even when termiticide residues were found in the air.
- There was a lack of precautions to limit exposure during or after applications, and some people had large inventories of pesticides - some of which had been banned for years.
In 1992, the National Home and Garden Pesticide Use Survey of all 48 contiguous states and Washington DC revealed:
- 85% had at least one pesticide on premises
- 63% had 2-5
- 22% had more than 5 pesticides in storage
- The smaller the container, the longer it had been stored
- Some respondents did not know how to dispose of them
- Many reported pouring them down the sink or in trash
- The 2 major pest concerns were ants and roaches, followed by mosquitoes and fleas.
- Kitchens, persons and pets were the most frequently treated sites.
- People were treated with pesticides in 13% of households at least once a year (includes repellants)
- No safety precautions were used with 16% of sprayer usage
- 28% considered holding the breath a safety precaution for foggers and 23% for ready-to-use sprayers.
- Protective clothing was worn by only 30% where hose-end or compressed air sprayers were used. Only 30% mixed these chemicals outdoors.
- 20% had been commercially treated for indoor pests such as roaches, ants or fleas.
- Indoor pesticide use was most intensive in kitchen, least intensive in living and sleeping areas.

To summarize these studies, people apparently have a casual attitude about pesticides and their risks: 85% choose to use and store pesticides inside, 60% of the time they take no precautions when applying them, 75% of the time they don't recall learning of precautions from labels or suppliers, and they fail to inquire of previous owners about the kind and frequency of pesticide usage.

PESTICIDES USED OUTSIDE

Americans admire a healthy, green, weed-free yard. This may come with a price tag according to the May-June 2000 issue of *Audubon Magazine*. We pour 136 million pounds per year of pesticides on our home lawns and gardens. This is three times more per acre than the average farmer. Organophosphates,

Dursban, Diazinon, and herbicides such as 2,4-D (a chlorinated phenoxy herbicide) and Round-Up (which contains Gyphosate, an aliphatic herbicide) are neurotoxic to man, birds and fish. You should know your pest, the risk to humans and wildlife, and choose the safer alternatives. "Kicking the pesticide habit isn't mission impossible. Just ask one of the 6000 certified organic farmers, or the City of Arcata, CA, which after 15 years of using non-toxic pest control, banned all pesticide use on city property as of this past February."

Use of non-toxic pesticides is important because adults play and work outside; and children and pets play outside and breathe the air close to the ground. Lawn and garden pesticide usage continues to increase. The EPA estimates that more than 40% of all lawns are treated with pesticides. These pesticides affect weeds, insects (good and bad), people, birds and animals.

There are 34 pesticides commonly used for lawn care according to the EPA. Diazinon, an organophosphate, and 2,4-D, a chlorophenoxy herbicide, are the two most commonly used. Diazinon, a neurotoxin, is extremely toxic to birds, and has been responsible for massive killing of waterfowl. 2,4-D, which also acts as a neurotoxin, can cause brain demyelination and is a possible carcinogen.

These pesticides become part of our homes as we and our pets carry them inside, to reside for extended periods of time in our carpets. Our pets can even absorb them through their paws and suffer central nervous system, liver and kidney damage.

It is imperative for golfers to be prudent about pesticide exposure on golf courses because these chemicals can be absorbed through some shoes. At least 2 or 3 weeks should elapse between treatment and playing time. Living beside or on a golf course can also be hazardous, due to pesticide drift. A buffer zone of 1-5 miles should be allowed for wind displacement.

Of the 18 pesticides commonly used for lawn care, the EPA has found 13 in ground water. This poses a serious risk of contamination of our drinking water supplies.

Weed control needs to be less toxic to protect today and preserve tomorrow. Fertilizer needs to be organic and weed control should utilize fatty acid herbicides. Pulling weeds is good exercise and ecologically correct.

CATEGORIES OF PESTICIDES

ORGANOPHOSPHATES

Organophosphates are the most extensive category of organic compounds used as pest control chemicals. They may be grouped either by the form of phosphoric acid (from which they are derived) or structurally (aliphatic, heterocyclic or phenolic). These groupings cross each other's boundaries.

Organophosphates include malathion, chlorpyrifos (Dursban) and diazinon (Spectracide).

N-METHYL CARBAMATES

N-Methyl Carbamates include bendiocarb (Ficam) and carbaryl (Sevin and Dicarbam).

ORGANOCHLORINES

Organochlorines include chlordane (Chlordan), DDT (chlorophenothane), dieldrin (Dieldrite), dicofol (Kelthane), lindane (gamma BHC or HCH, Isotox), mirex (Dechlorane), and TDE (DDD, Rhothane). Many of these have been banned, while others are still the active ingredients of various home and garden products; and their residues persist for a long time.

SYMPTOMS & SIGNS OF POISONING

Pesticides can be mutagenic, tetratogenic and carcinogenic. They can affect numerous body systems and be absorbed into the blood and tissue to live out their lives inside the human body.

Organophosphates poison primarily by phosphorylation of the acetylcholinesterase enzyme at nerve endings. This enzyme is critical to normal control of nerve impulse transmission from nerve fibers to muscles and also to other nerve cells in autonomic ganglia of the brain. At sufficient dosage, loss of enzyme function allows accumulation of acetylcholine at cholinergic nerve effector junctions, skeletal nerve muscle junctions and autonomic ganglia. Exposure can reduce or deplete the enzyme detoxification mechanism causing pesticide sensitivity and severe reactions upon repeated exposure.

Symptoms of acute organophosphate poisoning develop during exposure or within 12 hours (usually within 4 hours) of contact. Early symptoms include headache, nausea, dizziness, anxiety and restlessness. These may progress to muscle twitching, weakness, tremor, vomiting, incoordination, abdominal cramps, diarrhea, hypersecretion (sweating, salivation, tearing, rhinorrhea, and bronchorrhea), blurred and/or dark vision. Tightness in the chest, wheezing and productive cough may progress to pulmonary edema. Bradycardia may progress to arrest of sinus rhythm, or be superseded by tachycardia and hypertension. Toxic myocardiopathy has been a prominent feature of severe organophosphate poisoning. Toxic psychosis, manifested as confusion or bizarre behavior, may be evident. Unconsciousness, incontinence, convulsions, and depression of respiration may occur in life threatening cases. Ingestion of large quantities can lead to paralysis of muscles of the head, neck, limbs and thorax requiring mechanical pulmonary ventilation to sustain life.

Symptoms of N-methyl carbamate poisoning include malaise, muscle weakness, dizziness and sweating. Headache, salivation, nausea, vomiting, abdominal pain, diarrhea, miosis, incoordination, slurred speech; dyspnea, bronchospasm, chest tightness leading to pulmonary edema, blurred vision, muscle twitching, and spasms may also occur. These symptoms tend to be of shorter duration than from organophosphate poisoning.

Symptoms of organochlorine poisoning include sensory disturbances, headache, dizziness, nausea, vomiting, incoordination, tremor and mental confusion. More severe cases report myoclonic jerking movements, convulsions, coma and respiratory depression.

TESTING FOR EXPOSURE

Blood and urine tests can sometimes detect the presence of pesticides immediately after exposure. Red blood cell and plasma acetylcholinesterase

(ASC) tests can detect organophosphate or carbamate exposure. In the case of N-methyl carbamate exposure, the red blood cell or plasma ASC tests must be performed within an hour or two of exposure. Some organochlorine pesticides or their products (DDT, dieldrin, mirex, heptachlor epoxide, beta isomer of benzene hexachloride, kepone, and oxychlordane) can persist in blood and tissue for weeks or months after absorption, but others are likely to be excreted in a few days.

Specific urine metabolites tests related to individual carbamate exposures can be performed, but are complex and not generally available. The alkyl phosphates and phenols to which organophosphates are hydrolyzed in the body can often be detected in the urine during pesticide absorption and up to 48 hours thereafter. These analyses are sometimes useful in identifying the actual pesticide.

Certain organophosphates and organochlorines can be stored in fatty tissue. Fatty tissue biopsies can sometimes detect organochlorine or organophosphate exposure.

Pesticides can be absorbed through eyes, skin or by inhalation. A physician should treat pesticide exposure. Ingested food-grade charcoal, dry heat sauna, intravenous vitamin C, glutathione, and oxygen can be useful in treating pesticide exposure.

> > < <

OTHER CHEMICALS IN OUR AIR

FORMALDEHYDE

Formaldehyde is a colorless gas with a pungent odor. It outgasses into indoor air from adhesives in particleboard and plywood, insulation, carpeting, upholstery, kerosene heaters and tobacco smoke. It is released into outside air from the incomplete combustion of fossil fuels, gasoline or diesel, and methanol powered automobiles. Formaldehyde resins are being used in wrinkle proof and crease resistant fabrics. It is widely used in plastic production, the photography industry, dying and tanning of leather, artificial silk, and in the rubber and explosives industries.

Formaldehyde combined with methanol is used in the production of numerous disinfectants. It is also a powerful antiseptic, germicide, fungicide and preservative.

Formaldehyde is a potent eye, upper respiratory and skin irritant. Evidence from several studies also indicates that it is a central nervous system depressant. It also has the potential for causing asthma, and studies suggest it is a potential human carcinogen.

Some of the symptoms associated with formaldehyde exposure are eye irritation, increased thirst, depression, coughing, sneezing, shortness of breath, headache, and skin rash. Young children who have suffered formaldehyde exposure can develop high fever, nausea, severe diarrhea and vomiting. Infants are particularly at risk for formaldehyde exposure.

Because of its widespread use, scientific evidence suggests that formaldehyde contamination of indoor residential and work place environments can result in serious health problems. Formaldehyde has been implicated as a cause of air quality problems and the sick building syndrome for a long time. Several factors affect the rate and amount of formaldehyde off-gassing including atmospheric conditions (higher temperature and humidity cause more outgassing), the manufacturing process used, air exchange rate, age of the material, and the method of treatment after installation. Infiltration of outside formaldehyde contaminated air into indoor air seems to be affected by the outside wind speed and the differences in outside/inside temperature. Thus a windy, cold, dry winter day would result in lower concentration of indoor formaldehyde contamination; but a warm spring or fall day with low wind and little temperature differential between inside and outside would produce greater contamination.

The type of formaldehyde resin correlates to the amount of formaldehyde in indoor air. There are two types of formaldehyde resins (phenol and urea) which are widely used as adhesives. Phenol formaldehyde adhesives are used in exterior grade plywood. Urea adhesives are used in particleboard and hardwood plywood paneling, foam, carpeting, upholstery and permanent press clothing. Emissions of formaldehyde from phenol resins are only a fraction of those from urea. Thus, urea formaldehyde resins are more likely to be the major source of indoor formaldehyde levels.

Initially the major source of formaldehyde is the excess that is bound to water. As a result, old wood products are less toxic because the passage of time and evaporation has already resulted in the release of formaldehyde.

OSHA has now set the acceptable level of formaldehyde in indoor air at .7 ppm; however studies show indoor formaldehyde levels vary from .04 to 1.0 ppm. Long-term exposure to low levels of formaldehyde can create myriad symptoms and hypersensitivity in individuals, resulting in intolerance of even a minimal exposure of less than .03ppm.

Time and outgassing or volatility of formaldehyde reduces indoor levels; however, time is not a solution to an immediate problem. The best solution is, thus, source removal. Secondly, a bake-out for a day or two reduces levels of formaldehyde. This is best accomplished in an unfurnished building as it can crack paint, damage computers, warp wood, and break caulking seals. Ozone generators can be used for 6-8 hours to reduce indoor levels of contaminants, then aired for 24 hours. Precautions must be taken because plants, animals and people can suffer ill effects if exposed to ozone. Overuse can create worse indoor air contamination problems.

Carpet can be steam cleaned, and formaldehyde filters can be installed in central or room air purifiers. Ventilation or increasing the flow of outside air can reduce indoor levels.

Paints and sealers can reduce the rate of emissions but lack effectiveness on new wood products. They seal out moisture and stop hydrolysis of resin; however, they are ineffective in preventing passage of volatilizable formaldehyde trapped in adhesives. Special coatings are available that are

36   *Less-Toxic Alternatives*

capable of reducing formaldehyde emissions by as much as 99 percent if they are tolerated by the hypersensitive.

The best solution is the use of products that are low in formaldehyde resins or do not contain them at all. Good indoor air quality can be achieved through the exclusive use of less toxic products and proper air filtration, purification and ventilation. There are wood products that are free of formaldehyde and green label carpets with no VOC's or formaldehyde. The use of solid wood provides an even better option *(see less-toxic building products - page 113).*

RADON

The EPA found at least 20% of all homes it surveyed were contaminated with dangerously high levels of radon, a radioactive gas formed from decaying uranium found naturally in soil and rocks. The permeability of the soil below the house affects radon concentrations in the home, and the EPA estimates that the average soil contains 1.0 ppm. It is the differential in the pressure that drives radon from high pressure in the ground into the lower pressure of buildings. Uranium concentrations in shale tend to be low, while phosphate rock contains 10-50 ppm. Clay soil retards radon movement, while sandy soil increases it. Porous construction material (such as cinder blocks) allows more movement from the soil through them. Deep-water wells may allow radon to enter the water supply. One-story houses usually have higher concentrations than multi-level homes because radon diffuses as it rises.

There is no health hazard when it is safely dispersed into the atmosphere; however, if released into a building where people spend long amounts of time, continued exposure can be detrimental.

This colorless, odorless gas – a suspected cause of lung and nasal cancer – can seep into a house in various ways including: well water, porous cinder blocks, foundation cracks, sump pumps, loose-fitting drains and pipes, or diffusion through the foundation and concrete walls.

The health effects of radon are well documented through years of research, and the EPA estimates that radiation exposure inside buildings may account for 10% of all lung cancer deaths in the United States.

Radon itself is not the culprit. Tissue damage results from the by-products produced when radon decays. In the decay process, radioactive elements throw off sub-atomic particles, and energy rays become more stable and have a lighter structure. Uranium decays into radium, then radon. Radon further decays into different forms of polonium, bismuth and lead. When these radon decay particles are inhaled, they further decay into alpha particles in the lung and become the primary cause of tissue damage.

Test kits are available for determining the level in your home *(see page 230).* Tests indicate that first-floor measurements, instead of basement, provide the best estimate of personal radon exposure.

Basement walls and floor can be sealed or concrete placed over cinder blocks. Ventilation fans can bring fresh air into upper stories and move radon contamination out through the basement vents. Prior to construction, vent pipes can be installed in the soil below the slab to keep radon from entering the home. A layer of crushed stone can also be placed beneath a plaster cover to reduce radon migration. Electronic precipitators may also help capture charged radon decay particles. There are also experts who specialize in radon migration.

Radon can also leak from cracks in Fiestaware (popular in the 1930s and 1940s) or bright orange colored plates. Gamma rays are emitted from uranium based paints on some older dinnerware.

For further information on radon, send $1 for each of the following pamphlets to: Superintendent of Documents, U.S. Government Printing Office, Washington, DC 20402:
  "A Citizens Guide to Radon: What it is and What to Do About It"
     (Stock #055-000-00258-4)
  "Radon Reduction Methods: A Homeowner's Guide"
     (Stock #0505-000-00259-2)
  "Radon Reduction in New Construction"

EMF (ELECTROMAGNETIC FIELD)

The effect of EMF is another area of concern in the home and workplace. It is important to know the location of substations, transmission lines, and transformers near your home. The location of fuse boxes and electric wiring in the walls, floors and ceilings of structures can be important. Care should be taken in the selection, use and placement of all electrical products including electric clocks, hair dryers, electric blankets, microwaves, TVs, computers, and even your heating/air conditioning systems.

> > < <

CHEMICALS IN THE WORKPLACE

There are many opportunities for chemical exposure in the office or workplace. Toxic fumes may be released by:
- Air fresheners and odor absorbers
- Office arrangement in relationship to other employees or production areas
- Building and remodeling materials including particleboard
- Carbonless papers which contain alkyl phenol novalac resin
- Chemicals generated by the use of office equipment
- Chemicals in papers, correction fluids, and glues
- Cleaning products, disinfectants, furniture polishes and floor waxes
- Computer laser printers which expose you to ozone, styrene, butadiene, and EMF
- Cosmetics, perfumes and other personal care products used by other employees and customers
- Cubicles and sectioned work stations that trap air and increase exposure to hydrocarbons and formaldehyde
- Energy source for heating / air handling system
- Excessive exposure to glare, electromagnetic radiation and chemical outgassing from computers and their cases
- Formaldehyde and other chemicals in carpets

Less-Toxic Alternatives

- Furnishings and draperies
- High voltage lines
- Industrial or laundry chemicals
- Lubricants and solvents used for servicing office equipment
- Particleboard, plastics and stain-resistant materials in furnishings and cubicles
- Pest management in offices
- Pesticide and herbicide spraying along roadways
- Photocopiers which expose you to isocyanates, xylene and phthalates
- Policies regarding smoking and other factors affecting the air you breathe
- Vehicle pollution on highways

American industry uses an estimated 500,000 chemicals to produce many of the benefits of modern living today. Twenty million Americans work with one or more of these chemicals which can damage the nervous system. However, by 1982, the National Institute for Occupational Safety and Health had thoroughly assessed the behavioral effects of only a few dozen chemicals. In 1988 there were 850 known neuro-toxic chemicals that caused loss of memory, inability to concentrate, sexual dysfunction and whose symptoms might be indistinguishable from Parkinson's disease or ALS (Lou Gehrig's disease). At that time, regulatory standards existed or had been recommended for only 167 of those chemicals.

Office workers are regularly exposed to central nervous system depressants such as styrene (computer monitors), ozone (laser printers), benzene (copy machines), 1,1,1-Trichloroethane (white out), plus alcohols and glycol ethers in inks. Many of these common products also serve as respiratory irritants, and can adversely affect other body systems.

Workers exposed frequently to methyl n-butyl ketone (a solvent used as ink thinner and machine cleaner) have suffered varying degrees of nerve damage to the lower limbs.

Continued exposure to paint solvents can impair intellectual capacity and affect coordination. Toluene, a paint additive and solvent, and trichloroethhylene, a degreaser and dry cleaning agent, can not only cause peripheral neuropathy, but their usage can create addiction.

Methylene chloride, a solvent and spray can propellant, can produce hallucinations. It is also an active ingredient in paint strippers and pesticides, and has been blamed for the death of a pest-control worker who died while spraying pesticides in a poorly ventilated crawl space. This is a chemical that is considered harmless outdoors.

Fumes from aerosol paint cans have also been responsible for numerous deaths and serious neurological damage among children and teenagers who thought huffing (sniffing the fumes) would simply produce a cheap high. There have been numerous reports in some major metropolitan areas of otherwise healthy teenagers found dead with a spray paint can beside them.

Acetone, used in cellulose production, can produce vertigo/dizziness. Carbon disulfide, used in rubber vulcanizing, can cause numbness and tingling in the lower limbs, psychosis, and memory loss. Frequent exposure to

1,2-dibromo-3-chloropropane, a soil fumigant, can induce sterility. Methyl bromide, a popular termiticide, is a known neuro-toxin. Anesthesiologists and dentists routinely inhale halothane, chloroform, cyclopropane and nitrous oxide.

Workers and professionals can be exposed to these neuro-toxins daily. According to Edward Bergin, a program analyst with the Occupational Safety and Health Administration (OSHA), the EPA and OSHA have a difficult job regulating the one-half million chemicals in use in industry today. Only a small percentage have been adequately tested because 1,300-1,500 compounds enter the market each year, and the regulating agencies (EPA and OSHA) are not given enough authority, money, and manpower to perform the task.

The fact that many chemical companies do their own product testing is another complicating factor that can lead to fraudulent behavior. What isn't known about chemicals and their synergistic effect is greater than what is known. The consequences of these facts are indoor pollutants that can cause irreversible damage to the health of the unsuspecting worker.

Even if no spray or volatile organics are introduced into the indoor air, the structure itself can be a source of contaminants. Chemical companies manufacture nine billion pounds of formaldehyde each year, making it a common contaminant of indoor air. It is found in some glues, cleaners, carpets, fabrics, and wood products like plywood, pressboard, and chipboard. Formaldehyde is a potent eye, upper respiratory and skin irritant; and a probable carcinogen. Significant amounts of trapped formaldehyde are released from new products into indoor air. The hydrolytic decomposition of formaldehyde occurring over the years also maintains undesirable levels of it in closed buildings. This continuing release of formaldehyde into the air can make it a major contributor to indoor air pollution and the sick-building syndrome.

Unlike other contaminants that are found in water and outdoor air, there is no regulation that requires monitoring of homes or office buildings for indoor pollutants. Virtually all cases of unhealthy indoor air or sick-building syndrome have been discovered by the human body's adverse response to this pollution. In many instances the building was new or recently remodeled, and the occupants may have expressed innumerable complaints. When air in the structure was sampled, one culprit was often a formaldehyde level above the standard .1 parts per million. Removal of the formaldehyde-containing agents or increased ventilation sometimes improved the air pollution problem. However, if the occupants' symptoms were severe and the structure contained excessive levels of numerous pollutants, the decision had to be made to declare the structure unfit for occupancy, and close the building.

Even the ductwork of our workplaces can be a source of indoor air contamination. Fungi, bacteria, and dust mites can invade the heating and cooling systems to create illness and sensitivity responses. In such cases it becomes necessary to have the ductwork and the entire climate-control system professionally cleaned with the offending contaminants removed.

To preserve the integrity of your workplace, products should be chosen

Less-Toxic Alternatives

which are low in formaldehyde, petrochemicals, volatile hydrocarbons and tung oil. Solid wood, tile, latex paint, pesticide alternatives and the use of natural fibers and products help preserve the healthy atmosphere of indoor living. Individual air purification equipment and select office materials can aid in the creation of a less-toxic work environment.

The future of our world is in your hands. You can affect air quality by the choices you make. Your voice in promoting improved air quality should not be stilled.

AWARENESS ACTIVATES

Bad workplaces may affect the cardiovascular system, central nervous system, eyes, kidneys, liver, and respiratory system

> > < <

ENVIRONMENTAL TESTING & EVALUATION
Isolate the incitant – Protect your greatest treasures.

Testing is available to determine contaminants present in indoor air. Tests for EMF, formaldehyde, volatile organic compounds, lead, microbials, pesticides, mold, radon, and others are available from air quality firms. Some testing services are available from your local utility companies, health department or your County Extension Agents *(also see page 228).*

> > < <

CHEMICALS IN OUR FOODS

One of the primary ways chemicals enter our bodies is through the food we eat. Natural food of the early twentieth century has been replaced by processed, enriched, chemically altered and genetically engineered products, which sometimes bare little resemblance to the original. The use of pesticides, antibiotics, hormones, dyes, and preservatives has vastly altered the composition of many products. Not only do we get a large dose of natural vitamin C in our morning orange juice; our breakfast may subject us to a chemical cocktail of pesticides, antibiotics, antioxidants, anti-microbials, steroids, hormones, dyes, and preservatives plus artificially produced vitamins and minerals. Can you really be sure what is in that beautiful salad at the restaurant, or even in the turkey sandwich you had for lunch?

PESTICIDES

Highly toxic chemical pesticides are the main contaminants of food. A pesticide is used to kill insects and pests on food crops, and it is usually blended with an equally toxic herbicide that kills weeds. According to Lawrie Mott of the National Resource Defense Council, pesticide usage increased tenfold from 1950 to 1990, while the number of crop insects doubled. The United States Department of Agriculture reported that 439 billion pounds of pesticides were scheduled for use on ten major food crops during 1991: 226 million pounds on corn, 112 million pounds on soy beans, and 37 million pounds on cotton. In

September 1999 it was reported that U.S. farmers used 1 billion pounds of pesticides.

Many pesticides sold today have not been fully tested by the EPA, especially for their long-term health effects. Until 1970, pesticides did not have to pass stringent health or safety standards before being placed on the market. Congress initiated more stringent health requirements for registering pesticides in 1972, including long- and short-term effects on human health and environment. The EPA has faced a difficult task of reregistering and retesting over 600 active ingredients in products registered before 1972. The EPA estimates it will not have this expensive and arduous review process completed until after the turn of the century.

The EPA's job is made more difficult by the lack of information on active ingredients in pesticides. No information was required for many years on inert ingredients, even though they are far from inactive. This information is essential to determine a pesticide's health risk. The EPA considers only 300 of the 1200 known inerts safe, while 100 others are of toxicological concern.

In the late 1980s, the National Academy of Science reported that only about one-fifth of all pesticides sold in the United States had been adequately tested for cancer risk, about one-half for their role in causing birth defects and about ten percent for adverse effects on the nervous system. In a 1988 report, Unfinished Business: A Comparative Assessment of Environmental Problems, a group of seventy-five EPA experts ranked pesticide residues among the top three environmental cancer risks. Tested or not, health risk or not; these pesticides still remain on the market, and pose serious risk to the young, the old, and people with health problems.

Pesticides are extensively present in food. The EPA estimates that 100 percent of non-organic grocery store food contains pesticides. These residues are known or suspected carcinogens, and may affect central nervous system disorders.

In the late 1980s, the Food and Drug Administration (FDA), and the California Department of Food and Agriculture (CDFA) detected pesticide residues in 63% of all strawberries, 55% of all peaches, and 53% of all celery. In 1998, Consumers' Report stated that 77% of the non-organic produce they sampled had pesticide traces, while 25% of the organic produce had traces of less-toxic pesticides.

According to the September 1999 issue of Fitness Magazine, the foods with the highest amount of pesticides were apples, spinach, peaches, pears, strawberries, grapes, potatoes, celery and green beans. The ten least contaminated were corn, cauliflower, sweet peas, asparagus, broccoli, onions, pineapple, bananas, cherries and watermelon. The Environmental Working Group in Washington, DC, found seven different pesticides on a single sample of apples.

In the early 1990s, the five most commonly detected pesticides in food were known or suspected carcinogens. Organochloride pesticides such as chlorophenothane (DDT), benzene hexachloride (BHC), and dieldrin have already been banned from usage in the United States. However, because of their persistence in the soil, they are still part of the food chain.

Captan, considered by the EPA to be a probable human carcinogen, is still in legal use, and thirty-three percent (33%) of the strawberries sampled by the FDA between 1982 and 1985 had Captan residues *(see strawberry below)*.

Chlorothalonil, classified by the EPA as another probable human carcinogen, was found on one-half of the celery sampled by the FDA in conjunction with the CDFA in the early 1990s.

Organophosphates are another class of pesticides present in the food chain. These pesticides attack the central nervous system by inhibiting the enzyme acetylcholinesterase. This causes over-stimulation of the central nervous system, thereby creating stomach upset and other nervous system symptoms. Three or more organophosphates were found to be among the five most common pesticide residues on one-half of all foods sampled in one study.

Number of pesticide products	20,000
Number of active ingredients they contain	700
Pounds of active ingredients sold	6.077 Billion
Most heavily used pesticides	
Herbicides	61%
Insecticides	21%
Consumer spray units sold	200 million
Pesticide products cost to users	$8.260 Billion
Percentage of pesticides used by:	
Agriculture	75%
Industry, commerce & government	18%
Consumer home and garden	6%
Pounds of pesticides applied on 10 major crops	439,000,000
Corn (lbs.)	226,000,000
Soybeans (lbs.)	112,000,000
Number of pesticides approved for use on:	
Apples	110
Bell Peppers	50
Broccoli	70
Tomatoes	100

(Sources: Womach, "Pesticide policy issues in the 103rd Congress." CRS issue Brief, June 15, 1993; Chemical & Engineering News, June 29, 1993.)

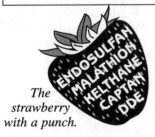

The
strawberry
with a punch.

The bugs are active and well
The fish and birds are dead or dying…
And we are sick.
Are there any alternatives?
Yes! We can cancel the pesticide monster,
and protect our environment.
> > < <

ANTIBIOTICS

In February 1987, the Centers for Disease Control stated that sixty percent (60%) of all cattle, ninety percent (90%) of all pigs and veal calves, and one-hundred percent (100%) of all poultry ate antibiotic-spiked feed. Some environmental groups now estimate that one-half of all antibiotics produced in the United States are used in animal feed.

Antibiotics such as penicillin and tetracycline are used to control infection or disease in the host. Because of continual exposure to specific antibiotics, bacteria in the animal can become resistant to these antibiotics. If a person becomes ill after consuming meat containing resistant bacteria, treatment with these antibiotics may not destroy the bacteria, alternatives may be difficult, and serious illness may ensue.

A National Academy of Science report in May 1987 concluded that many bacteria-laden chickens passed USDA inspection. Americans for Safe Food claim that at least one-half of all chickens contain salmonella. Visual inspection of birds will not detect the bacterial, and chemical tests that detect it are not used because they are too slow.

With the emergence of widely publicized cases of food poisoning from improperly cooked meat at restaurants in the mid-1990s, many restaurant chains have established new policies regarding meat preparation. Grocery stores have also mounted an effort to educate the American public regarding the handling and preparation of meat (especially poultry) in an effort to curb the spread of these antibiotic-resistant bacterial diseases.

When one considers the dangers of handling and eating foods containing antibiotic-resistant bacteria, and the presence of those antibiotics in the meat itself, food becomes much less appetizing.

> > < <

HORMONES

Animals are frequently fed hormones such as progesterone, estradiol, and testosterone to increase muscle and weight; but these chemicals (which are already present in the body in their natural form) may also increase cancer risk. This certainly causes concern in individuals who eat meat, eggs, milk and poultry.

Because of the delicate hormonal balance that exists in the human body, the addition of these residual hormones makes maintenance of a correct hormonal balance more difficult while creating a serious health risk. The Food & Drug Administration (FDA) has therefore advised that no one consume more than one percent of these hormones. The United States Department of Agriculture requires a fourteen-day waiting period between a hormone dose and slaughter, in the hope that the animal has eliminated the hormone.

In Puerto Rico, very young prepubescent children were experiencing changes attributed to puberty: girls were developing breasts and boys' voices were lowering. These changes were finally linked to hormones present in chicken feed.

> > < <

Less-Toxic Alternatives

DYES

Artificial food coloring added to numerous gelatins, cereals, meats, pudding, and canned fruits and juices is usually made from coal tar or petroleum. Dyes in our foods may make them attractive, but they add undesirable chemicals that can create multiple sensitivity reactions.

Food colorings have also been linked to hyperactivity in children. Any eye appeal that they give food may be combined with a potential life-threatening sensitivity response to the colorings. Tartrazine, a yellow dye, has been known to cause reactions from hives to laryngeal edema. Red dye #3 has been named as a possible carcinogen. Red dye #4 can effect the adrenal glands and bladder. Yellow #10 can be contaminated with carcinogen beta-naphthylomia. Many food dyes have already been banned in Europe, and American manufacturers must be forced to seriously consider the risks involved in their usage.

> > < <

PRESERVATIVES

Sulfites added to salads, potato chips, soups, relishes, and wines may spark serious asthma attacks in steroid-dependent asthmatics. Butylated hydroxyanisole (BHA) and butylated hydroxytoluene (BHT) are common preservatives found in breakfast cereals, donuts, potato chips, meats, meat products, fats and oil. These can cause eczema, hives and asthma in sensitive individuals. Many preservatives are listed in the following section.

> > < <

WHAT TO LOOK FOR ON LABELS

It is important to read labels on all food products in order to avoid additives, preservatives and dyes that can be harmful to your health. David Steinman in "Diet for a Poisoned Planet" classifies common food additives into three categories: Usually Acceptable, Caution and Unacceptable. This list includes some of his designations plus additional pesticides and chemicals often found in our foods.

USUALLY ACCEPTABLE

These additives appear safest for most people but may not be tolerated by everyone. Some allergic reactions have been reported from some of these. Avoid those containing sodium if on a low-sodium diet.

Alginates and propylene glycol alginate – derived from seaweed

Alpha tocopherol (vitamin E) – derived from vegetable oils

Ascorbic acid (vitamin C) – antioxidant (gravies, jams, toppings)

Ascorbyl palmitate – antioxidant (fats and oils)

Beta-carotene (precursor of vitamin A) – used to color foods

Calcium propionate and sodium propionate – antimicrobial/mold inhibitor (bread, baked goods)

Calcium stearyl lactylate and sodium stearyl lactylate (bread dough, egg whites)

Carbon dioxide – preservative (meats, meat products, nonalcoholic beverages)

Casein and sodium caseinate – a complete protein containing amino acids (ice cream, dairy products)

Citric acid and sodium citrate – a fruit flavoring used to brighten colors, as an emulsifier and to control acidity

Erythorbic acid – an antioxidant similar to ascorbic acid but without vitamins (meats and meat products)

Ferrous gluconate – food coloring and flavoring

Fumaric acid – derived from plant tissues – antioxidant, imparts tartness

Furcelleran – derived from seaweed – stabilizer and emulsifier

Gelatin – derived from animal tissues – thickener and stabilizer

Ghatti – derived from plants – emulsifier

Glycerin (glycerol) – food additive (candies, meat coatings, margarine, shortenings)

Guar gum – derived from plants – stabilizer and thickener

Gum arabic – stabilizer and prevents sugar crystallization

Gum tragacanth – derived from plants – thickener and stabilizer

Invert sugar – combination of glucose and fructose – very sweet

Karaya – flavoring derived from trees in India

Lactic acid – fermentation of plant tissues and dairy whey – preservative and flavor enhancer (cheese, condiments)

Lactose – a culture medium and nutrient

Lecithin – common antioxidant and emulsifier

Locust (carob) bean – flavoring extracted from carob tree seed

Mannitol – texturizer and sweetener

Potassium sorbate – mold inhibitor/preservative (tortillas, English muffins, fish, cheese, gelatins, jams, nuts)

Sodium ascorbate – antioxidant (meats and poultry)

Sodium benzoate – preservative (fats/oils, frostings, puddings, gelatins, gravies)

Sorbic acid (acetic acid, hexadienic acid, hexadienoic acid and sorbistat) – mold and yeast inhibitor

Sorbitan monostearate – emulsifier, defoamer and flavor-dispersing agent

Sorbitol – sweetener

Vanillin and ethyl vanillin – vanilla substitute

CAUTION

These products are known to cause more problems and exposure should be kept at a minimum:

Artificial flavoring

Carageen – stabilizer and emulsifier

Chlorine monoxide – water chlorination

Corn syrup (dextrose) – simple sugar – flavoring and antimicrobial (preserves, toppings)

Ethylene – fruit ripening

EDTA (Ethylenediaminetetracetic acid) – preservative – can rob your body of essential minerals

Green # 3 used in beverages and candy – one of the safest food colorings but can cause or promote bladder tumors

Heptyl paraben – preservative (alcoholic beverages) – avoid if pregnant
Hydrochloric acid – preservative (sweet sauces, toppings, food processing)
Hydrogen peroxide – preservative (baked goods, grain products)
Hydrolyzed vegetable protein – not safe for children – contains MSG
Methyl paraben – preservative (vegetables and vegetable juices)
Modified food starch – may contain aluminum sulfate which is suspect
Monoglycerides and diglycerides – synthetically prepared – do not eat regularly
Paraffin – food wax
Phosphates – essential for proper parathyroid function but can be harmful at
    high levels
Phosphoric acid – flavoring for colas – will remove rust from chrome or auto
    batteries, therefore its safety in humans is suspect
Polyester – food packaging
Polyethylene – food packaging film
Propionic acid – antimicrobial (baked goods)
Propyl paraben – preservative (vegetables, vegetable juices, fats and oils, baked
    goods)
Sodium carboxymethylcellulose (CMC) – cotton by-product derivative –
    thickening and stabilizing compound – has caused cancer in animals
Yellow Number 5 – used in beverages, baked goods and pet food – has been
    implicated in behavioral disturbances in children – not good for hyperactive
    children or anyone sensitive to aspirin

UNACCEPTABLE
    These products are generally used in nutritionally inferior junk food
products and should be avoided. The food dyes and colorings should definitely
be eliminated.
Ammonium chloride – preservative (bakery goods)
Ammonium hydroxide – food additive
Aspartame – the FDA has received the longest list of complaints for these
    products (trade names NutraSweet and Equal)
Benzene hexachloride – pesticide (fruits and legumes)
Benzoic acid – preservative (fats and oils, nonalcoholic beverages, sugar
    substitutes, and artificial flavors)
BHA (butylated hydroxyanisole) – preservative/antioxidant that prevents food
    from changing color or flavor or becoming rancid (meats, meat products,
    fats and oils)
BHT (butylated hydoxytoluene) – preservative similar to BHA (cereals, meats,
    meat products, fats, and oils.
Blue Number 1 – in candy, baked goods and soft drinks – potential carcinogen
    – chromosomal damage (banned in France and Finland)
Blue Number 2 – in baked products, candy, soft drinks, and pet food – potential
    carcinogen – brain tumors (banned in Norway)
Brominated vegetable oil (BVO) – emulsifier (in many soft drinks) – can inhibit
    baby's natural defenses because it reduces histamines

Carbon tetrachloride – agricultural fumigant

Chlorine gas – processing of meat, fish and vegetables

Chlordane – pesticide (vegetables)

Citrus red number 2 – used to color orange skins – probable carcinogen – may cause chromosomal damage

DDD (DDT analogue) – pesticide (fruits and vegetables

DDT (chlorophenothane) – pesticide (fruits, vegetables, cotton) – in soil

Dieldrin – pesticide (vegetables, fruits)

Endrin – pesticide (corn, cabbage, cotton, field crop insecticide)

Endosulfan – pesticide (potatoes, cottonseed)

EDB (Ethylene dibromide) – fumigant (grains and fruits)

Formaldehyde – preservative (gelatin capsules, vitamin A & E)

Formic acid – preservative (brewing alcoholic beverages)

Heptachlor – pesticide (soil insects for corn and cotton)

Hexachlorobenzene – fumigant (wheat and other grain seed)

Methyl bromide – fumigant (produce and soil)

Monosodium glutamate (MSG) – flavor enhancer (beef, chicken, salad dressings, soup, many oriental foods, hydrolyzed vegetable/plant protein and autolyzed yeast) – many people are allergic to this

Nitrite or Sodium Nitrite – preservative in meats – probable carcinogen

Nitrogen – antioxidant (fats and oils)

Phenol – food additive

Potassium metabisulfite – preservative (fruits and fruit juices)

Propyl gallate – antioxidant often combined with BHA or BHT (fats and oils) – probable carcinogen

Red dye number 3 – carcinogen and chromosomal damage (was banned in 1990 but some may still be around in candy, desserts and pastries)

Red dye number 40 – (recently developed) used in beverages, candy, desserts and pet food – probable carcinogen (lymphomas)

Saccharin – banned by FDA but still widely used in artificial sweeteners – every packet of Sweet-N-Low has 40 milligrams of saccharin

Salt (sodium chloride) – can cause high blood pressure and increase risk of heart attack and stroke – best to limit use

Sodium bisulfite – preservative (salads, baked goods, seafood, vegetables, vegetable juices)

Sodium chloride – preservative (fats and oils, cheese, meats, condiments)

Sodium chlorite – preservative (grain products)

Sugar (sucrose) – sweetener – has no nutritional value

Sulfur dioxide, sodium bisulfite and sulfites – preservatives – dangerous for asthmatics

TBHQ (Tertiary butylhydroquinone) – often used with BHA or BHT – toxic at extremely low doses – childhood behavioral problems

Yellow Dye Number 6 – used in candy, carbonated beverages, desserts and sausage – may cause chromosomal damage / probable carcinogen –kidney tumors (banned in Norway and Sweden)

Less-Toxic Alternatives

MAKING THE RIGHT CHOICES

We must all exercise self-protection because of the complexity of the problem with chemicals in our foods. The person who has elevated levels of pesticides in the blood and fat must strive to reduce additional exposure or face increased health risk. The presence of these chemicals in the body is a contributing factor to developing serious illnesses including environmental illness and the chemical sensitivity so characteristic of the condition. It is, therefore, important to minimize ingestion of these chemicals in food. Careful selection must be exercised if regular grocery store food is used. Organ meats must be avoided because they contain concentrations of chemicals. Foods from foreign countries and the southern and eastern parts of the United States may contain more fungicides and pesticides than foods from the western states. Washing fruits and vegetables removes some pesticides, as does removing the outer leaves of lettuce. Peeled fruits usually contain fewer pesticides since the peeling process removes some of the chemicals.

Some pesticides, dyes, hormones, antibiotics and other chemicals will remain in the regular grocery store food in spite of every effort to remove them. Organically grown, less-chemically contaminated foods are, therefore, the safest alternative for everyone, especially at-risk individuals. Organically grown fruits, vegetables and meats may either be purchased from an organic producer or grown in your own garden. The choice becomes one of life and illness maybe even death for those with environmental illness.

A number of nationally distributed foods are now available without artificial coal tar food dyes or other additives. These include Cheerios, Grape-Nuts, Nutri-Grain, Dannon Yogurt, Pepperidge Farm products, real fruit juices, gelatin desserts, and Popsicles made with fruit juice. The wise consumer safeguards the health of the family *(see Organic Food Suppliers on page 220).*

> > < <

CHEMICALS IN OUR WATER

Your water is a lifeline! Two-thirds of the human body is fluid, and any contaminates in the water you drink are quickly dispersed throughout the body's systems. Water is a nutrient that is essential for life, but not all water is safe. Various chemicals can contaminate our water; and, for the environmentally sensitive, even those chemicals used in the treatment of our water can be hazardous to your health.

Water contamination is not new. During World War II, President Roosevelt considered the Delaware River a threat to national security because it was so polluted. He feared that gasses from the water might cause corrosion at a nearby radar installation. Just as the population has increased, water contamination has increased steadily since World War II – paralleling the chemical and technological revolutions. Home and industrial waste disposal; plus chemical and petroleum production, usage, and storage are major contributors to water contamination.

The increased use of nitrate fertilizers and pesticides in agriculture further adds to the problem. In the late 1980s, the EPA estimated that seventy-seven percent (77%) of the 1 billion pounds of pesticides produced each year in the United States were used for agriculture. Pesticides have high potential for leaching into groundwater because of their persistence in the soil and water solubility. Sandy soils and shallow water tables make groundwater contamination a major concern.

Irrigation of farm land concentrates natural salts and minerals at the land's surface; then, when rain or irrigation water returns to the groundwater below, the minerals and salts may be two to four times more concentrated. Selenium and arsenic, common earth minerals, are toxic at certain levels; thus this multiple concentration caused by irrigation can create serious health hazards.

Landfills and hazardous waste sites also have high potential for water contamination. In 1982 an EPA study of 929 hazardous waste sites revealed that drinking water was contaminated at 128 sites, and contamination was suspected at 213 additional sites. This same study reported confirmed or suspected groundwater contamination at two-thirds of the hazardous waste sites.

According to the Council of Economic Priorities in 1980, eight out of ten Americans lived near these toxic waste sites, and forty-nine percent (49%) of Americans drank groundwater. These toxic sites can and do contaminate groundwater. In 1984 the EPA's National Water Quality Inventory reported 4400 incidents of groundwater contamination in twenty-one states; causing closure of private, public, or industrial wells and forcing users to find alternative water sources.

Underground storage tanks for petroleum, gasoline and chemicals can lead to groundwater contamination. In the early 1990s, the Texas Water Commission estimated that there were 50,000 to 100,000 underground storage tanks in Texas; while the EPA estimated a total of three to five million nationwide. Recent laws in some areas have forced the removal of old tanks from some service station sites; however, there are many other tanks that may be lost, forgotten or conveniently overlooked by unscrupulous businessmen and officials.

Twenty-five percent (25%) of the American households dispose of their residential wastewater through cesspools and septic systems. Though they may individually be of minimal significance, these disposal methods become important if drinking water wells and septic systems are located in close proximity. Contamination of the drinking water with bacteria, nitrates, and viruses can occur; and serious health problems ensue.

The U.S. Public Health Service regulated viruses and bacteria in the public drinking water as early as the beginning of the twentieth century. The standards were overwhelmingly successful in curbing the spread of disease; but fifty years later, traces of approximately 65,000 chemicals used in homes and industry began appearing in drinking water. Recognizing this threat, the drinking water standards were revised in 1962 to include limits on organic chemicals. At that time the Environmental Protection Agency succeeded the U.S. Public Health Service as administrator of drinking water standards.

The number of chemicals in use continued to grow, and chemical carcinogens were found in the Mississippi River, which was the water supply for New Orleans. The presence of these chemicals and a heightened public awareness led to the Safe Drinking Water Act of 1974. This Act was supposed to establish specific standards for maximum levels of a contaminant, guidelines for treatment technologies to cleanse the drinking water, and monitoring requirements for chemical detection in water systems.

Seven hundred organic, inorganic, biological, and radiological contaminants have since been detected in water supplies in the United States. Yet, by 1986, the EPA was regulating only twenty-three contaminants. Understanding of the health risks from long- and short-term chemical exposure, and advances in analytical testing capabilities led to the realization that drinking water standards were grossly inadequate. Because of the EPA's slow regulatory pace, the United States Congress passed amendments to the Safe Drinking Water Act in 1986. Fifty-three additional drinking water contaminants were required to meet contamination standards, and the EPA was also required to review and revise existing standards.

An increasing number of organic and synthetic volatile chemicals have been added to the list of microbiological contaminants such as giardia and viruses, and inorganic chemicals such as arsenic and lead. Many cities have been required to provide new and better filtration in order to meet the standards of the Act and its revision; thus adding a financial burden which strains their limited budgets. While some larger metropolitan systems were equipped to meet the Act's requirements, thirty-five percent (35%) of the community water systems were cited for failure to meet the established standards for maximum contaminant levels. These smaller community systems are not equipped to monitor such a large number of volatile and synthetic organic chemicals; thus they must contract with outside agencies to conduct periodic testing for them in order to stay in compliance and avoid EPA sanctions. As the number and intensity of these hazardous chemicals increase, compliance becomes even more difficult; and health risk increases.

Even if compliance is met and the standards are achieved, the danger of exposure to carcinogens in drinking water still exists. The EPA regulated only six pesticides as late as 1991; and regulation of pesticides in groundwater has evolved slowly, due to the belief that pesticides would break down in the soil or be bound to it. Such is not the case. The EPA reported in 1985 that 17 unregulated pesticides had been found in the groundwater of 23 states. This measure of exposure to carcinogenic chemicals appears intolerable.

The EPA's standards for carcinogens allow a high risk for cancer. The EPA standard for a substance as a cancer risk is in the range of one in ten thousand to one in one million. A one in ten thousand risk would allow 24,000 additional cancer cases in the entire population. Furthermore, these risk numbers apply to each contaminant separately. Thus, the risks are additive for each additional contaminant which is present in the water supply and in the body. Since we daily drink water containing many of these contaminants, these standards appear to fall far short of health assurance and protection.

Woburn, Massachusetts, was an example of drinking water contamination, industrial pollution, and risk involved when volatile organics are present in drinking water. The incidence of childhood leukemia in Woburn was more than twice as high as expected. Within a half-mile radius of the city it was 7.5 times higher than expected. The health hazard was high levels of trichloroethylene, tetrachloroethylene and chloroform – chemical that had contaminated the wells supplying water to the community. This case points out the risk of well water consumption and the tremendous need to continually test samples of well water and small municipal water supplies.

Another contaminant that can be present in well water is radon gas, a carcinogenic uranium derivative. The EPA estimates that as many as 1,000 to 10,000 public water systems have excessive amounts of radon. Water suppliers can remove radon from the water. The danger lies in untested and untreated well water, or with small municipalities that lack the equipment or facilities to deal with this and other contaminants.

Industrial and agricultural pollution occurring on land can contaminate groundwater and thus drinking water; but this problem is also creating major concern for our oceans, their inhabitants, and our oceanic food sources. Fishermen reported hauling in lobsters and crabs with ulcerous lesions all along the shoreline from Portland, Maine, to Morehead City, North Carolina; and oysters in Chesapeake Bay have experienced a fungal disease. According to a report in the August 1988 Time magazine, shellfish beds in Texas had been closed eleven times in the previous eighteen months due to pollution. In Louisiana, 35% of the state's oyster beds had been closed because of sewer contamination. Pesticides and chemicals have filled New York's marine waters.

In the 1980s there were reports of health risks with certain ocean fish including bluefish, flounder, and striped bass. At times lakes and rivers are also closed to fishermen and fish contamination warnings issued due to fish kills from chemical pollutants, industrial runoffs and accidental spills.

According to an article in the July 1992 issue of the American Journal of Public Health, 9% of all bladder cancers and 15% of all rectal cancers may be attributable to long-term consumption of chlorinated water. This translates into approximately 6500 cases of rectal cancer and 4200 cases of bladder cancer per year. The increased cancer risk appears to result from carcinogenic compounds generated when chlorine gas reacts with organic contaminants in water to form chloroform and other harmful chemicals.

Chlorine, chloroform, and other harmful chemicals can also cause skin problems when you shower or swim. Studies have shown that higher doses of volatile organic compounds are absorbed through the skin while showering/bathing and swimming in contaminated water than are absorbed through the intestines from drinking the same water. The American Journal of Public Health, Vol. 74, No. 5 reports that skin absorption constitutes an average of

64% of the daily dose of volatile organic compounds from chlorinated household water. This increases to up to 91% skin absorption for children.

The Center for Environmental Epidemiology at the University of Pittsburgh reported in Environmental Science and Technology that 50% of the dissolved chloroform (a carcinogenic chlorinated volatile organic chemical) escapes into the air in showers before the water even reaches the floor. The remaining chloroform may be absorbed through the skin. This exposure exceeds the daily dose from drinking water by 600%.

The pollution of our lifeblood of water is devastating and cumulative. Dangerous minerals, chemicals, and pesticides enter the water and are concentrated when we eat fish and shellfish. Laws and agencies exist to protect our water supply and our food supply; however, the contaminants are numerous, pollution vast, and the public has not been sufficiently impressed with the magnitude of the problem.

Water pipes can also pose a health hazard if deteriorated, improperly installed or of improper material.

WATER CONTAMINANTS

Filtration Systems and Common Water Contaminants They Remove			
Contaminant	Reverse Osmosis	Charcoal & Carbon Block	Distillation
Arsenic	Some	Some*	Yes
Asbestos	Yes	Yes	Yes
Bacteria	Some	Some	Yes
Benzene	Yes	Yes	No
Chlorine	Some**	Yes	No
Fluoride	Some	Some	Some
Heavy Metals	Yes	Some	Yes
Lead	Yes	No	Yes
Mercury	Yes	Yes	Yes
Minerals	Yes	No	Yes
Nitrates	Yes	No	Yes
Pesticides	Some	Most	Some
Salts	Yes	No	Yes
Sulfates	Yes	No	Yes
Toluene	Some	Yes	No
Trichloroethylene	Some	Yes	No
Trihalomethanes	Some	Yes	No
Viruses	Some	Some	Yes
Xylene	Some	Yes	No
*Organic arsenic complexes only **Chlorine compounds only			

WARNING: None of these units are recommended for the removal of viruses and bacteria. Chlorination, ozonization and ultraviolet radiation are used to remove harmful bacteria. Therefore, the filtration methods listed here are to be used with chlorinated water or well water that tests free of bacteria.

WATER FILTRATION

Water filtration reduces health risks. Common drinking water contaminates can include: alcohols, chemicals used in dry-cleaning fluid (trichloroethlene, 1-1-1,trichlorethane, tetrachlorethylene), pesticides and herbicides, solvents such as toluene and benzene, styrene, trichloroethane and trihalomethanes.

Contact and exposure must be minimized because probable carcinogens are present in contaminated water. Filtered or bottled water is a necessary alternative. Environmentally sensitive individuals should also avoid chlorinated tap water, plastic bottled water, and untested well water.

Activated carbon makes strong absorption bonds with volatile organic chemicals in cold water; however, in hot water, such bonds are weakened and toxic chemicals may not be captured. Thus the by-products of chlorination (i.e. trihalomethanes), volatile organic chemicals, pesticides, etc. may be flushed out of the carbon when hot water runs through it. The dangerous by-products of chlorination do not have the warning taste and odor of chlorine; thus the user can be given a false sense of security.

If one desires to filter both hot and cold water, a whole house filtration system should be installed on the point-of-entry water supply line. However, if only cold water is to be filtered, individual sink units can be installed.

The first step toward correcting drinking water contamination is to be aware of the pesticides, herbicides or toxic products you use which lead to contamination. Secondly, you must be aware of your own sensitivities and those of your family. Then, to reduce individual health risks, you should have your drinking water tested by a professional to determine its specific contaminants. Water testing is often available through your County Extension Agent and water test kits can be secured from various mail-order sources, some of which are listed under Environmental Testing in Part IV.

After you receive an analysis of your water you can compare the results with your sensitivities to determine your filtration needs. Select the water filtration method or methods that will best resolve the problem. Your product selection must reflect non-toxic construction. These methods must then be incorporated into a cost-efficient system to meet your needs. The following narrative and the table of water contaminants (*above*) will help you determine which filtration unit or combination of units is best for your particular situation.

REVERSE OSMOSIS

These units reduce suspended and dissolved solids in water. They can reduce the concentration of chlorine, and are effective in reducing heavy metals such as lead, mercury, copper, and arsenic. They are effective in the reduction of nitrates, herbicides and pesticides; and can reject bacteria and viruses. However, they waste water, are slow and expensive to operate.

ACTIVATED CARBON

Activated carbon units are excellent for removing chlorine, some man-made chemicals, and unpleasant odors and tastes. Carbon can remove organic chemicals such as benzene, carbon tetrachloride, trichloroethylene and trihalomethanes. It is also effective in removing most pesticides such as chlordane. Activated Carbon is NOT effective in removing heavy metals, nitrates and iron.

It is extremely important to keep these filters clean as they can breed bacteria. Also, when the carbon becomes saturated, high concentrations of contaminants can flush through the filter. This can result in water being more contaminated than it was before filtration.

A Ceramic Carbon Block does everything an activated carbon filter does; plus it removes asbestos, bacteria, rust and sediment from water.

DISTILLATION

Distillation is effective in removing heavy metals such as lead and mercury, viruses and bacteria, nitrates, sulfates, and some chemicals. However, volatile organic compounds that have boiling points lower than water, boil off with the water and enter the clean water. One mode called a fractional distiller avoids this problem by separating the volatile chemicals from the water. Most distillers have small capacities and a holding tank is required if this method is to be extensively used.

OTHER WATER TREATMENT DEVICES

Other devices that meet specific water treatment problems include:

WATER SOFTENERS use ion exchange to remove minerals such as calcium and magnesium from the water. These softeners use sodium to capture the calcium or magnesium. This can be a problem for those needing to avoid excess sodium intake. This treatment method could be combined with one that removes sodium from the water.

IRON & HYDROGEN SULFIDE FILTERS use sand or artificial resins treated with manganese dioxide to remove iron, manganese and hydrogen sulfide from water. The manganese oxidizes the iron, which is then filtered out by the sand or resin.

ION EXCHANGE SYSTEMS remove inorganic chemicals from water by passing water through a resin bed which exchanges ions in the bed for ions in the water. This system is based on the theory of the attraction and repulsion of charged particles. Ion exchange systems can be designed to remove either positively charged minerals such as cadmium, lead, sodium or calcium; or negatively charged compounds such as nitrates, sulfates, chromium, radium or arsenic. Contaminants are attracted to the opposite charged resin bed. When the contaminant reaches the bed, another ion is released in exchange for the contaminant. Resin beds must be replaced when full. Also water containing both nitrates and sulfates does not allow nitrates to be filtered by this method. An additional filtration method would be required.

IRON FILTERS use sand or artificial resins treated with manganese dioxide to remove iron, manganese, and hydrogen sulfide (rotten egg) odor from water. The manganese oxidizes the iron that is filtered and removed by the sand or resin. These filters are particularly useful when there is no need for a water softener, and when iron levels are between 3 and 10 ppm or mg/liter *(see pages 156 for drinking water filtration and page 122 for swimming pool and spa water filtration).*

> > < <

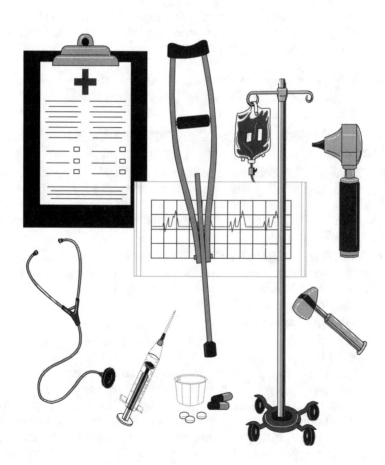

Part II: Diagnosis & Treatment Options

A detailed history with symptom response provides the physician with much needed information, helping him determine which laboratory analysis and diagnostic tools will uncover the disease process. After evaluation of all factors, a treatment program can then be initiated and illness attacked.

Diagnosis

Allergy skin testing (scratch or intradermal) or blood (RAST, Elisa/ACT) testing can aid in the diagnosis of many traditional allergies or sensitivities to pollens, molds, dust/dust mites, foods, danders, smuts, terpenes and fabrics.

Nutritional analysis, vitamin and mineral assessment of both essential and toxic minerals, or a rotary elimination diet may provide useful information for treating food sensitivities.

Chemical panels to determine levels of xenobiotics can be helpful in linking cause and effect. Chemical challenges in a testing booth can aid in the diagnosis of chemical sensitivities.

A brain SPECT (Single Proton Emission Computerized Tomography) Scan can also be helpful in the diagnosis of chemical exposure and in correlating memory deficits, depression, and headaches as they relate to chemical exposure.

Other diagnostic tools may include blood testing to determine lack of specific enzymes; RAST testing for IgE, IgG levels of allergy or sensitivity response; or ELISA/ACT testing for delayed sensitivity reactions.

Interpreting Lab Results

Your physician may order laboratory studies to better understand your physical condition. Blood testing may evaluate electrolytes, serum, iron, blood sugar, protein, liver enzymes, kidney and heart function, and anti-nuclear antibodies. Physician also frequently order thyroid, adrenal and immune system function tests. Normal (desirable) ranges are listed on the report forms and vary between laboratories. These tests may include any of the following.

Routine Blood Tests

WBC (WHITE BLOOD COUNT): An abnormally low count may indicate immune suppression, and an abnormally high count may indicate infection. The WBC includes LYM (Lymphocytes) and GRA (Granulocytes). The Granulocytes may be further broken down by studies of Neutorphils,

Eosinophils and Basophils. These are all tests that help your physician evaluate your overall health and disease process.

RBC (RED BLOOD COUNT): A low count may indicate anemia – possibly caused by poor diet, internal bleeding, etc.; whereas a high count may indicate lung disease. This may be further broken down for HGB (Hemoglobin) and HCT (Hematicrit).

PLT (PLATELETS): This disk-shaped structure is found in all mammalian blood and is a chief factor in clotting.

ANA (ANTINUCLEAR ANTIBODIES): Screens for several auto-immune diseases, SLE (Systemic Lupus Erythematosus), Sjogren's syndrome, ulcerative colitis, and juvenile rheumatoid arthritis.

RA (RHEUMATOID ARTHRITIS): Screens for rheumatoid arthritis, but is not always 100% accurate.

CBC (COMPLETE BLOOD COUNT): In a complete blood count, MCV is Mean Corpuscular Volume, MCH is Mean Corpuscular Hemoglobin, and MCHC is Mean Corpuscular Hemoglobin Concentration. Depressed B12, copper, manganese, zinc, B6 or folic acid may mimic depressed iron.

SAMPLE HEMATOLOGY REPORT (CBC)			
PARAMETER	RESULT	NORMAL	RANGE
- WBC	3.5 K/uL	4.0	11.0
- LYM#:	0.4 K/uL	1.0	4.0
MID#:	0.3 K/uL	0.2	1.1
GRA#:	2.8 K/uL	2.0	7.7
- LYM%:	13.0 %	20.0	45.0
MID%:	7.9 %	1.0	10.0
+ GRA%:	79.0 %	45.0	70.0
RBC	4.42 M/uL	3.90	6.50
HGB:	13.8 g/dL	12.0	17.5
HCT:	39.8 %	36.0	54.0
MCV:	90.2 fL	82.0	98.0
MCH:	31.2 pg	27.0	33.0
MCHC:	34.6 g/dL	32.0	36.0
+ RDW:	16.3 %	12.0	15.0
PLT:	298 K/uL	150	400
MPV:	7.3 fL	7.0	11.0

Note: Report appearance will vary between laboratories.

Less-Toxic Alternatives

BLOOD CHEMISTRY TESTS

SAMPLE BLOOD CHEMISTRY TEST							
TEST	RESULT	NORMAL RANGE	LL[	NORMAL		]HH	UNITS
NA	143.	136. – 145.	[		*	]	mmol/L
K	5.2 H	3.5 – 5.1	[			]*	mmol/L
CL	106.	98. – 107.	[		*	]	mmol/L
TIRON	138.	65. – 175.	[		*	]	µg/dL
CHOL	197.	0. – 200.	[			*]	mg/dL
TRIG	79.	0. – 250.	[	*		]	mg/dL
UA	5.6	3.5 – 7.2	[		*	]	mg/dL
ALT	18.	5. – 30.	[		*	]	U/L
AST	29.	7. – 31.	[			*]	U/L
AMYL	64.	25. – 125.	[	*		]	U/L
CK	100.	38. – 174.	[		*	]	U/L
LDH	124.	63. – 155.	[		*	]	U/L
ALP	73.	53. – 128.	[	*		]	U/L
GGT	60. H	2. – 30.	[			]*	U/L
TBILI	1.1 H	0.0 – 1.0	[			]*	mg/dL
DBILI	0.3 H	0.0 – 0.2	[			]*	mg/dL
MG	1.6	1.3 – 2.1	[	*		]	mEq/L
CA	8.8	8.5 – 10.5	[*			]	mg/dL
PHOS	3.0	2.7 – 4.5	[*			]	mg/dL
GLU	88.	70. – 105.	[		*	]	mg/dL
TP	6.9	6.5 – 8.3	[*			]	g/dL
BUN	14.	7. – 18.	[		*	]	mg/dL
CREAT	0.9	0.7 – 1.3	[	*		]	mg/dL
ALB	3.9	3.5 – 5.0	[*			]	g/dL
BC	16.						
GLOB	3.						
AG	1.					H=HIGH NORMAL	

A major screening of the various elements vital to bodily function may include the following.

<u>ALBUMIN & GLOBULIN</u>: These primary blood proteins are indices of overall health and nutrition. The Albumin/Globulin Ratio measures the relationship between these two proteins. Globulin fights disease.

<u>ALKALINE PHOSPHATASE</u>: This liver and bone enzyme may increase in reaction to drugs or with rickets, liver disease, myocardial or pulmonary infarction. It may decrease in patients with excess Vitamin D, scurvy, hypothyroidism, malnutrition, pernicious anemia, etc.

BILIRUBIN: This is a measure of liver health. Low levels are usually not significant, but high levels may indicate liver disease or another disorder that affects bile flow or production.

BUN (UREA NITROGEN) & CREATININE: BUN is a liver waste product, excreted by the kidneys, that is affected by high protein diets or strenuous exercise (which raise the level) and pregnancy (which lowers it). Creatinine, another waste product, indicates how the kidneys are functioning, but is not affected by high protein diets. Further evaluation is necessary when high values are recorded for BUN or the BUN/Creatinine Ratio.

CALCIUM & INORGANIC PHOSPHORUS: These minerals are stored primarily in bones and are important for proper blood clotting and nerve, muscle and cell activity. The parathyroid and kidneys control them. Low calcium can cause bone problems. High calcium or low phosphorus levels need further evaluation.

CHOLESTEROL & TRIGLYCERIDES: These fats in the blood are, when elevated, associated with heart disease. They are best taken after a 10-hour fast. Cholesterol testing usually breaks it down into two types (HDL and LDL) and provides comparisons.

GGT (GAMMA GT): Increased levels are associated with liver disease or damage.

GLUCOSE: This is a measure of the sugar level in blood. High fasting levels may indicate diabetes, while below normal levels may indicate hypoglycemia due to metabolic malfunction.

IRON: This is an essential constituent of hemoglobin and other respiratory enzyme components. It transports oxygen to tissues and aids in cellular oxidation. Ranges higher or lower than normal may indicate different types of anemia, including anemia resulting from chronic disease.

LD (LACTATE DEHYDROGENASE): A enzyme present in all body cells that can be elevated by any problem that damages cells such as heart attack, anemia, hepatitis, etc.

POTASSIUM: A mineral that is important for proper function of nerves and muscles, especially the heart. The kidneys control it. Any deviation from normal range requires medical evaluation, especially if patient is taking a diuretic or heart medication.

PROTEIN: This measure of total blood protein can fluctuate up or down due to nutritional deficiency, fighting disease, bleeding, etc.

SGOT or AST: This enzyme is found in muscle, liver and heart cells. Damage to those cells by a heart attack, alcohol, liver disorder or other injury can produce high values. Elevations can indicate liver stress or disease. Muscle enzyme elevations can be indications of muscle fatigue, excessive exercise, muscle wasting or heart muscle problems.

SODIUM & CHLORIDE: Major body salts that are important for nerve, muscle and most cell function. Regulated by kidneys and adrenal glands.

URIC ACID: This is normally excreted in urine. Elevated values can be a result of gout, arthritis, kidney problems or some diuretics.

IMMUNE STUDIES

These studies are usually recommended for patients suffering from the symptoms of chronic illnesses such as allergies, chemical sensitivity, environmental illness, chronic viral or bacterial infections, and immune disorders. They help evaluate the status of the immune system and its response to various forms of treatment. (All of the following that contain Ig refer to a form of immunoglobulin). Testing may include:

IgG: Most abundant immunoglobulin group. Achieves high concentrations in both vascular and extravascular spaces. They are responsible for most of the body's immunity. It may be active in fighting infection for three weeks.

IgA: Second most abundant antibody class and important in external secretory system. First to respond to inhaled substances through mucous secretion. It is found in the intestines and respiratory systems.

IgE: A reactive antibody that is responsible for common pollen, dust and mold reactions.

IgD: Newly discovered antibody that may be implicated in penicillin hypersensitivity.

IgM: Largest antibody molecules and seem to be of greatest importance during the first few days of a primary immune response.

T-CELLS (T-LYMPHOCYTES): The mastermind of the immune system. There are both helper and suppressor t-cells. These cells encounter antigens and process them, then instruct B-cells and plasma cells in the production of the proper immunoglobulin.

B-CELLS (B-LYMPHOCYTES): The cells that direct the production of immunoglobulins. Low levels indicate an inability to properly perform their task, and may also indicate a disease process.

BLASTOGENIC INDEX: Tests for proper lymphocytic function by challenging both T-cells and B-cells.

TOTAL COMPLEMENT: System of 11 soluble and cell-bound proteins, reacting in chain-like sequence and setting the stage for the body's protective mechanisms against invading substances.

ENDOCRINE STUDIES: These tests evaluate hormones that are secreted into the blood or lymph by one organ or structure and have a specific effect on another. Thyroid system hormones are often tested (usually involving four hormones (T_3, T_4, T_7 and TSH). These tests may also include Estrogen, Progestrone, Luteinization Hormone (LH), Follicle Stimulating Hormone (FSH), Testosterone and Prolactin.

URINALYSIS TESTS

A urine specimen is usually analyzed for the following:

GLUCOSE: A measure of sugar in urine. Abnormally high levels may indicate diabetes.

KETONES: A by-product of metabolism. Abnormally high levels may be sign of diabetes or malnutrition.

PROTEIN: Elevated protein (e.g. albumin) in urine may indicate kidney disease or be the result of intense physical or emotional stress.

BLOOD: Red blood cells in urine may indicate urinary tract infection, kidney stones, tumor, injury or menstrual blood contamination. White blood cells, bacteria and yeast are also indicative of urinary tract infection.

NUTRIENT DEFICIENCY TESTS

Blood or urine can be used to test for several essential vitamins, minerals and amino acids. Normal or reference ranges depend on specimen source and can vary between labs. The proper range will be listed on the lab report.

SAMPLE RED BLOOD CELL ELEMENTS TEST							
NUTRIENT ELEMENTS							
Nutrient Element	**Result µg/g**	**Reference Range**	**Percentile**				
			2.5th	16th	50th	84th	97.5th
Calcium	13	8 – 31		*********			
Magnesium	40	36 – 64		**********			
Potassium	67	65 – 95		************			
Phosphorus	464	480 – 745	******************				
Copper	0.68	0.52 – 0.89				***	
Zinc	12.7	8 – 14.5			*********		
Iron	807	745 – 1050		************			
Manganese	0.026	0.007 – 0.03				**************	
Chromium	0.029	0.012 – 0.07		*******			
Selenium	0.21	0.19 – 0.38	************				
Boron	0.075	0.005 – 0.11				*********	
Vanadium	0.0002	.0001 – 0.002		*********			
Molybdenum	0.0006	.0005 – 0.002		************			
POTENTIALLY TOXIC ELEMENTS							
Toxic Element	**Result µg/g**	**Reference Range**	**Percentile**				
			95th		99th		
Antimony	0.0004	< 0.005	**				
Arsenic	0.004	< 0.01	******				
Cadmium	0.002	< 0.005	******				
Lead	0.028	< 0.09	*****				
Mercury	0.009	< 0.01	*************				

RBC and whole blood tests can evaluate many essential and toxic minerals.

Calcium, Chloride, Phosphorus, Potassium, Sodium and Chloride are often included in normal blood chemistry tests and are discussed above.

Other essential or important elements studied include: Barium, Boron, Chromium, Cobalt, Copper, Germanium, Iodine, Iron, Lithium, Magnesium, Manganese, Molybdenum, Rubidium, Selenium, Sodium, Strontium, Sulfur, Vanadium, Zinc, and Zirconium.

Blood testing for B vitamins, along with A, E and K can aid in assessing nutritional status. Some of these elements are further discussed later in this section under Supplements.

TOXIC ELEMENT TESTS

For those who may have experienced or suspect environmental exposures, the following toxic elements are often tested through blood or hair testing: Aluminum, Antimony, Arsenic, Beryllium, Bismuth, Cadmium, Lead, Mercury, Nickel, Platinum, Silver, Thallium, Thorium, Tin, Titanium and Uranium. Reference ranges vary depending on lab and type of test.

SAMPLE GVST / VOLATILE PANEL				
Compound	Results	Pop. Avg.	Detection Limit	Units
Benzene	< 0.5	< 2.5	0.5	mg/ml (PPB)
Dichloronethane	< 0.5	< 1	0.5	mg/ml (PPB)
Toluene	< 0.5	< 1	0.5	mg/ml (PPB)
Ethylbenzene	< 0.5	< 1	0.5	mg/ml (PPB)
N. P.-Xylenes	< 0.5	< 1	0.5	mg/ml (PPB)
O-Xylene	< 0.5	< 1	0.5	mg/ml (PPB)
Styrene	< 0.5	< 1	0.5	mg/ml (PPB)
1,2,4-Trinethylbenzene	< 0.5	< 1	0.5	mg/ml (PPB)
1,3,5-Trinethylbenzene	< 0.5	< 1	0.5	mg/ml (PPB)
Chloroform	< 0.5	< 1	0.5	mg/ml (PPB)
1,1,1-Trichloroethane	< 0.5	< 1	0.5	mg/ml (PPB)
1,1,2-Trichloroethane	< 0.5	< 1	0.5	mg/ml (PPB)
Trichlorethene	< 0.5	< 2.5	0.5	mg/ml (PPB)
Tetrachloroethylene	< 0.5	< 1	0.5	mg/ml (PPB)
1,2-Dichlorobenzene	< 0.5	< 1	0.5	mg/ml (PPB)
1,3-Dichlorobenzene	< 0.5	< 1	0.5	mg/ml (PPB)
1,4-Dichlorobenzene	< 0.5	< 1	0.5	mg/ml (PPB)
Bromodichloronethane	< 0.5	< 1	0.5	mg/ml (PPB)
Carbon Tetrachloride	< 0.5	< 1	0.5	mg/ml (PPB)

Results: parts per billion of the analyzed compound / Population Average: The arithmetic mean derived exclusively from the population segment tested by this lab.

A GVST or Volatile Panel may also be ordered to reveal levels of toxic chemicals. Other toxicological panels are available to evaluate many other xenobiotics including pesticides.

> > < <

Treatment Options

Individuals need to be knowledgeable about various treatment options and, with their doctor's help, choose those options that are best suited for them. EPD (Enzyme Potentiated Desensitization), NAET (Nambudripad Allergy Elimination Techniques), muscle testing, acupuncture, and immunotherapy are options for treating sensitivities. Immunotherapy often provides the most effective, long-term relief for the allergic patient. Food sensitivities are usually most effectively treated by a combination of rotary/diversified elimination diet and immunotherapy. Inhalant allergies respond most effectively to environmental controls and immunotherapy.

Medications for the allergic patient include Nasalcrom (Cromolyn Sodium), Seldane, Hismanal, Sudafed and Benadryl. Alternative and homeopathic treatments are also available. Vitamins, minerals and herbs can often promote health and reduce symptoms. IV therapy in combination with deep-heat-chamber chemical detoxification can be helpful in reducing the toxic body burden.

Environmental controls and the use of less-toxic products within your environment are vital to controlling allergens and contaminants. Less-Toxic Alternatives for many common toxins are listed in Part III.

> > < <

Supplements

Knowledge is power – power to control decisions that influence your environment and health, and mold your future.

Knowledge is helpful to the experts who assist you in achieving your health goals. Your medical, surgical, employment and environmental history are essential to health professionals as they make decision that affect your health. Your assistance and active participation is vital as they make decisions that can be the difference between illness, health and length of recovery.

Sometimes conventional treatments do not achieve the desired goals. Individuals can also be allergic to medication, or the need to take one medication can interfere with the success of another. Knowledge of the effects and interactions of your medications, vitamins, minerals, amino acids and herbs; and the role they can play in the creation and maintenance of a healthy mind and body is essential to the health conscious individual.

Many people who think they eat a balanced diet, and therefore receive all the essential vitamins and minerals, fall short of their goal. Food is not always grown in soil full of nutrients. Years of pesticide usage, overuse of land, and use of commercial fertilizers can rob the soil of nutrients. Food additives, preservatives, and the processing of foods can rob the diet of adequate vitamins and minerals. Also a person's ability to digest and efficiently absorb nutrients affects availability of essential vitamins, minerals and amino acids.

Prevention's 1994 Complete Book of Natural and Medicinal Cures (Rodale Press) quotes Neil Stone, M.D., (Chairman of the American Heart Association's Nutrition Committee and Associate Professor of Medicine at Northwestern University) as saying: "Perhaps five of the ten leading causes of death in the United States are nutritionally caused and, as such, diseases like heart disease, cancer and stroke can often be prevented."

"There are four ways in which diet can produce disease," explains John Potter, M.D., Ph.D. (Professor of Epidemiology at the University of Minnesota). "We eat too much, we eat too much of the wrong things, we don't eat enough of the right things, and we eat things in our foods like preservatives and pesticide residues that the body can't handle well – or at least not in the quantities we consume."

Also most of us experience stress, find ourselves in a time bind, which leads to fast food consumption and the consumption of too much fat, meat, and not enough fiber. Potter says that we need to think about the ways our ancestors ate. They were gatherers, hunters, and ate more berries, fruits, roots, leaves, nuts and seeds with only an occasional piece of meat. He also stresses that milk came from mom and that there were no ice cream and potato chips.

Genetic engineering and molecular biology have provided tools to obtain information at the molecular level of food. Researchers like Dick Huston, Ph.D. (a Biochemist who heads the Interdisciplinary Functional Foods for Health Program at the University of Illinois) discovered that broccoli contains sulforaphane, a substance that may help in cancer prevention. Brussels sprouts and mustard greens contain indols that may reduce the risk of breast cancer. Garlic and onions contain organosulfides that may prevent blood clots and tumor growth.

According to Gary Frazer, M.D., Ph.D. (Professor of Medicine and Epidemiology at Loma Linda University) "foods are no longer fats, proteins and carbohydrates, but bio-chemically active substances that can be of value in fighting disease."

You must eat right, knowing the benefits of the foods; but you also need to know the benefits of vitamin and mineral substances to assist your body with all the stresses of job, family and disease.

Dr. Jeffrey B. Plumberg, Ph.D. (Former Associate Director of the U.S. Department of Agriculture's Human Nutrition Center on Aging at Tuffs University) encourages proper eating habits, but insists that supplementing with vitamins and minerals should be considered as a low cost form of health insurance."

Aerobic activity is concerned with every cell receiving maximum oxygen for maximum cellular growth and health. In *The Complete Book of Nutraerobics* (Harper & Row, 1983), Jeffrey Bland, Ph.D. (Professor of Nutritional Bio-chemistry at the University of Puget Sound) presents a program of nutraerobics, which reminds us that aerobics is more than exercise and adequate cellular oxygen. Aerobics is exercise and nutrition and life style. Nutraerobics, achieving maximum cellular efficiency, requires exercise, diet, knowledge and commitment.

> > < <

VITAMINS

Vitamins and minerals are classified as micro-nutrients and are central to human nutrition. Vitamins are organic, meaning they contain the element carbon, and are found in plant and animal substances in small amounts. We obtain them by eating the plants and animals that make them. Most vitamins cannot be manufactured in our body, with the exception of some of the B vitamins that can be made by our intestinal bacteria, and an occasional biological conversion of a precursor into an active form (such as beta-carotene conversion to vitamin A).

Vitamins function principally as co-enzymes for a variety of metabolic reactions and biochemical mechanisms within our many body systems. Vitamins, themselves, are not part of our body tissues – they are not building blocks, but helpers in our body's metabolism. We can't live on vitamins, but must have food and certain minerals to best absorb any vitamin supplements we take. Vitamins are essential for growth, vitality and health; and are helpful in digestion, elimination and resistance to disease. Deficiencies can lead to a variety of both specific nutritional disorders and general health problems.

Water-soluble vitamins are B and C, which are mostly found in vegetables and are not stored in the body to a large degree. These may be easily lost during the cooking and processing of foods. Fat-soluble vitamins A, D, E and K are found in the lipid component of both vegetable and animal source foods. These can be stored in body tissues, so we can function for longer periods of time without obtaining them from our diet.

Vitamin supplements may be used as a preventative approach to improve or maintain health. They can be especially helpful after surgery or an illness. If soil was rich in vitamins and minerals – and none were lost in cooking or processing – we could probably get enough in our diet, and there would be no need for supplementation. However, due to our stressful way of life with consumption of fast foods, sugar, alcohol, and caffeine, a need for supplementation may arise. It is up to each individual, with the help of his physician, to assess one's own situation and achieve a supplementation program best fitted to existing needs.

VITAMIN A – BETA CAROTENE or RETINOL

Importance: This is a very important vitamin for the eye and helps maintain the health of the cornea, which is the covering of the eye. It counteracts night vision problems and weak eyesight. It is necessary for the growth and repair of tissues, bones and teeth. It stimulates growth at the base layer of the skin cells. Vitamin A helps both external skin cells and the mucous membrane cells that line the eyes, mouth, nose, throat, and lungs; thereby reducing susceptibility to infections and protecting us from air pollution. It may even aid the immune response by aiding T-helper cell activity. Vitamin A helps protect the body from free radical damage. It helps promote the cellular integrity of the mucous membrane lining of the intestinal tract, respiratory system and bladder. It helps them reach maturity and gives them structural integrity. It may also be helpful in preventing ulcers and arteriosclerosis. Vitamin A, along with adequate protein intake, generates healthy hair. It is absorbed primarily from the small intestine; and is a fat-stored vitamin that can be stored in the liver, kidneys, lungs, eyes and fatty tissue

Deficiencies: Vitamin A deficiency may result in night blindness and lack of tearing, increased susceptibility to infections, frequent fatigue, insomnia, loss of smell, decrease in appetite, and retarded growth. Vitamin A deficiency can reduce both t-lymphocyte and b-lymphocyte responses. Deficiency causes rough, dry, scaly skin (especially on the back of the arms); decreased skin tone and skin aging. Vitamin A deficiency can also be related to periodontal disease (defective teeth and gums), kidney stone formation, ear problems and acne. Vitamin C seems to be lost most rapidly from the body when there is a vitamin A deficiency.

Dangers: Because it is stored in fat, too much vitamin A can be detrimental to health. This can lead to swelling of the brain with resulting headaches.

Sources: Preformed vitamin A (retinol) is found in all kinds of liver, fish liver oil, egg yolk and milk. Pro vitamin A (beta carotene) is converted in the body from several carotene pigments found in foods – mainly yellow and orange vegetables and fruits as well as some green, leafy vegetables. Beta carotene is the most available pigment and yields the most vitamin A. Its absorption is reduced with the use of alcohol, mineral oil, exercise, cortisone medication, excessive iron intake and by a vitamin E deficiency. Its storage is decreased during times of excessive stress and illness.

Supplementation: An adult can safely take approximately 10,000 IUs of vitamin A daily. Supplementation is more efficient when there are sufficient body levels of zinc. (If sufficient vitamin C and E are present in the body, less vitamin A is needed as C and E protect fat-stored A.)

VITAMIN B1 – THIAMINE

Importance: Thiamine helps all the cells in our body function normally. It has a key metabolic role in the cellular production of energy by helping the body break down the macro-nutrients of carbohydrates, protein and fat. It helps in the initial steps of fatty acid and sterol production, and is necessary for the metabolism of ethanol. It is important to the health of the nerves and nervous system – possibly because of its role in the synthesis of acetylcholine.

Thiamine is linked to individual learning capacity and to growth in children. It is important to the muscle tone of the stomach, intestines and heart because of the function of acetylcholine at the nerve synaptic junction. It stabilizes the appetite, and it is conceivable that adequate thiamine levels may help prevent the accumulation of fatty deposits in the arteries. Thiamine has been helpful in decreasing the sensory neuropathy that accompanies diabetes and in lessening the pain of trigeminal neuralgia. It has a mild diuretic effect. It is eliminated through the skin and may thus help repel insects such as flies and mosquitoes. It can be used in the treatment of muscle tension, diarrhea, fever, infections, cramps and headaches.

Deficiency Symptoms: When there is a lack of B1, the nerves are more sensitive to inflammation. Thiamine was originally used to treat beriberi, which produced the symptoms of edema (swelling in the feet and legs spreading to the body), weight loss and muscle wasting. Some of the earliest symptoms of thiamine deficiency could be fatigue and instability, gastrointestinal disturbances, constipation, insomnia and burning chest pain. If unchecked, more severe thiamine deficiency symptoms could include mental confusion, muscular weakness and fatigue, enlargement of the heart, memory loss, confusion, depression and nerve degeneration. It may also involve degeneration of the brain and affect general orientation. Thiamine is lost in cooking and is depleted by the use of sugar, caffeine, tannin from black teas, nicotine, alcohol and birth control pills. Thiamine needs are increased with higher stress levels, fever, diarrhea, and during and after surgery.

Sources: Good sources of thiamine include wheat and rice germ and bran, rice husks, enriched wheat flour and brown rice. The milling of flour and the use of refined grains decrease the amount of available thiamine. Other good sources include brewer's yeast, black strap molasses, spinach, collard greens, brussels sprouts, asparagus, cauliflower, peanuts and other nuts, seeds, legumes, cooked beans and peas, potatoes, green peas, raisins, oranges, avocados and milk. Pork has a high amount of this vitamin.

Supplementation: Adequate supplementation is approximately 10 milligrams a day.

VITAMIN B2 – RIBOFLAVIN

Importance: Riboflavin is easily absorbed from the small intestine into the blood, which transports it to the tissue. Intestinal bacteria produces small amounts of riboflavin. Riboflavin functions as a precursor or building block for two coenzymes that are important in energy production: flavin mononecleotide (FMN) and flavin adenine dinucleodite (FAD). FMN and FAD carry nitrogen to cells throughout the body to help produce energy. B2 helps each cell utilize oxygen, thereby aiding cell respiration.

Riboflavin is necessary for carbohydrate, fat and protein metabolism; aids in the formation of antibodies and red blood cells; and is necessary for cell respiration – helping each cell utilize oxygen most efficiently. It helps maintain good vision, and supplemental riboflavin is commonly used to treat and help prevent vision problems, eye fatigue and cataracts. It is essential for healthy hair, skin and nails. B-2 is used in the treatment of alcohol problems, ulcers, digestive difficulty and leg cramps.

Deficiency Symptoms: Riboflavin is found in many foods that contain other B vitamins, but not in very high amounts; therefore dietary deficiency is fairly common. It may be the most common nutrient deficiency in America. Symptoms of vitamin B-2 deficiency include sensitivity and inflammation of the mucous membranes of the mouth, cracks or sores in the mouth and lips, purplish tongue, dermatitis with a dry yet greasy or oily scaling, dizziness, trembling, sluggishness and nerve tissue damage. Deficiency may result in itching and burning eyes, bloodshot eyes, and a higher incidence of cataracts. Hair loss, weight loss, growth retardation, general lack of vitality and digestive problems may also exist with B-2 deficiency.

Sources: Milk products contain some riboflavin. It is also found in brewer's yeast, liver, oily fish, nori seaweed, eggs, shellfish, millet, dark green leafy vegetables, and apples, figs, berries, grapes and tropical fruits. Riboflavin is very stable, but is sensitive to light – especially ultraviolet light. Therefore foods that contain even moderate amounts of riboflavin, such as milk, need to be protected from sunlight.

Supplementation: Riboflavin supplementation is usually between 25 to 50 milligrams daily, but can approach 100 milligrams if the need arises. Ten mg. daily is considered the best level of supplementation.

VITAMIN B3 – NIACIN

Importance: Vitamin B3 really consists of two different compounds – nicotinic acid and niacinamide. It is one of the more stable of the B vitamins and is resistant to heat, light, air, acid and alkaline. It is readily absorbed from the small intestine and can be manufactured from the amino acid tryptophan. About 50% of daily niacin results from the conversion of tryptophan to niacin with the help of vitamin B6. That conversion cannot take place if we are deficient in B1, B2, B6, Vitamin C and iron. When niacin is not present in sufficient amounts, extra protein is needed. Originally touted as a cure for pellagra, it (along with B1, B2, tryptophan and other nutrients) is responsible for successfully treating pellagra.

Niacin is helpful in the metabolism of some drugs and toxicants, and can be involved in more than 50 metabolic reactions. Niacin and its two coenzymes play a key role in glycolysis, are important in fatty acid synthesis, and are needed in the formation of red blood cells and steroids. Vitamin B3 stimulates circulation and may reduce blood cholesterol levels in some people. It is important to the healthy activity of the nervous system and to normal brain function. It has proven useful in treating Bells' palsy and trigeminal neuralgia. It is an important vitamin needed for the synthesis of sex hormones such as estrogen, progesterone and testosterone. Niacin is helpful in maintaining the healthy functioning of the nervous system, and supports the tissues of the digestive tract.

The flushing form of niacin is called nicotinic acid. Its most beneficial effect has been on the cardiovascular system. It may be beneficial in treating leg cramps caused by circulatory deficiencies. It can be useful for headaches, especially migraine, and in treating Meniere's disease. Nicotinic acid may also be useful in reducing blood pressure.

Deficiency Symptoms: A niacin deficiency affects every cell, but especially those with rapid turnover such as the skin, gastrointestinal tract and nervous system. Niacin deficiency can produce photosensitivity, a sore, red tongue, tender gums, canker sores, nausea, vomiting and diarrhea. It can also result in the neurological symptoms of irritability, insomnia, headache, tremors, extreme anxiety and depression. Although pellagra was once a common indication of deficiency, those deficiencies are now rare. However, a low protein diet (especially corn-based) may produce symptoms.

Dangers: When taken in high doses (50 mg. or more), niacin produces a temporary, harmless flushing sensation. However, large doses over a prolonged period can cause liver damage.

Sources: Some of the best sources of vitamin B3 are liver and other organ meats, poultry, fish, peanuts and peanut butter, brewer's yeast, cooked dried beans, green peas, wheat germs, avocados, dates, figs, prunes and milk.

Supplementation: Adequate intake of niacin may be from 25 to 50 milligrams a day. More may be needed during pregnancy and other growth periods. Athletes require more B3 than less active people because niacin's need is increased by exercise. Stress, illness and tissue injuries also increase the body's need for niacin.

VITAMIN B5 – PANTOTHENIC ACID

Importance: Pantothenic acid is closely involved in adrenal cortex function. It increases adrenal function and supports the adrenal glands in the production of cortisol. It aids in the utilization of other vitamins, and in the production of red blood cells. It helps the body heal wounds and fight infection by building antibodies. Pantothenic acid is important to healthy skin and nerves and could be useful for treatment of neuritis, MS, and epilepsy. It is also important in the metabolism and release of energy from protein, carbohydrates and fats. It is useful for treating fatigue and in blood sugar metabolism. It also increases gastric motility or peristalsis.

Deficiency Symptoms: A deficiency of B5 could result in increased allergies, decreased immunity, muscle cramping, abdominal stress, digestive disturbances and vomiting. Other symptoms of depletion may include fatigue, painful and burning feet, skin abnormalities, retarded growth, dizzy spells and restlessness. More severe depletion could result in increased cardiovascular and respiratory problems. Much pantothenic acid is lost in the processing and refining of grains. Up to 50% can be lost in cooking. Sugar and antibiotics reduce its absorption.

Sources: B5 is found in organ meats, fish, eggs, cheese, sweet potatoes, green peas, avocados, cauliflower, broccoli, collard greens, mushrooms, bananas, oranges, cantaloupe, cooked soybeans, peanut butter, brown rice, whole wheat bread and wheat germ.

Supplementation: The basic requirement for adults is 5.5 milligrams.

Less-Toxic Alternatives

VITAMIN B6 – PYRIDOXINE

Importance: Pyridoxine and its coenzyme form pyridoxal-5-phosphate have a wide variety of metabolic functions in the body. It is especially in amino acid metabolism and in the central nervous system where it supports the production of gamma-amino-butyric acid (GABA). Because it is involved with the central nervous system, it may be helpful in treating Parkinson's and MS, plus autism and hyperactivity in children. It elevates the immune system by helping in the formation of antibodies. B6, along with magnesium, aids in the prevention of kidney stones. It promotes healthy skin and may help decrease skin problems and dandruff. B6 can be helpful in managing stress, and may help counteract low blood sugar. Pyridoxal 5 Phosphate may be important for treating fatigue, allergies, viral infections, chemical sensitivities and carpal tunnel syndrome.

B6 is needed to maintain adequate intercellular magnesium levels, and helps maintain the balance of sodium and potassium in the body; thus its diuretic effect may be helpful in treating PMS, It is also needed for production of norepinephrine, acetylcholine and parahistadine. B6 helps amino acids cross the intestinal mucosal barrier; and, combined with Pyridoxal 5 Phosphate, helps build, break down, and change one amino acids into another. B6 is especially related to the production of choline, methionine, serine and cystine; and is essential for the conversion of tryptophan to niacin. It can also reduce muscle spasms, leg cramps, hand numbness and stiffness, and nausea.

Deficiency Symptoms: A deficiency of B6 may result in anemia, nervousness, insomnia, mouth disorders, skin eruptions and dermatitis, loss of hair, muscle weakness and loss of muscle control, arm and leg cramps, learning disabilities and water retention. Estrogen and birth control pills decrease levels of B6. Sugar, a high protein diet, radiation, aging and digestive problems increase the need for B6.

Sources: The best sources are meats, whole grains (especially wheat, wheat germ), fish, egg yolk, soy, bananas, avocado, cauliflower and potatoes.

Supplementation: The basic dosage of B6 is 10 to 15 mg. daily. But, for short periods of time, 50-100 mgs. of pyridoxal 5 phosphate can be taken daily. B6 absorption is aided by magnesium, zinc and B2.

VITAMIN B12 – COBALAMIN

Importance: Cobalamin is called the red energy vitamin. Because of its importance in the formation and regeneration of red blood cells, it helps prevent anemia, stimulates energy and encourages appetite and growth in children. It contributes to the health of the entire nervous system because it nourishes the myelin sheath. It may be helpful in treating trigeminal neuralgia, osteoporosis, fatigue (when given with folic acid), shingles, asthma and skin disorders. It is vital to the growth and repair of all our body's cells. B12 can also be helpful in treating amenorrhea if a person is deficient in B12, and should be given whenever gamma globulin IVs are given.

Deficiency Symptoms: Symptoms of deficiency may not show up for several years because B12 is stored in the kidney, liver and tissues. Some signs of B12 deficiency include vulnerability to colds, anemia and fatigue, bruising, poor absorption of food and poor appetite, and growth failure in children. If untreated a deficiency can lead to nerve disorders, neuritis, brain damage, degeneration of the spinal cord, lack of balance, and possibly Alzheimer's disease. Laxatives, antacids, stress, stomach problems, and the natural aging process can reduce B-12 absorption.

Sources: B-12 is not actually produced by plants and animals, but is created by bacteria in soil and in the digestive tracts of animals, including humans. It is found in animal protein foods, meat, fish, eggs, milk, cheese, and fermented soybean products such as miso and tempeh. Hydrochloric acid, calcium and the thyroid hormone aid its absorption, which takes place in the ileum.

Supplementation: Only minimal amounts (3 to 4 micrograms) of B12 are required in most adults to prevent deficiency. Anyone who does not consume animal products should take a multivitamin containing B12 at least every other day.

VITAMIN C – ASCORBIC ACID

Importance: Vitamin C is an essential, water-soluble vitamin that is easily absorbed by the intestine; then stored in the adrenal and pituitary glands, brain, eyes, ovaries and testes. It is used in the formation and maintenance of collagen, the intercellular "cement" which is the basis of connective tissues, bones, skin, ligaments, discs, capillary walls, teeth and gums. It gives strength to and helps maintain healthy blood vessels, and gives support and shape to the body. It helps wounds, scars and fractures heal; and prevents scurvy. Vitamin C builds resistance to infection and aids in the prevention and treatment of the common cold. It aids the metabolism of folic acid, and the metabolism or conversion of tyrosine to tryptophan and serotonin. Vitamin C stimulates adrenal function and the release of norepinephrine and epinephrine. It helps in cholesterol metabolism, thyroid hormone production, and helps prevent free radical damage. It may activate neutrophils and increase the production of lymphocytes. Vitamin C helps the absorption of iron and is a major antioxidant nutrient. It may help prevent the formation of cataracts and glaucoma. It prevents the conversion of nitrates found in tobacco smoke, smog, bacon, lunch meats and some vegetables into cancer-causing substances. Vitamin C may relieve the bronchospasms caused by inhalation of noxious stimuli.

Deficiency Symptoms: Symptoms may include soft, bleeding gums or tooth decay; swollen, painful joints or muscular weakness; slow-healing wounds and fractures; bruising, skin hemorrhages, capillary weakness, nosebleeds, or anemia; and loss of appetite or impaired digestion. Stress, birth control pills, estrogen, alcohol, smoking, cortisone, antibiotics, aspirin, pain medications, environmental toxins, and sulfa drugs all cause us to use vitamin C more rapidly.

Sources: Ascorbic acid is found in citrus fruits, rose hips, acerola, cherries, red and green peppers, broccoli, Brussels sprouts, tomatoes, asparagus and sprouts. It is an essential nutrient which must be obtained from the diet or through supplementation. It is destroyed by cooking, is easily oxidized in air and is sensitive to heat and light. Baking soda also destroys it. Copper, present in water or cookware, diminishes the vitamin C content of foods.

Supplementation: The body stores only about 5 grams of vitamin C, but we need at least 200 milligrams a day to maintain our body storage. It is used by the body within two hours and is out of the body in 3 to 4 hours. It is best to supplement with 2 to 4 grams per day. Vitamin C should be taken in 500 mg. increments every 3-4 hours with hesperidin and rutin.

CHOLINE

Importance: Choline is an integral part of the neurotransmitter acetylecholine. It aids in the transmission of electrical impulses between nerve endings. It is important to the health of the myelin sheath. It is often referred to as the memory vitamin and crosses the blood/brain barrier into spinal fluid to be directly involved in brain chemical metabolism. Choline may be useful in the treatment of nerve conduction problems, muscle twitching, memory deficiencies, dizziness, insomnia, headaches, glaucoma, tinnitus, and heart palpitations. It may even be useful in treating Alzheimer's disease, where it could increase brain function and perhaps slow the disease's progression. Choline also helps regulate the function of the kidneys, liver and gall bladder. It is important in the utilization of fats and helps control cholesterol buildup in the body, thus supporting weight loss.

Deficiency Symptoms: Choline is very sensitive to water and may be destroyed by cooking and food processing. It is diminished by the intake of alcohol and various drugs including estrogen and sulfa antibiotics. Severe deficiency may result in cirrhosis and fatty degeneration of the liver, hardening of the arteries, heart problems, high blood pressure and hemorrhaging kidneys.

Dangers: High doses of choline could aggravate epileptic conditions because of the nerve stimulation potential.

Sources: Choline can be synthesized from glycine. The highest amount of choline is present in lecithin (a soy product). Other good sources include egg yolk, brewer's yeast, wheat germ, fish, peanuts, liver and other organ meats.

Supplementation: There are no specific dietary requirements for choline, however the range can be from 500 to 1000 mg. daily.

VITAMIN D – CALCIFEROL

Importance: Vitamin D is also known as the sunshine vitamin because it is manufactured in the skin when in contact with ultraviolet light from the sun's rays. It is also a fat-soluble vitamin that is absorbed through the intestinal wall. Calciferol is taken from the blood to the liver where it is utilized and stored. It is also stored in the skin, brain, spleen and bones.

Vitamin D is most important in regulating calcium metabolism in the body and thus the normal calcification of bones. It helps increase the absorption of calcium from the intestine and decreases its excretion from the kidneys. Vitamin

D influences our utilization of the mineral phosphorus. It helps the teeth absorb calcium and phosphorus, stimulates the reabsorption of calcium and phosphorus from bones, and helps maintain the normal blood level of those two minerals. Its function is closely tied to that of the parathyroid gland. It functions more like a hormone because it is produced in one part of the body, the skin, then released into the blood to affect other tissues such as bones. When Vitamins D and A are taken together, they can reduce the incidence of colds and have helped muscle spasms, especially when related to anxiety. Vitamin D has also been used in the treatment of diabetes, cataracts, visual problems, allergies, sciatic pain and skin problems. It also helps maintain a stable nervous system and normal heart action.

Deficiency Symptoms: Decreased vitamin D may lead to rickets, tooth decay, softening of bones, improper healing of fractures, lack of vigor, muscular weakness, inadequate absorption of calcium and retention of phosphorous in the kidneys. People with gastrointestinal disease such as ulcerative colitis may be deficient in Vitamin D. Even though calcium supplementation could be adequate, if there is not enough vitamin D in the body, there will be poor calcification; therefore, those with osteoporosis or osteomalasia should be sure they are getting enough vitamin D along with their calcium supplementation. Mineral oil binds Vitamin D in the intestine and reduces its absorption.

Sources: Pro-vitamin D is found mainly in animal foods. D3 or natural vitamin D is found in fish liver oil. Egg yolk, butter and liver contain some.

Supplementation: Supplementing with vitamin D improves calcium absorption and reduces bone loss. It is best utilized with vitamin A, however most of the need for vitamin D is met through foods and sunlight exposure. The recommended supplementation of vitamin D is 400 IUs, and it is wise for adults to limit their supplementation to that amount.

VITAMIN E – TOCOPHEROL

Importance: Vitamin E is a yellow, fat-soluble vitamin; but is not stored quite as readily as other fat-soluble vitamins. Alpha-tocopherol is basically stable in heat and acids, and is absorbed from the intestines. It is also absorbed through the skin when used as an ointment or oil application.

The primary function of vitamin E is as an antioxidant. Its key role is to protect us from the oxidation of polyunsaturated fats and other oxidized fats such as the hydrogenated oils of margarine. Hydrogenated oils generate free radicals that lead to cellular and tissue irritation, damage, then inflammation. As an antioxidant, it helps stabilize cell membranes and protects the tissues of the skin, eyes, liver, breast and testes. This cellular protection is especially important to the vascular lining.

Vitamin E can have some anti-clotting properties and protects the red blood cell membranes from oxidated damage. It has recently been shown to reduce platelet aggregation and platelet adhesiveness to collagen; therefore it may be helpful in the prevention of atherosclerosis.

Vitamin E along with vitamin C, beta-carotene, glutathione or L-cystine, and the mineral selenium help protect us against the effect of free radical damage. Vitamin E modifies and stabilizes blood fat so that the blood vessels, heart and entire body are more protected from free radical-induced injury.

Vitamin E has also been used to enhance immunity in the treatment of viral disease and to reduce the neurological pain from shingles (a viral infection of the nerves and skin). It is also helpful in preventing eye problems such as poor vision or cataracts. Leg cramps and circulatory problems associated with diabetes may be helped with vitamin E treatment.

Deficiency Symptoms: Intestinal absorption is somewhat reduced by chlorine, inorganic iron and mineral oil. Unsaturated oils and estrogen deplete vitamin E. The inorganic form of iron also depletes vitamin E absorption and the two should not be taken together. Chlorine, ferrous chloride and rancid oils also deplete or destroy vitamin E.

Dangers: Large does of E should be avoided in people with high blood pressure because, although unproven, it has been thought to raise blood pressure. Excess intake is usually eliminated through urine and feces within a few days after excess supplementation is stopped.

Sources: Vitamin E, in its various tocopherol forms, is found in both plant and animal foods. There is a small amount found in egg yolk, butter, milk fat and liver; but the best sources are vegetable, seed or nut oils. The oil component of all grains, seeds and nuts contain tocopherol. The vitamin E content of most foods is related to the content of linoleic and linoleic acids. Safflower oil is one of the best sources of alpha-tocopherol.

Supplementation: A good supplementation with 100 IUs of 100% natural alpha tocopherol (which is 4 times as strong as synthetic alpha tocopherol – which would require 400 IUs) is probably sufficient. Natural alpha tocopherol is derived from soybeans, while the synthetic form is a petroleum by-product. Supplementation of 400 IUs of vitamin E palmatates and acetates (synthetic water-dispersible forms of vitamin E that have a good level of activity) are often easier to take because they can be combined with other vitamins. Supplemental estrogen and air pollution increase the need for vitamin E. It should not be taken with iron. However, selenium may increase the potency of vitamin E.

FOLIC ACID – FOLATE

Importance: Folic acid aids in amino acid metabolism and is essential for the formation and maturation of blood cells through its action on bone marrow. Folic acid, along with B12 and vitamin C, assists many amino acid conversions. Folic acid is necessary for DNA & RNA synthesis, which is important for the growth and division of cells in the body. It is thus more essential in times of rapid cell multiplication and growth, such as during pregnancy. Vitamin A and folic acid can help prevent cervical dysplasia. Folic acid is used rapidly by the skin and in those who have psoriasis.

Deficiency Symptoms: Folic Acid deficiency is one of the most common deficiencies of the B vitamin family and generates a picture similar to a B12 deficiency. Low levels of folic acid impair cell and tissue growth and repair; and result in anemia, poor nutrient absorption, weakness, fatigue, irritability, weight loss, headache, gastrointestinal disorders, diarrhea, heart palpitations, forgetfulness and possibly even a feeling of paranoia. Folic acid deficiency can sometimes be noted by cracks at the corners of the mouth, sore and inflamed tongue, and premature graying of the hair. A deficiency of folic acid and decreased nucleic acid synthesis during pregnancy can hamper cell division and result in low birth weight and growth problems in infants. Birth control pills can reduce absorption by 50%. Sulfa drugs, estrogen and dilantin may interfere with its absorption.

Sources: The best sources of folic acid are dark fresh green, leafy vegetables including spinach, kale, beet greens, chard, asparagus, romaine lettuce, Brussels sprouts, and broccoli. Bean sprouts of lentils, mung and soy are particularly good sources; as are wheat germ and whole wheat bread. It is also found in cooked red beans, beets, liver, kidney, brewer's yeast, and fruits such as avocados, bananas, oranges, pineapple, cantaloupe and berries. Folic acid's potency is lost during food processing because it is sensitive to light, heat, cooking and long-term storage.

Supplementation: Most Americans do not get adequate amounts in their diet, normally consuming only about half the recommended daily amount. People who are especially stressed or fatigued or have any loss of adrenal gland function may benefit from supplementation of folic acid. Illness and alcohol use create a greater need for folic acid. Those who suffer from cirrhosis and epileptics on any type of drug therapy require more folic acid. High dosage of Vitamin C may also cause the need for additional folic acid. The RDA of folic acid is 400 mcg. Daily and vitamin supplements usually contain that amount. 180-200 mcg are needed daily to replace tissues stores.

INOSITOL

Importance: Inositol is a member of the B vitamin family that is closely associated with choline. It helps emulsify (break down) fats, and reduce blood cholesterol. Inositol as phosphatidyl inositol has its primary function in cell structure and integrity. With choline it is important in brain cell nutrition. Inositol is especially important for the cells of the bone marrow, eye tissue and intestines. It may help promote healthy hair and skin and has been used to treat eczema. For sleep, 500 mg. of inositol before bedtime has a mild anti-anxiety effect. Inositol has also had some therapeutic success in improving nerve function in diabetic patients with pain and numbness due to nerve degeneration.

Deficiency Symptoms: An inositol deficit may result in eczema, hair loss, high blood cholesterol and constipation.

Sources: Inositol is found in lecithin, but in lesser amounts than choline. The body can produce its own inositol from glucose.

Supplementation: The therapeutic dosage is usually 500 milligrams daily. The need for inositol increases with coffee consumption.

PABA – PARA AMINO BENZOIC ACID

Importance: PABA is also a member of the B vitamin family and is part of the folic acid molecule. It is made by our intestinal bacteria. PABA aids in the assimilation of pantothenic acid, supports folic acid production by intestinal bacteria, and aids in the metabolism and utilization of amino acids. It is supportive of blood cells – particularly the red blood cells. PABA is important to the skin, hair pigment and is a very useful as a sunscreen. Vitiligo, a skin depigmentation condition, can be helped by supplementation of PABA. PABA can be useful in the treatment of fatigue, irritability, depression, nervousness, headache and graying hair. It is important to intestinal health and can be used to treat constipation and other digestive symptoms.

Deficiency Symptoms: A deficit of PABA may cause extreme fatigue, irritability, depression, nervousness, headaches, constipation, digestive disorders, eczema and premature graying of the hair. High amounts of sulfa drugs can cause a deficiency of PABA.

Dangers: High does of PABA can irritate the liver, and can also cause nausea and vomiting. People can be sensitive to PABA, especially in sunscreens.

Sources: Liver, brewer's yeast, wheat germ, whole grains, rice, eggs and molasses.

Supplementation: 50-1000 mg. daily (usually 150-300 mg.)

> > < <

MINERALS

Our natural minerals come from the earth, and it is important to obtain those essential minerals. If a mineral nutrient is not in the soil, it will not be in the water or food obtained from that soil. Our food may be lacking in minerals because of the loss of top soil, continual replanting without enriching the soil, and by the farmers' use of fertilizers that contain only nitrogen, phosphorus and potassium (without the addition of other important micro-minerals. Mineral deficiency is more common than vitamin deficiency because our bodies do not manufacture minerals, and foods may be enriched with only vitamins and not minerals. Minerals are harder than vitamins to liberate from foods during digestion; thus lower amounts are absorbed, even when the digestive system is functioning properly. With digestive difficulties, trace minerals such as chromium and zinc may be absorbed poorly and deficiencies may arise. Most minerals are destroyed by heat, and those soluble in water are often lost or leached out during cooking and processing.

There are approximately 17 essential minerals – 8 are macro minerals: calcium, potassium, sodium, phosphorus, chloride, sulfur, magnesium and silicon. The trace minerals that are known to be essential are iron, copper, zinc, cobalt, iodine, manganese, chromium, molydenium, selenium, boron 10 and vanadium. The uses, sources and functions of many of these minerals will be discussed in the following pages. Certainly the healthy approach is to get the majority of them from foods; but it is also necessary to assess your body's mineral content, state of health and lifestyle; then, after consultation with your physician, supplement accordingly.

CALCIUM

Importance: Calcium is the most abundant mineral in the human body and one of the most important. It constitutes about 1.5 to 2% of our body weight. Almost all of our approximately 3 pounds of calcium is contained in our bones, about 1% in our teeth, and the rest in other tissues and the circulation.

Calcium has some very important life supporting functions, the best known of which is the development and maintenance of bones and teeth. Calcium is one of the most important minerals used in the treatment of osteoporosis, although estrogen used in menopausal replacement therapy can certainly do its part in reducing the likelihood of this disease. Calcium may also help in the reduction of headaches, irritability, insomnia and depression associated with menopause.

Calcium circulating in the blood is needed for muscle contraction in muscular activity and in regulating the heart beat. Calcium along with magnesium is often used to reduce heart irregularity – calcium stimulates contraction, magnesium supports the relaxation phase, while sodium and potassium are important in generating the electrical impulse. Calcium plays an important role in cell division and blood clotting, and is important to normal kidney function. It also helps regulate the passage of nutrients in and out of cell walls.

In the nervous system, calcium is important to nerve transmission. It helps maintain proper nerve and muscle function, and influences nerve and cell membranes in the release of neurotransmitters including acetylcholine. Additional calcium may help protect us from the toxicity of cadmium or mercury exposure by competing for absorption. It has also been shown to lower blood pressure, reduce blood cholesterol levels, and reduce the incidence of colon cancer.

Deficiency Symptoms: Calcium deficiency in the blood can cause a wide range of symptoms: toxemia in pregnancy, anxiety, hyperkinesis, and otosclerosis. Mild calcium deficiency can cause nerve sensitivity, parathesias, muscle twitching, brittle nails, tooth decay, irritability, confusion, depression and insomnia. As it progresses, calcium deficiency can result in back, arm, leg, foot and other muscle cramps/spasms; bone softness, brittleness or deterioration (osteoporosis); rickets; heart palpitations/spasms; numbness, tingling and finally sustained contraction of the muscles. Calcium and vitamin D deficiency in puberty has even been linked to multiple sclerosis.

Many other nutrients, vitamin D and certain hormones are important to calcium absorption, function and metabolism. Calcium and phosphorus are both necessary for normal bones. Magnesium, silicon, strontium, and possibly boron, and the protein matrix are all part of our bone structure.

Vitamin D is needed for much calcium to be absorbed from the digestive tract. Along with the parathyroid hormone and calcitonin (secreted by the thyroid), vitamin D helps maintain normal blood calcium levels. Vitamin D may not be quite as necessary when calcium chelates such as calcium aspartate or calcium citrate are used. Besides vitamin D, vitamin A and C can help support the normal membrane transport of calcium. Gastric hydrochloric acid also helps calcium absorption.

During infancy and childhood we absorb 50 to 70% of the ingested calcium, whereas an adult absorbs only 30 to 50% of dietary calcium. Exercise has been shown to improve absorption and circulation of calcium, whereas lack of exercise and stress diminish its absorption. A diet containing proper, not excessive, amounts of protein, fat and acid foods may also help calcium absorption.

Calcium absorption becomes less efficient as we age. Many things in our diet can affect its absorption including chocolate and antacids. When the diet is too high in phosphorus, we can lose extra calcium through urine because the phosphorus content in the blood causes calcium to be pulled from the bones; therefore care should be taken to avoid excessive ingestion of phosphorus from soft drinks.

Sources: Milk and cheese are good sources of calcium. Most green, leafy vegetables are also good sources, but some contain oxalic acid, which impedes calcium absorption. Foods high in oxalic acid such as spinach, rhubarb, chard and beet greens are not particularly good sources. Broccoli, cauliflower and many peas and beans supply some calcium. Molasses, citrus fruits, figs and raisins are also good sources. Pinto, aduki and soybeans, almonds, Brazil nuts, hazelnuts, sunflower seeds and sesame seeds are good sources of calcium (though their phosphorus content is high). Exposure to sunlight increases the manufacture of vitamin D by the body, which in turn increases our absorption of calcium.

Supplementation: Many factors affect calcium absorption. Between 30 to 80% of calcium may be excreted and not utilized by the body. Adequate supplementation may approach 1000 milligrams (1 gram) daily. It is best taken between meals and before bedtime when the stomach is more acidic. Supplement calcium with a balance of magnesium, zinc and manganese. It is important to take ½ as much magnesium as calcium. Taking calcium with vitamin D and hydrochloric acid also helps its absorption. Calcium aspartate (50-90% absorbed), calcium citrate and chelated calcium such as calcium gluconate are good forms of supplemental calcium. Calcium carbonate is one of the lesser-absorbed forms of calcium. If a person has atherosclerosis or forms calcium oxalate kidney stones, supplementing with calcium can be hazardous and should be taken only under the direction of a physician.

CHROMIUM

Importance: Chromium is an essential, tri-bound trace mineral. It is a necessary part of the glucose tolerance factor, which is composed of chromium, niacin, and three amino acids (glyciene, cysteine, glutamic acid). The blood has about 20 parts per billion of chromium. It is stored in the brain, muscles, spleen, kidneys, testes and skin. Chromium regulates carbohydrate metabolism by enhancing the insulin function and improves the uptake of glucose into the cells. Elevated chromium tissue stores above 6 mg. are associated with decreased symptoms of both diabetes and arteriosclerosis. It is shown to mildly lower cholesterol while raising HDL.

Deficiency: An estimated 20 to 25 percent of the population is deficient in chromium. It is difficult to absorb and absorption decreases with age. Ten to twenty percent of the glucose tolerance type chromium is absorbed. It is lost in the refining of whole grain and sugar. The US has low levels of soil chromium, which decreases the amount available in food production. An elevated sugar or elevated fat diet can decrease chromium levels and make you prone for diabetes. Decreased chromium levels can produce anxiety, fatigue and can slow wound healing.

Source: Brewer's yeast is the best source with 44 parts per million, black pepper has 10 parts per million and molasses has 2 parts per million. Other sources include beef, liver, whole wheat, potatoes, apples, butter, bananas, spinach, beets, oysters, other shellfish and fish. The body does not produce chromium, so foods or supplementation must supply it.

Supplementation: 200-300 micrograms per day is an acceptable supplementation. It is better absorbed when combined with niacin, glycine and cysteine. Do NOT take chromium with milk.

COPPER

Importance: Copper is an essential trace mineral. It is present in all body tissues in the amount of 75-100 mg. with highest concentration in the brain, liver and muscles. Copper is important as a catalyst in the formation of hemoglobin. It is part of the cytochrome system for cell respiration. It works with C to form collagen. It is found in the superoxide dismutase system, thus playing a role in the metabolism of oxygen free radicals. Copper is important to the synthesis of phospholipids, thus contributing to integrity of the myelin sheath. Copper and zinc aid in converting the thyroid hormones T_3 to T_4. It also helps control levels of histamine.

Deficiency: A deficiency can result in reduced cellular immune response and reduced activity of whole blood cells. Copper deficiency is commonly found with iron deficiency and anemia. Symptoms include fatigue, paleness of skin, edema, hair loss, diarrhea and dermatitis. Low copper can affect collagen formation and tissue health and healing. Skeletal defects related to bone demineralization and irregular heart rhythm can result from copper deficiency.

Sources: 30% of copper intake is rapidly absorbed in the body from the stomach and upper intestines. Whole grains, wheat, shellfish, peas, beans, nuts, dark green leafy vegetables, black pepper and yeast provide our bodies with copper.

Supplementation: 2 mg. Zinc supplementation should be in a ratio of 15 mg. zinc to 2 mg. copper. Supplementation should be carefully considered

Less-Toxic Alternatives

being guided by laboratory tests under the direction of a physician. Copper toxicity is easily achieved due to copper water pipes. Estrogen and birth control pills can increase copper absorption. Symptoms of toxicity include depression and schizophrenia. Learning disabilities can be related to elevated copper levels. Supplementing with zinc, manganese, vitamin C and B may decrease elevated copper levels. EDTA can also be used.

IRON

Importance: Iron a is trace mineral found in every cell in the body, almost all of which is combined with protein. There is about one-tenth of a teaspoon in a 150 pound person (60 parts per million). Its primary function is the production of hemoglobin. Three-fourths of the body's iron is active – 70% in hemoglobin (the oxygen carrier), 5% in myoglobin (muscle), and the rest in iron cofactors and enzymes. Iron is stored in the liver, spleen and bone marrow; with these stores released for extra hemoglobin. When the body needs more iron, it increases its availability through iron-curing proteins called iron-transferrin (iron bound to tranferrin), which go to the bone marrow to form hemoglobin. There are 20 trillion red blood cells in the body, composed of 30% hemoglobin. The body produces about 115 million red blood cells a minute. About 90% of the needed iron is available from old blood cells, which are recycled by the spleen at the end of their 120-day life span. Myoglobin is an iron protein compound that contains oxygen and carries it to the muscles and heart. It provides our ability to work by increasing oxygen in muscles during activity. Twenty-five percent of the body's iron is stored bound to ferritin. Good serum ferritin is 15 to 200 micrograms.

Deficiency: Decreased iron will reduce hemoglobin and myoglobin, resulting in decreased oxygen to the tissues and muscles. Deficiency can result in fatigue, weakness and anemia (small, pale red blood cells). The cytochrome system (important in the oxidative process) depends on iron enzymes, which may also work within the mitochondria to produce energy.

Poor GI absorption plus decreased iron diets can lead to iron deficiency. We absorb only about 8 to 10 percent of the iron we consume. Milling of grain causes a 75% loss of its iron contents. Phytates in whole grains and oxalates in certain vegetables bind iron and reduce its absorption. Antacids, copper, phosphates in soft drinks, oxalates in spinach, caffeine, tannic acid, soy protein and fast GI motility decrease absorption. The average person loses about 1 milligram of iron per day, but thirty to forty milligrams can be lost in a menstrual period. Blood tests to check for iron deficiency include a ferritin, a total iron-binding capacity, a serum transferin, and an iron saturation test.

Thyroid problems and lead toxicity can create anemia. Red blood cells need calcium, protein, vitamins E and C to stay healthy. Depressed iron leads to paleness, sore tongue and possibly canker sores. Hair loss, itchy scalp, brittle nails, apathy, depression and irritability can also be signs of low iron. Low intake, poor absorption, parasites and decreased stomach acid can also cause low iron.

Sources: Pork, lamb, chicken, shell fish, salmon, egg yolks, whole grains, wheat, millet, oats, peas, beans, green peas, tomatoes, strawberries, kelp, brewer's yeast, Brazil nuts, and unsulfured molasses (1 tablespoon equals 3 milligrams of iron). Vegetables have non-heme iron, while meats have heme iron of which 10 to 30% is absorbed. When you eat both, more non-heme iron is absorbed. Iron absorption takes 2 to 4 hours. Vitamin C and citrus fruits increase iron absorption because they create the ferric form, which is better absorbed. Iron cookware and manganese also help increase iron absorption.

Supplementation: An adult should have about 10 mg. a day. Iron supplements need to be taken between meals and should be chelated such as iron aspartate, ferrous succinate or humorate. Even though absorption increases with Vitamin C, it may take months to replenish an iron deficiency. Iron can rob your body of vitamin E so it should not be taken at the same time as supplementation with that vitamin. Do not take Calcium with Iron because it may be rendered unavailable for absorption. A deficiency or need should be medically documented before supplementation is undertaken. A high meat diet and taking multivitamins plus iron supplements may cause iron toxicity because we excrete very little iron. Elevated iron can increase the risk of heart disease.

MAGNESIUM

Importance: Magnesium is a very important intracellular macro-mineral. It is involved in many enzymatic reactions, many of which contribute to the production of energy and cardiovascular function. Magnesium and calcium are earth-alkaline minerals. Magnesium is the iron of the plant world – as iron is to hemoglobin, magnesium is to chlorophyll. There are only several ounces in the body. About 65% is in the bones and teeth; and the remaining 35% in the blood, fluid and other tissues. The highest concentration of magnesium is in the brain. It is even present in significant amounts in the heart.

Magnesium is considered the anti-stress mineral, and it is a natural tranquilizer. Its function is to relax skeletal muscles and the smooth muscles of blood vessels and the GI tract. While calcium stimulates muscle contractions, magnesium relaxes them. Because of its influence on the heart, magnesium is considered important in preventing coronary artery spasms. Magnesium can help myocardial infarctions. It has a mild affect on lowering blood pressure, and can also help reduce the symptoms of mitral valve prolapse including palpitations and arrhythmia.

Magnesium also modulates the electrical potential across cell membranes. It helps in the release of energy, and fatigue can often be reduced with the use of magnesium and potassium supplementation. It can be an aid in the prevention of kidney stone formation and in treating PMS. Magnesium, combined with vitamin B6, is also given as part of the treatment for autism and hyperactivity in children.

Deficiency Symptoms: Magnesium deficiency is fairly common. Early symptoms can include fatigue, anorexia, irritability, insomnia, nervousness, muscle tremors or twitching. Tachycardia can result from a mild magnesium deficiency. Numbness, tingling and tetany or prolonged muscle contractions can be symptoms of a more severe deficiency. Decreased levels of magnesium can be related to high blood pressure, kidney stones, heart disease and heart attacks due to coronary artery spasms. A deficiency in magnesium may also result in calcium depletion. Alcohol, caffeine, excess sugar, diuretics, birth control pills and drinking too much water cause magnesium loss and increase the need for magnesium. Stress also increases magnesium excretion. Temporary magnesium depletion may make the heart more sensitive to electrical abnormalities and vascular spasm; this can even lead to cardiac ischemia. Deficiency is usually more common after burns, serious injuries or surgery, and in diabetes, liver disease or malabsorption problems.

Sources: Almost all of our magnesium comes from the vegetable kingdom, primarily from dark green leafy vegetables since it is the iron of the plant world. Many nuts (almonds, pecans, cashews and Brazil nuts), seeds and legumes have high amounts of magnesium; as well as soy, tofu, whole grains and hard water. However, magnesium can be lost in the processing and refining of foods, with nearly 85% of the magnesium in grains lost in the milling process. Soaking and boiling foods can leach magnesium into the water. As with calcium, oxalic acids in vegetables such as spinach can form insoluble salts with magnesium, causing it to be eliminated rather than absorbed.

Supplementation: If you take 1000 milligrams of calcium daily, you should take 500 milligrams of magnesium. Magnesium, chelated with amino acids, is probably the most absorbable form. Magnesium oxide is probably better absorbed than magnesium carbonate. The newly available salts of magnesium such as magnesium aspartate or citrate do have a good percentage of absorption. Because magnesium also requires an acidic stomach, it should be taken between meals and at bed time. A diet that is too high in protein, fat, phosphorus or even calcium can reduce magnesium absorption; therefore it is best to take some magnesium by itself on an empty stomach. Usually about 40 to 50% of the magnesium we consume is absorbed, but this can vary from a low of 25% to a high of 75%.

MANGANESE

Importance: Manganese is an essential mineral. The body contains 15 to 20 milligrams: one-half of which is in the bones. The remainder being in the liver, pancreas, pituitary gland, adrenal gland, and kidneys. It activates the enzyme that enables the body to utilize biotin, B1, C and choline. Chromium, zinc and manganese are important to glucose metabolism. Manganese helps pancreatic function, is important to the digestion and utilization of food, and the synthesis of fatty acids and l-dopamine. Manganese activates the arginine enzyme system, which forms urea – the end product of protein and ammonia breakdown cleared by the kidneys. It is important to the growth and development of proper bone structure, and in the formation of mucopolysaccharides, which are needed for healthy joint membranes. It is an antioxidant, and is part of the superoxide dismutase system in the brain and other tissues. It also protects the mitochondia – the energy factory of the cell.

Deficiency: Decreased manganese can lead to decreased strength, ataxia, dizziness, weakness, irregular heart beats, skin problems and weight loss.

Sources: Nuts, whole grain bran and germ, egg yolk, seeds, legumes and spinach. Soil effects the amount of manganese in food, and 90% is lost in refinement.

Supplementation: We need 4 to 5 milligrams a day. Optimal absorption occurs when it is taken in the absence of all other minerals or food, and in its protein-chelated form. Lecithin can increase our body's absorption of manganese. Antacids, zinc, cobalt and soy protein all interfere with manganese absorption into the blood from the intestines. We must carefully manage each mineral's supplementation because one can interfere with the absorption of another: magnesium and zinc can decrease copper; zinc, cobalt and soy interfere with magnesium; iron and manganese interfere with each other's absorption.

PHOSPHORUS

Importance: Phosphorus is the second most abundant mineral next to magnesium. One percent of our total body weight is phosphorus. It is present in every living cell, but most abundant in the bones and teeth. The proper overall body level of calcium to phosphorus is 1-to-1. In the bones it is present in calcium phosphate, in an amount one-half that of total calcium. These minerals are in constant turnover, even in the bones.

Phosphorus is vital to tooth and bone formation, with most deposited in bones, then teeth, then other cells – including red blood cells. Phosphorus is important in energy production and exchange, in the utilization of carbohydrates and fats, and in protein synthesis. It is also a component of phospho-lipids. It helps maintain membrane fluidity and permeability, aids muscle contraction, regulates the heartbeat and aids nerve conduction. It is important in treating bone fractures in osteoporosis and minimizes bone calcium loss.

Deficiency Symptoms: Iron, aluminum, magnesium and antacids deplete phosphorus absorption. Low calcium to phosphorus ratio increases the risk of elevated blood pressure and colon and rectal cancer. A phosphorus deficiency can contribute to stiff joints, paresthesia, bone pain, weakness and anorexia.

Sources: Proteins have 10 to 20 times more phosphorus than calcium. Since phosphorus is part of all cells, it is readily found in food. Beets, fish, chicken, turkey, milk, cheese, and eggs all contain substantial amounts. Most red meats and poultry have 10 to 20 times more phosphorus than calcium, whereas fish generally have 2 to 3 times as much phosphorus as calcium. Seeds and nuts also contain more calcium than phosphorus. Dairy products, fruits and vegetables are generally more balanced.

Supplementation: If needed, 800 milligrams a day is usually adequate supplementation. The typical American diet is too elevated in phosphorus. Calcium and phosphorus compete for absorption in the intestines, but phosphorus is absorbed more efficiently with about a 70% absorption rate.

84

This can result in reduced body stores of calcium. The kidneys and parathyroid regulate the amount stored in the body; while calcium, vitamin D and parathyroid hormone regulate the metabolism of both phosphorus and calcium.

POTASSIUM

Importance: Potassium is a significant body mineral that is important to the functioning of cells. Potassium, sodium and chloride are the three main blood minerals or electrolytes. Potassium is the primary positive ion within the cell. 98% of potassium is found within the cells, and magnesium helps maintain potassium within the cells. Elevated sodium in the diet with low potassium influences the vascular volume and tends to elevate blood pressure.

It regulates the water and acid base balance in the cells. It enters the cells easier than sodium. When potassium leaves the nerve cell, it initiates the sodium-potassium exchange across the cell membrane. It changes the membrane potential and allows nerve impulses to progress. It is important in the synthesis of proteins to amino acids and in carbohydrate and glucose metabolism. It is crucial to cardiovascular and nerve function.

Sources: Oranges, apples, raisins, whole grains, spinach, lettuce, broccoli, lima beans, tomatoes, potatoes, seeds, nuts, fish and salmon are good sources of potassium. The body should contain 9 ounces of potassium to 4 ounces of sodium. The packaging of foods and use of convenience foods with excessive salt intake makes maintaining the proper balance very difficult. About 90% of potassium in foods is absorbed in the small intestine.

Deficiency: Potassium is easily lost in cooking and processing and is heavily lost in sweat. Alcohol, coffee, sugar, diuretics, laxatives, and cortisone can all deplete potassium stores. It is important that we avoid increased sodium and decreased potassium. Diarrhea, vomiting, and GI problems can cause decreased potassium. Depressed potassium can lead to elevated blood pressure, congestive heart failure, arrhythmia, fatigue, depression, bone fragility, muscle weakness, insomnia, loss of GI tone and impaired glucose metabolism. Potassium deficiency is a very common deficiency.

Supplementation: Using potassium salt will help maintain proper electrolyte balance. It is important to have a 2-to-1 potassium to sodium balance in your diet. The RDA for potassium is 2-2.5 grms. per day.

SELENIUM

Importance: Selenium is an essential nutrient. Its main function is as a component of the glutathione-peroxidase enzyme system. It protects cell membranes and the intercellular structural membrane from lipid peroxidation. It also protects us from the toxic effect of heavy metals. It aids in preventing cardiovascular disease, stroke and arteriorsclerosis. It can reduce cancer risk. It works together with vitamin A for antioxidant protection and immuno-stimulating effects. There is less than 1 milligram in our bodies, which is found in the liver, kidneys, pancreas, and the testes. It aids in sperm production and motility but is lost in semen. It aids red blood cell metabolism, and can slow aging and tissue degeneration. It has immuno-stimulating properties, and can aid antibody formation in response to vaccines.

Deficiency: Decreased selenium can be associated with elevated cancer rates. But elevated sodium-selenite is toxic. Soils can be low in selenium – Ohio is the lowest and South Dakota is the highest. Deficiency can be involved in infections, cervical dysplasia and can lead to breast and GI cancer. A deficiency may be associated with eczema, rheumatoid arthritis, psoriasis and cataract formation.

Sources: Brewer's yeast, butter, liver, fish, shellfish, lamb, wheat germ, whole grains, barley, oats, whole wheat, brown rice, molasses, nuts, Brazil nuts, vegetables, garlic, onions, mushrooms, broccoli, radishes, and swiss chard – if the soil they are grown in has adequate selenium. It is lost in the processing of white rice and white flour.

Supplementation: 200 mcg. daily. Take Selenium with vitamin E, to enhance its absorption; but not with C, which may inactivate it.

SODIUM

Importance: Sodium is the primary positive ion in the blood and body fluids. It is found in every cell but is mainly extra-cellular, with sixty percent outside the cells, 10% inside cells and 30% in the bones. Ninety to a hundred grams of sodium are in the body – mostly in combination with chloride. The kidneys and adrenal glands regulate sodium in cells, and it is closely tied to the movement of water in the body. Sodium, potassium and chloride are the body's electrolytes. Sodium works closely with potassium to regulate the fluid balance inside and outside the cell. Potassium and sodium work with the kidneys to regulate the acid-base balance. The membranous shifting of potassium and sodium create the electrical charge that helps muscle contract and nerve impulses to be generated. Sodium is important in the production of hydrochloric acid and aids in transporting amino acids to the blood.

Deficiency: The body normally loses 8 grams of sodium a day; but an excess can be lost in sweating, vomiting and diarrhea. When sodium and water are lost together, the extra cellular fluid volume is depleted, which can lead to increased hematacrit, decreased blood pressure and muscle cramps. Failure to replenish salt loss can result in nausea, vomiting, swelling, headache, muscle weakness, loss of appetite, poor concentration and poor memory.

Sources: Sodium is found in seafood, beef and vegetables such as celery, beets, carrots, kelp, and sea-vegetables. Lunchmeat, cheese, pickles that are salt-cured, crackers and chips yield too much salt. Sodium can also be contained in baking soda and MSG. Americans today normally consume 6 to 12 grams of salt, which is 40% sodium and 60% chloride. The sodium-potassium ratio is very important to blood pressure and a healthy lifestyle. Too much salt in the diet may lead to or be related to elevated blood pressure. A low sodium diet with adequate calcium, magnesium and chloride is usually implicated to maintain proper blood pressure. Almost 100% of sodium intake is absorbed in the stomach, and it is estimated that Americans consume 90% more sodium than is needed.

86

Supplementation: We should get 2 grams of sodium daily, and calcium should exist in a 2-to-1 ratio to sodium. This ratio can be aided by the use of potassium salt. When sodium and water are lost together, it needs to be replenished with one-fifth teaspoon of salt per quart of water.

ZINC

Importance: It is found in only small amounts in the body (33 parts per million – 2 to 2.5 grams total), second to iron. It is found in the body in the heart, spleen, lungs, brain, adrenal glands, nails, hair, teeth, retina and semen. Zinc is involved in the production of 100 enzymes, and in probably more body functions than any other mineral. It helps utilize and maintain body levels of vitamin A, is important in energy production, helps the liver detoxify alcohols, and is part of the alkaline-phosphatase enzyme that helps contribute phosphates to bones.

It improves antibody response to vaccine and improves cell-mediated immunity. It aids in the production of t-lymphocytes. It is important to insulin activity, taste, male sexual organ function and can decrease prostrate enlargement. It may have anti-inflammatory effect on joints and arterial lining. Because it enhances wound healing, it should be taken before and after surgery. It can be used in healing burns and may help acne. 150 milligrams a day has been used to help with leg and gastric ulcers. It can decrease the incidence of colds and enhance the sense of taste. It can decrease dental carries by strengthening enamel. Zinc can lower sodium and cadmium toxicity. Zinc with B6 can help schizophrenia. Zinc with manganese can help treat senility.

Deficiency: American soil is somewhat depleted of zinc. Zinc is also decreased in food processing as 80% of the zinc is lost in making white flour. Much zinc is lost in the water during cooking, and we absorb only 20 to 40 percent of what is ingested. It is absorbed to a lesser degree when bound with phytates in grains or oxalates in vegetables. Calcium, phosphorus and copper also affect its absorption. Decreased zinc can result in hair loss, brittle nails, stretch marks, poor growth and loss of appetite in children. Birth control pills, alcohol, diuretics, diet, stress, aging, parasites and sweating deplete zinc, and increase your need for it. Vegetarians and people who eat only grains may be deficient in zinc. GI surgery and poor pancreatic function decreases zinc in the body.

Sources: Animal foods, fish, poultry, whole grains, nuts, Brazil nuts, pumpkin seeds, black pepper and ginger root are good sources of zinc.

Supplementation: 30 milligrams of zinc daily. It should be taken first thing in the morning or 2 hours after meals. Magnesium, vitamin A, B and C can be taken with zinc. Zinc supplementation can cause decreased copper absorption, therefore supplement zinc with some copper and iron so that a deficiency isn't created in either mineral.

> > < <

AMINO ACIDS

Protein is an essential part of nutrition. Water makes up the principal part of the body's physical composition, and protein makes up 20% or about 1/5 of body weight. Protein is found in muscles, especially the heart and brain, and in the hair, nails, skin and eyes. It is important for immune function, metabolism, and the oxygen carrying capacity of the blood. Proteins combine nitrogen, carbon, oxygen and hydrogen and are comprised of 22 naturally occurring amino acids. Twenty main amino acids and some minor ones are required to build body proteins. There are 8 essential amino acids we cannot synthesis that must be obtained from the diet, and 12 non-essentials that we use to build body proteins. If protein, vitamins and minerals are deficient in our diet; a deficiency may be created in non-essential amino acids and the proteins produced by those amino acids. Production and conversion of many non-essential amino acids are found in the liver. Vitamin B6 is required to generate the non-essential amino acids.

PROTEIN REQUIREMENTS
Recommended Daily Allowances for Dietary Intake of Protein
Reflecting Average Health and a Variety of Common Foods

	Age (years)	Weight (kg)	Weight (lb)	Height (cm)	Height (in)	Protein (g)
Infants	0.0-0.5	6	13	60	24	kgx2.2
	0.5-1.0	9	20	71	28	kgx2.0
Children	1-3	13	29	90	35	23
	4-6	20	44	112	44	30
	7-10	28	62	132	52	34
Males	11-14	45	99	157	62	45
	15-18	66	145	176	69	56
	19-22	70	154	177	70	56
	23-50	70	154	178	70	56
	51 +	70	154	178	70	56
Females	11-14	46	101	157	62	46
	15-18	55	120	163	64	46
	19-22	55	120	163	64	44
	23-60	55	120	163	64	44
	51 +	55	120	163	64	44
Pregnant						+30
Lactating						+20

Source: *Recommended Dietary Allowance*, 9th ed. Committee on Dietary Allowances, Food and Nutrition Board, National Research Council, Washington, D.C.; National Academy of Science, 1980.

Less-Toxic Alternatives

Amino acids are an important part of nutrition. Supplementation should be done under the care of a physician after blood and urine tests have revealed an individual's need for supplementation of amino acids. They can help protect us from the environment and maintain healthy heart, muscles, brain and neurotransmitter function.

ESSENTIAL AMINO ACIDS

MINIMUM ESSENTIAL AMINO ACID REQUIREMENTS FOR THE AVERAGE AMERICAN

| | Minimal Requirements | | |
| | Infants | Men | Women |
Essential Amino Acid	mg/kg/day	g per day	g per day
Histidine	32		
Isoleucine	90	0.70	0.45
Leucine	120	1.10	0.62
Lysine	90	0.80	0.50
Methionine			
In absence of cystine		1.10	
In presence of 15 mg cystine per kg	85		
In presence of 50 mg cystine per kg	65		
In presence of 200 mg cystine			0.35
In presence of 810 mg cystine	0.20		
Phenylalanine			
In absence of tyrosine		1.10	
In presence of 175 mg. tyrosine per kg	90		
In presence of 1100 mg. tyrosine	0.30		
In presence of 900 mg tyrosine			0.22
Threonine	60	0.50	0.30
Tryptophan	30	0.25	0.16
Valine	93	0.80	0.65

Source: Robinson, C. *Fundamentals of Normal Nutrition.* New York: Macmillan, 1983.

ISOLEUCINE
Importance: Isoleucine is found in high concentration in muscles. It is used for energy production, and it may decrease twitching and tremors.
Sources: Fish, meat, cheese, wheat germ, seeds and nuts.

LEUCINE
Importance: Leucine is essential for growth as it stimulates protein synthesis. It can help produce energy, stabilize blood sugar and can be helpful in healing wounds involving skin and bones.
Sources: Poultry, red meat, dairy products, wheat germ and oats.

LYSINE
Importance: Lysine helps in the absorption of calcium from the intestinal tract. It promotes bone growth and, in combination with vitamin C, yields hydroxy-lysine to make collagen, which is the matrix of skin, bones, cartilage

and connective tissues. It is popular in the treatment of herpes. Lysine and arginine can be used in a three-to-one lysine-arginine ratio to stimulate growth hormones. A deficiency can lead to suppressed immune response and urinary calcium elevation.

Sources: Grain, cereals, peanuts, fish, meats, dairy products, beans, eggs, fruits and vegetables. We need 75 mg. per day, but for short periods up to 1000 mg. per day can be used.

METHIONINE

Importance: Methionine is the least abundant sulfur amino acid. It helps prevent skin and nail problems and may help prevent fat buildup in the liver. It reduces histamine release, helps prevent and relieve fatigue, and can help lower an elevated copper level. It is also an anti-oxidant as it converts to cysteine.

Sources: Least abundant in foods such as legumes, soy and peanuts; but higher in dairy products, eggs, fish and meat. Also in nuts, seeds, rice, corn.

PHENYLALANINE

Importance: It can cross the blood-brain barrier and affect brain chemistry. It is a precursor of tyrosine, so phenylalanine can be linked to the production of norepinephrine, epinephrine and dopamine. Phenylalanine metabolism requires the presence of B6, B3, Vitamin C, copper and iron. In combination with B6 it is sometimes used to treat depression. It can be used for musculoskeletal problems: i.e. osteoarthritis, low back pain, rheumatoid arthritis, headache and neck pain.

Sources: Readily available in most foods but highest in meats, milk, oats and wheat germ.

THREONINE

Importance: Necessary for the formation of tooth enamel, elastin and collagen. Need increases with stress. It is a precursor of glycine and serine. It is an immune-stimulating amino acid, and a deficiency can be reflected in a weakened cellular immune response.

Sources: Readily available in dairy, eggs, wheat germ, nuts, beans, seeds.

TRYPTOPHAN

Importance: Vitamin B6, C, folic acid and magnesium are needed to metabolize tryptophan. It is a precursor for vitamin B3 or niacin and the vital neurotransmitter serotonin, which influences our moods and sleep. It has been used as an antidepressant and can be effective in treating manic-depression and depression associated with menopause. It can be used to treat Parkinson's, epilepsy, schizophrenia and insomnia. It can be used for relief of pain, especially dental pain. People with asthma or systemic lupus erythromytosis should not take tryptophan.

Sources: Corn, many cereal grains and legumes. Although not particularly high in any foods, it is readily available in eggs, dairy products, some nuts and seeds. It must often be taken as a supplement to increase its blood level. Other amino acids such as tyrosine and phenylalanine compete with tryptophan for absorption.

Less-Toxic Alternatives

VALINE

Importance: Valine may be metabolized to produce energy that spares glucose. A deficiency may affect the myelin covering of nerves. Valine supplementation may be helpful in muscle building.

Sources: Found in substantial quantities in most foods.

SEMI-ESSENTIAL AMINO ACIDS

Histidine and arginine are considered semi-essential amino acids.

HISTIDINE

Importance: It is involved in a wide variety of metabolic processes that are involved in blood cell production. It is vital to the production of histamine and has been used in the treatment of allergic disorders, peptic disorders, anemia, and cardiovascular disease where it has a mild hypotensive effect. It also acts as a metal chelating agent. It may be needed in malnourished or injured individuals. It can protect the body from radiation damage and is important to the health of the myelin sheath. The injured or malnourished individual may have a definite need for supplementation with this amino acid.

Sources: It must be obtained from the diet. It is found in most animal and vegetable proteins, particularly poultry, pork, cheese, wheat germ.

ARGININE

Importance: A semi-essential amino acid that is usually synthesized by adults in adequate amounts so supplementation is not needed. However, supplementation may be needed during periods of high stress and energy growth periods that occur in childhood and pregnancy. Arginine deficiency can exist in humans as a result of high protein demands such as following trauma. It is essential to the metabolism of ammonia that is generated from protein breakdown and transports nitrogen used in muscle metabolism. It influences several hormone functions, and stimulates the pituitary gland to produce and secrete human growth hormone in young males. Arginine increases the size and activity of the thymus gland, thus stimulating t-lymphocytes. This has a positive effect on immune system.

Sources: It is present in most proteins including meats, milk, nuts, cheese and eggs. It is particularly high in nuts, grains and chocolate. However, if these foods are eaten in excess, it contributes to an increase in herpes simplex attacks. L-lysine must be in a 3-to-1 balance with arginine.

NON-ESSENTIAL AMINO ACIDS

Non-essential amino acids are normally made by our body and are found in body proteins. They are supposedly not needed in our diet because they can be made by the body; however it is very possible that metabolic deficiencies in biochemical systems may exist in some individuals and supplementation may be needed.

ALANINE

Importance: Alanine is an important part of muscle tissues. Glucose can be made from alanine in the liver or muscles whenever energy is needed. It may help maintain proper blood-sugar level. Alanine deficiency has been seen in people with hypoglycemia. Alanine stimulates lymphocyte production, and may help people who have immune suppression. It is also an inhibitory neurotransmitter in the brain and may decrease excitation of the brain such as is found in epilepsy.

Sources: Protein foods such as beef, pork, turkey, cheese, wheat germ, oats, yogurt and avocado.

ASPARTIC ACID

Importance: It is very active in many body processes including the formation and disposal of ammonia and urea from the body. It is found in very high levels in the body, especially in the brain where it performs an excitatory function. It has been found in increased levels in people with epilepsy and in decreased amounts in some cases of depression.

Aspartic acid may help protect the liver from some drug toxicity and the body from radiation. It may also increase resistance to fatigue. It is employed to form some mineral salts such as potassium, calcium and magnesium aspartate. Since aspartates are easily absorbed, they can help transport these minerals across the intestinal lining into the blood to their proper cellular destination. Aspartic acid has an effect on the thymus gland, and can be said to have a mild immuno-stimulating effect.

Sources: Readily available in most protein foods.

CYSTEINE / CYSTINE

Importance: Cysteine, the sulfur amino acid, is formed from homocystine, which comes from the essential amino acid methionine. Cysteine can be converted to cystine and taurine. Cysteine, together with glutamic acid and glycine, can form glutathione. It is a powerful and useful antioxidant that can help protect against harm from heavy metals, chemicals, and smoke. Cysteine is especially important in binding and ridding the body of lead, mercury and cadmium. Cysteine helps neutralize the aldehydes produced by the liver as we metabolize alcohol, fats, air pollutants and some drugs. It can also help promote tissue healing after surgery or burns.

Sources: Poultry, yogurt, oats and wheat germ, egg yolks, red peppers, garlic, onions, broccoli and Brussels sprouts.

GLUTAMIC ACID / GLUTAMINE

Importance: Glutamic acid is converted to glutamine and is synthesized from arginine, ornithine, and proline. Glutamic acid is important to brain function and is the only amino acid metabolized in the brain. The conversion of glutamic acid to glutamine helps clear the body of potentially toxic ammonia. Glutamic acid plus B6 and manganese is a precursor of gamma-amino-butyric acid – an important neurotransmitter in the central nervous system. Research has shown that L-glutamine taken in doses of 500 mg. four times a day can decrease the craving for alcohol and sugar. Glutamic acid has been used in the treatment of fatigue, Parkinson's, schizophrenia and muscular dystrophy. Glutamine can be used in the repair of the lining of the GI tract and is the most abundant amino acid found in the muscles of the body.

Sources: Abundant in animal and vegetable protein.

GLYCINE

Importance: Glycine can be formed from choline and from the amino acids threonine and serine. Glycine is one of the few amino acids that helps spare glucose for energy by improving glycogen storage. It is important in brain metabolism where it has a calming effect. Glycine is a simple amino acid needed in the synthesis of the hemoglobin molecule, and in collagen and glutathione synthesis. Glycine is useful in healing wounds and increasing immune antibody response. May help treat infection, immuno-suppression and fatigue.

HOMOCYSTEINE

Importance: Intermediary metabolite of the amino acid methoinine. Known mostly for its use in genetic enzyme problems. A buildup of homosysteine can cause problems of the vascular system, eyes and nervous system.

PROLINE, HYDROPROLINE & HYDROLYSINE

Importance: Important components of collagen and help in the formation of bone, cartilage and skin.

Hydrolysine is closely related to lysine and is important in the formation of collagen. It is found in gelatin and in digestive enzymes.

Sources: Proline is found in dairy products, eggs, meat and wheat germ. Hydroproline is converted from proline.

SERINE

Importance: Can be made in the tissue from glycine, but its production requires B3, B6 and folic acid. It is a constituent of brain proteins, including the myelin sheath. Aids in the production of immunoglobulins and antibodies. Elevated levels in sausage and lunchmeats may cause immune suppression and cerebral allergies.

Sources: Meats, dairy products, wheat, peanuts and soy.

TYROSINE

Importance: Tyrosine is easily made in the body from phenylalanine. It is very important to general metabolism and a direct precursor of adrenaline and thyroid hormones. Folic acid, niacin, vitamin C and copper are needed to support tyrosine metabolism. It is known as the antidepressant amino acid. It has mild antioxidant effect, and can be useful for heavy smokers.

NON-ESSENTIAL AMINO ACIDS (Not found in body proteins)

There are other important amino acids that are not found in body proteins, but are important in metabolic functions. These include: carnitine, citrulline, ornithine and taurine.

CARNITINE

Importance: Carnitine is found in the diet and can be made mainly in the liver and kidneys from lysine with the help of vitamin C, B6, B3, iron and methionine. It is stored primarily in the skeletal muscles and heart, where it transforms fatty acids into energy for muscular activity. It is also concentrated in the brain and sperm. Carnitine can help protect us from cardiovascular disease as it has been shown to reduce blood triglycerides because it increases fat utilization. Can also raise the HDL portion of cholesterol. Can help with weight loss and improves exercise capabilities. It is recommended for those with symptoms of fatigue, angina, muscle weakness, confusion, ischemia or arrhythmia and for those with elevated blood fat.

Sources: Mainly in red meats, with some in fish, poultry and milk.

CITRULLINE

Importance: Citrulline can be made in the body from ornithine and can be converted in the body to arginine. It promotes the detoxification of ammonia in the blood and may be helpful in relieving fatigue. It may also stimulate the immune system

GLUTATHIONE

Importance: A tri-peptide composed of three amino acids: cystine, glutamic acid and glycine. L-cysteine is usually supplemented to enhance glutathione's production by the liver. Found in all human tissues with highest levels in the liver, eye lenses, spleen, pancreas and kidneys. It is a chief anti-oxidant as it helps protect us against free radicals that can destroy cells. Peroxides release oxygen that can destroy bacteria and parasites; however, in unprotected cells, they can destroy the cell as well. Some chemicals that increase the production of oxygen are pesticides, plastics, benzene and carbon tetrachloride. Glutathione protects against these as well as heavy metals, cigarette smoke, smog, carbon monoxide, drugs, solvents, dyes, phenols and nitrates.

ORNITHINE

Importance: Ornithine can be made from arginine and can in turn form glutamic acid, citrulline and arginine. It is useful in ammonia metabolism. It may help stimulate the immune system, support wound healing, and regenerate the liver. Body builders can use it together with tyrosine as a growth hormone stimulant. A deficiency may occur in poorly nourished individuals.

TAURINE

Importance: Taurine is essential in newborns, however adults can produce the sulfur containing taurine from cysteine with the help of B6. Taurine functions in electrically active tissue such as the brain and heart, and helps stabilize cell membranes. It aids the movement of potassium, sodium, calcium and magnesium in and out of cells; and thus helps generate nerve impulses. Zinc seems to support the effect of taurine. It has been used to treat epilepsy, as it is an inhibitory neurotransmitter. It can be used in the treatment of ischemic heart disease, arrhythmia and hypertension. It also helps gall bladder function.

> > < <

HERBS

You should never try to treat medical conditions with herbs without consulting a physician, who can assist you in diagnosis and treatment.

An herb is a low-growing plant that has a fleshy or juicy stem when it is young, but may develop hard, woody tissue with age. The definition of an herb can include trees, shrubs, mushrooms, lichens, fruits, and vegetables that have medicinal purposes. Herbs are used in cooking to flavor foods and are commonplace in gourmet foods. They are also found in cosmetics. However, the most impressive use of herbs has been in the field of medicine. They have long been used in other cultures and by native Americans for their medicinal value.

Medicinal herbs were once considered Alternative Medicine, but are now thought of as a complimentary approach to aid the Western medical method. Herbs are commonly used in the holistic approach to the diagnosis and treatment of patients. Today herbs are known to be effective in treating many medical issues, and it can be helpful to know the benefits of using natural herbal medicines. However, we cannot always look to herbs as an alternative to medical science, especially in life-threatening situations.

"Most medicinal herbs contain many natural compounds that play off one another, producing a wide variety of results. Nature is still mankind's greatest chemist, and many compounds that remain undiscovered in plants are beyond the imagination of even our best scientist." according to botanist Walter Lewis, PhD and microbiologist Memory Elvin-Lewis, PhD.

Some herbs that regulate the body almost seem to have an inner intelligence, with the ability to perform many different functions. Certainly there are side effects of using traditional prescription medications as reported to the food and drug administration, but herbs do not have as many side effects and many contain protective compounds that enable them to keep their potency.

The effectiveness of herbs and their less-toxic affect on our bodies may be due to our long history of using medicinal plants. We have adapted ways to be more responsive to herbs.

Delicious Magazine (March 1999) quotes James Duke, Ph.D., author of the Green Pharmacy (Rodale) as saying "Herbs are popular because they're effective and cause few harmful side effects." He notes that ... "herbs are used not only to treat symptoms, St. John's Wort for depression, but also to help reduce the progression of some diseases such as the use of ginkgo to delay brain deterioration in patients with Alzheimer's disease."

Herbs can produce allergic reactions, and are not to be used by people with some specific illnesses. To avoid unfavorable interactions between drugs and herbs, your pharmacist, herbalist and physician must be aware of every drug, supplement and herb you are taking.

In the following pages we will look at the value of herbs in enhancing the effect of vitamins, minerals, and amino acids in treating viral, bacterial, and fungal infections.

CENTRAL NERVOUS SYSTEM

Some of the herbal allies used in combination with professional counseling and medical treatment of central nervous system problems are: oats, valerian, skullcap and shizandra.

Oatmeal can help those who are trying to quit smoking and it has been used for over a thousand years to help people addicted to opium. Valerian may also slow brain-cell damage from the overuse of alcohol. Gamma-linolenic acid, borrage or currant seed oils also help reduce the craving for alcohol.

Depression can be helped with St. John's Wort. Indian Ginseng and ligustrum have been used to help deal with anxiety. Valerian has been used in Europe to combat anxiety and reduce stress. It was also used during WW2 to treat those suffering shell shock. Motherwort increases blood circulation to the brain and has been used since the 17th century to prevent melancholy.

Headaches can be aided by ginger tea because it relaxes blood vessels in the head and reduces swelling in the brain. Lavender can also reduce muscle spasm, nervousness and headaches. Feverfew may help in the reduction in headache occurrence and severity by inhibiting the release of serotonin in the brain. It has been used as a treatment for headaches since about the 16th century.

According to the National Headache Foundation, people who have migraine headaches should avoid certain foods including: cheddar cheese, onion, pickles, cured meats, avocados, fresh bread, red wine, sour creams, nuts, chocolate, coffee, tea, cola and alcoholic beverages.

Valerian, skullcap, passionflower, chamomile, and hops may help insomnia. In India, gotu kola can be taken to reduce insomnia. Hops is another sleep promoting herb that works directly on the central nervous system and should take effect within 20 to 40 minutes when taken as a tea. Passionflower can also be used as a sedative.

Some herbs that can help increase memory or reduce memory problems are ginkgo, Siberian ginseng and gotu kola which all enhance mental abilities.

Skullcap, which has been used in China and Russia, has a sedative effect and has been known to stabilize nerve-related heart problems.

Ginseng and Siberian Ginseng can help in handling stress by sedating or stimulating the central nervous system according to your body's need. It also increases the brain's utilization of amino acids.

Kava is a muscle relaxant and can reduce muscle spasms more effectively than some anti-convulsant drugs. Licorice may increase energy storage in muscles.

Ginger has been known to reduce pain by lowering prostaglandin levels. It has long been used in India to treat inflammation and pain. Bromelain can also inhibit prostaglandins.

In China herbalists use bupleurum, ginseng and licorice to reduce or relieve pain resulting from inflammation. These three herbs stimulate the pituitary and adrenal glands to increase natural production of adrenal hormones such as cortisone, which reduces inflammation. Thymus atrophy, high cholesterol and decreased levels of the neurotransmitter serotonin and the pituitary hormone

Less-Toxic Alternatives

ACTH can be a side effect of the use of cortisone. Licorice can help prevent some of these side effects. Bupleurum and ginseng can reduce adrenal shrinkage caused by cortisone medication usage. Licorice, bupleurum and ligustrum can be used together to support adrenal glands during times of stress.

Rheumatoid arthritis can also be helped by the use of licorice and ginseng. Catsclaw and echinacea can also help reduce inflammation. Yucca root can also be helpful in treating arthritis. Some of the following can also be combined to treat arthritic pain and inflammation: guggul, turmeric, withania, and the mineral zinc.

CIRCULATORY SYSTEM

Hawthorne is the most reliable drug for maintaining heart blood flow, and Germany uses it in many pharmaceutical heart preparations. Motherwort can slow a rapid heartbeat and improve a heart's activity. Astragalus helps the heart develop a more regular rhythm, and has been used in China for this purpose for many years. Bromelain can help those with angina.

Five cloves of garlic per week have been shown to decrease arteriosclerosis or arterial plaque as it thins the blood and lowers cholesterol. Symptoms of decreased blood flow in arteriosclerosis which should be reported to a physician include dizziness, leg cramps while walking, changes in skin temperature, color, altered pulse, headaches and memory defects.

Turmeric helps prevent high cholesterol because it interferes with the absorption of cholesterol in the intestine. Skullcap, ginseng, Sanqi ginseng, and Shiitake and Reishi mushrooms are also used to decrease cholesterol.

Stress has an important effect on cholesterol. Researches from the San Antonio School of Aerospace Medicine show that blood cholesterol goes up after only one hour of emotional or physical stress, or overexposure to cold; and it can remain elevated for up to a week. The B vitamins in combination with valerian, skullcap, chamomile and California poppy can reduce stress.

About five grams per day of ginger can help prevent or reduce blood clotting caused by the consumption of saturated fats.

Powdered kelp and garlic as seasoning in place of salt can help lower blood pressure. Valerian, skullcap, lemon balm, motherwort may be helpful in reducing high blood pressure because it can go hand-in-hand with stress.

Siberian ginseng can raise blood pressure.

Hawthorne plus ginko biloba or horse chestnut plus butcher's broom may help varicose veins by making blood vessels stronger and less porous. Ginko and gotu kola are probably most effective when used together to improve circulation.

Siberian ginseng, ginseng and shizandra are three herbs that may improve mental efficiency, endurance, muscle strength, stamina and the general health of the cardiovascular system.

DIGESTIVE SYSTEM

People with irritable bowel symptoms may have food sensitivities especially to alcohol, caffeine and protein. Some of the best herbs to soothe the bowel, improve immunity and help prevent food allergies are chamomile, marshmallow and licorice.

Herbs that help control excess candida or yeast in the intestinal tract include cloves, cinnamon, allspice, tea tree, lavender, garlic, chamomile, black walnut husks, echinacea, valerian, berberine, barberry, and Oregon grape root.

Cascara is considered the gentlest herbal laxative. Licorice can also help those with an elimination problem.

Blackberry can help diarrhea. Chamomile, fenugreek and meadowsweet can also help light cases of diarrhea.

Garlic, onion, licorice, and chamomile have been found to help allergies by decreasing production of histamines and postaglandins.

Chamomile, marshmallow, licorice, slippery elm, calendula, garlic, wild yam and St. John's wort can help protect the stomach from it's own acid and help reduce inflammation and infection of the stomach lining.

Dandelion, hyssop, wild lettuce, chicory, sorrel, goldenseal, Oregon grape root, and blessed thistle can be helpful in treating indigestion.

Goldenseal and Oregon grape root fight intestinal infections due to the berberine they contain. Berberine can help fight e-coli, shigella and salmonella as well as giardia and other amoebas. Grapefruit seed extract can also be used to fight e-coil, candida and geotrichum infections.

IMMUNE SYSTEM

Improper diet, stress, illness, surgery, chemical exposure, and deficiencies in vitamins, minerals and amino acids lower natural immunity. Some diseases that can be related to the immune system are psoriasis, asthma, multiple sclerosis, Epstein Barr, cancer and chronic fatigue. But there are herbs to help boost the immune system and protect us from invaders and immune system disregulation.

Echinacea has been shown in many European studies to increase t-cell activity, interferon and natural killer cells. At the same time it destroys many types of viruses and bacteria. Echinacea works best if you take it for two weeks, then stay off for a week to ten days before resuming.

Other herbs that help immunity include astragalus, licorice, Chinese skullcap, and ginseng as they stop the development of certain viruses. Licorice and astragalus increase interferon production and can help prevent replication of viruses such as herpes and certain flu viruses. In addition, licorice root is effective against several types of bacteria including staph infections. Elderberries may also inhibit more serious viruses such as herpes and Epstein Barr. Calendula, chamomile, burdock, baptisia, red clover and marshmallow also have immune enhancing properties.

Eucalyptus, sage, licorice, lavender, tea tree, hickory, rose geranium, bergamot, lemon balm, hyssop and plantain have all shown an ability to inhibit some common forms of cold and flu virus. Sore throats can be soothed with marshmallow, licorice and slippery elm. Teas and syrups can be prepared and are frequently available in stores. Eucalyptus or peppermint essential oils can

Less-Toxic Alternatives

be used for laryngitis. Also, to prevent flu you need to increase immune system function with Siberian ginseng, echinacea, shizandra and astragalus.

Some people with chronic fatigue have been shown to have low levels of natural killer cells. Lentinan, a compound found in Shiitake mushrooms, has been shown to increase energy levels in people with chronic fatigue. Gamma linolenic acid has also been shown to alleviate symptoms in people with chronic fatigue and in those who suffer from MS or lupus. People with lupus must not take alfalfa. Pantothenic acid, vitamin C, B6 and magnesium can also be taken by those with chronic fatigue to help reduce symptoms.

There are many contaminates such as smog, smoke, chemicals, and cold air in today's world to irritate our lungs and lead to bronchitis and pneumonia. Therefore we need to do all we can to enhance the effectiveness of the immune system.

In order to fight existing lung congestion, some of the more popular herbal expectorants are mullein, thyme, horehound and elecampane. Eucalyptus oil helps combat nasal stuffiness. Yarrow, elderflowers and peppermint are fairly well known in the treatment of chronic sinus problems. Yarrow and elderflowers reduce inflamed sinuses, and, along with peppermint, help drain them.

Gotu kola, kelp and dandelion have affected tumor cells in laboratories.

The spleen, which is the largest lymphatic tissue in the body, helps destroy bacteria and cellular debris in the form of worn-out blood cells. Berberine, which is found in goldenseal, Oregon grape root and barberry enhances blood flow through the spleen. Astragalus and ligustrum may also improve spleen activity.

The liver is one of the more important detoxification organs. It also routes bile into the small intestine. As a cleansing organ, the liver can suffer from chemical exposure and be affected by many of the toxins that we eat, drink and breathe. Milk thistle is considered effective in cleansing the liver. Licorice, astragalus, shizandra and bupleurum also help neutralize liver toxins.

Laughter or positive imagery can also boost immunity, increase treatment effectiveness and promote health and a sense of well-being.

URINARY TRACT

The urinary tract must eliminate the toxins we inhale and ingest. Delay in urination can weaken the bladder. Tight pants, synthetic underwear and deodorant soaps can be irritating and invite infections. Cloudy urine, pain or burning on urination can be indicative of urinary tract infections. But herbs are ready to help promote and protect urinary tract health.

In Israel, research has shown that cranberries and blueberries increase urine acidity and contain compounds that keep bacteria from attaching to the bladder wall. Uva ursi works on bladder infections. Cranberry juice or cranberry capsules can help with bladder problems. Other herbs that fight urinary tract infections include rose hips (which has high vitamin C), garlic and nasturtium. Magnesium and B6 along with goldenrod and cranberries can help prevent formation of kidney stones.

Dandelion and corn silk have diuretic properties; however, because of their high levels of potassium, they do not decrease potassium levels in the body like some pharmaceutical diuretics.

THE SKIN

Many internal remedies for dermatitis start with the herb sarsaparilla, which can help because it binds toxins in the intestines. Milk thistle may help combat psoriasis. Licorice root can also help skin problems. Gamma linoleic acid, which is found in evening primrose oil, and compounds in licorice and chamomile can reduce skin inflammation.

Essential oils can be used for parasites such as lice. They should always be tested first. Place a drop on the inside of the elbow, and let it stay several hours to determine if there is any skin irritation. Keep all treatment for lice away from the eyes, and shampoo it off immediately at the first sign of irritation.

One possible essential oil combination is: combine 2 oz. vegetable oil; 20 drops tea tree essential oil; and 10 drops each essential oil of rosemary, lavender and lemon. Apply to dry hair and cover with shower cap or plastic bag. Wrap with a towel and leave for one hour, then shampoo and rinse hair several times to help cut the oil. This treatment may have to be repeated for several weeks to eliminate any new lice that may be hatching. Bedclothes, clothing and linens need to be washed. Anything that comes into contact with the person's head, such as the back of chairs and couches, needs to be vacuumed.

WOMEN'S HEALTH

Estrogen is an important issue for women past childbearing years. Each woman must decide for herself whether she will use estrogen-replacement therapy. However, the best therapy is probably one that relies upon natural hormones. It is very crucial to find the correct level of supplementation, but it can be done through various blood tests and muscle testing.

Too much estrogen is just as bad as too little. Stress, cortisone and some anti-depressant drugs enhance estrogen levels as do fatty or fried foods, sugar and alcohol.

Progesterone is an equally important female hormone. It can help you feel emotionally balanced in a number of ways. It reduces stress, uterine spasms, water retention and muscle weakness; and helps the body handle alcohol, sugar and food cravings.

Burdock roots, sarsaparilla, yellow dock, and dandelion can help prevent anemia. Chinese wild yams increase the assimilation of iron; as do carrots and most green vegetables.

Vitex is one of the most important herbs for treating gynecological problems.

Woman should also know that birth control pills, smoking and a deficiency in folic acid have an adverse effect on female organs.

Fibrocystic breasts may be helped by supplementation with vitamin E, but E should not be taken with iron. The use of coffee should be extremely curtailed or avoided.

Less-Toxic Alternatives

If, as a woman or teenager, you suffer from very heavy periods, certain herbs can be helpful to you. Scientists have known since the 1930s that shepherd's purse effectively decreases heavy periods. The Chinese have used agrimony to help regulate periods. Don quai has been shown to be helpful in increasing ovarian function, but those having heavy periods should not use it.

Vitamin E, B6 and magnesium seem to relieve certain PMS symptoms and lower prolactin and estrogen levels.

Licorice, black cohosh, fenugreek, hops, don quai, vitex, ginseng and vitamin E can aid in reducing menopause symptoms. Many menopause problems are thought to be due to the erratic activity of pituitary hormones such as LH (Luteinizing Hormone) and FSH (Folicular Stimulating Hormone), as they try to overcompensate for declining levels of estrogen and progesterone. Sometimes during menopause, FSH levels can become 20 times their original values.

Certain plants increase estrogen during menopause. Red clover sprouts, flax seeds, soy oil, alfalfa seeds and sprouts, whole grains, nuts and avocados can help increase estrogen levels.

Calcium supplementation and weight-bearing exercises are most important in protecting the bones during menopause and thereafter.

MEN'S HEALTH

Ginseng is supposed to improve virility, stamina and longevity for men as they increase in age. Siberian ginseng, shizandra, licorice, and ginseng are important nutrients to promote stamina and adrenal health while aging.

Saw palmetto berries and tinctures of nettle root, sarsaparilla, wild yam root, Echinacea root, and uva ursi leaves can be combined to reduce prostrate enlargement.

CHILDREN'S HEALTH

Valerian can be used for hyperactivity in children.

An herbal steam can help sore throat, congestion and swollen glands. Boil 1 quart water, remove from heat, then add 3 drops of eucalyptus, tea tree or lavender essential oil. Let the child breathe the steam.

FIRST AID

The best herbs to treat bruises, discourage swelling and promote quick healing are arnica, chamomile, lavender, St. John's wort, and witch hazel.

Contact with poison ivy can lead to misery for those sensitive to the plant and can cause an irritating rash. The plant's oil should be washed off as soon as possible. Jewel weed plant, comfrey and aloe vera help soothe skin that has been irritated by poison ivy; as well as oatmeal and Epsom salts baths. Simple peppermint oil can give many hours of relief from poison ivy's itch.

Honey lip balm for chapped lips: ¼ cup vegetable oil, ¼ oz. shaved beeswax, 1 tsp. honey, 10 drops lemon essential oil or 1 teaspoon vanilla extract. Heat oil in pan, add beeswax until melted. Stir in honey and essential oil or extract. Pour the balm into lip balm containers while it is still warm.

Insect repellant: 2 oz. vegetable oil or vodka, ¼ tsp. Citronella and eucalyptus essential oils, 1/8 tsp. each pennyroyal, cedar and rose geranium essential oils. Combine ingredients and apply mixture to all exposed skin, but keep away from eyes and mouth. This mixture should keep its strength for a year.

For bleeding: Powdered cayenne, the same pepper used in chili powder, will quickly staunch bleeding when sprinkled directly on the wound. It also contains a substance, capsaicin, which reduces the pain. Powdered kelp, a seaweed, was used by the British in WW2 to reduce bleeding on the battlefield.

> > < <

SUPPLEMENTATION SUMMARY TABLE

Carefully assimilate the information presented in the following four pages. It is not intended to be all inclusive. It is a tool to help you determine the vitamins, minerals, amino acids and herbs which might be helpful in the treatment of your particular health issues.

Some commercial brands contain chemicals, dyes, and fillers. These can present problems to some individuals. Carefully chose brands of supplements which are known to be free of known allergens and chemicals. Herbal supplements should be organically grown. Supplementation with products of uncertain origin or composition can defeat or reduce the benefits of their use.

Be selective. Choose supplements which have been prepared and marketed under strict conditions. Read all labels for content. You need to partake of a supplementation program only upon the advice of a licensed physician, pharmacist, nutritionist and/or herbalist.

Choice of medications or supplementations is complex. Individual uniqueness means individual response to all substances. Medications can react adversely with other substances. Also some medical conditions exclude some supplements from use.

Allow thoughtful, knowledgeable choices to improve your health.

> > < <

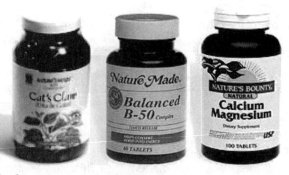

(For less-toxic supplementation alternatives, see page 223.)

PROBLEM	VITAMINS	MINERALS	AMINO ACIDS	HERBS
Adrenal Problems	B5, C, Folic Acid	Manganese, Zinc	Tyrosine	Bupleurum, Ginseng, Licorice, Lugustrum
Allergies	B5, B6, C, D, Quercitin	Copper	Histidine, Methionine	Chamomile, Garlic, Licorice, Onion, and more
Alzheimer's	B3, B12, Choline, Inositol			Ginkgo, Gotu Kola, Siberian Ginseng
Anemia / RBC Formation	B2, B3, B5, B6, B12, C, E, Folic Acid, PABA, Inositol	Calcium, Copper, Iron	Glycine	
Antioxidant (cellular protection)	A, C, E,	Copper, Manganese, Selenium, Zinc	Cysteine, Glutathione, Methionine	
Arthritis		Zinc	Phenylalanine	Cats Claw, Echinacea, Ginseng, Guggul, Licorice, Turmeric, Withania, Yucca Root
Asthma	B12, Quercitin			
Bells Palsy or Trigeminal Neuralgia	B1, B3, B12			
Bones/ Osteoporosis	A, B12, C, D	Calcium, Copper, Manganese, Zinc, CA/Phosphorus ratio	Lysine	
Candida		Zinc		Black Walnut Husks, Cloves, Garlic, Lavender, Oregon Grape Root, Pau d'arco
Cardiovascular System / Heart	A, B6, C, Choline, D, E, PABA	Calcium, Magnesium, Phosphorus, Potassium, Selenium	Carnitine, Histidine, Taurine	Astragalus, Bromelain, Garlic, Ginseng, Hawthorne, Motherwort, Siberian Ginseng, Shizandra, Skullcap

PROBLEM	VITAMINS	MINERALS	AMINO ACIDS	HERBS
Cholesterol	B3, C, Choline, E, Inositol,	Calcium, Chromium	Carnitine	Garlic, Ginseng, Sanqi Ginseng, Shiitake & Reishi Mushrooms, Skullcap, Turmeric, Gugulipid
Colds	C, D,	Zinc		Elecampane, Elderberry, Yarrow Eucalyptus oil, Horehound, Mullein, Peppermint, Thyme
Depression/Anxiety/ Psychological Problems	B6, PABA, Folic Acid, Inositol	Calcium, Chromium, Zinc	Aspartic Acid, Glutamine, Phenylalanine, Tryptophan, Tyrosine	Gingko Biloba, Kava, Motherwort, St. John's Wort, Valerian
Diabetes	B1, B5, D, E, Inositol	Chromium, Manganese, Potassium, Zinc	Alanine, Leucine	
Digestive System	A, B1, B2, B3, B5, Folic Acid, Inositol, PABA		Glutamine	Chamomile, Licorice, Marshmallow & others
Eyes, Cataracts, Glaucoma	A, B2, C, D, E, Choline, Inositol, Lutein	Selenium	Glutathione	
Fatigue	B5, B6, B12, C, PABA	Chromium, Iron, Magnesium, Phosphorus, Zinc	Alanine, Aspartic Acid, Carnitine, Citrulline, Glycine, Glutamine, Isoleucine, Leucine, Methionine	Ginseng, Lentimen, Licorice
Hair	A, B2, B6, Folic Acid, Inositol, PABA	Copper, Zinc		
Headaches	B1, B3, Choline, Folic Acid, PABA		Phenylalanine	Feverfew, Ginger, Lavender
Healing	A, B5, C	Chromium, Copper, Zinc	Cysteine, Glycine, Leucine, Ormithine	Arnica, Chamomile, Lavender, St. John's Wort, Witch Hazel

PROBLEM	VITAMINS	MINERALS	AMINO ACIDS	HERBS
High Blood Pressure / Hypertension		Calcium, Magnesium, Potassium, Sodium/ Potassium Ratio	Taurine	Garlic, Kelp, Lemon Balm, Motherwort, Skullcap, Valerian
Hyperactivity	B6	Magnesium		Valerian
Immune System	A, B2, B5, B6, C, E,	Copper, Selenium, Zinc	Alanine, Arginine, Citrulline, Glycine, Lysine, Ornithine, Serine, Threonine	Astragalus, Cat's Claw, Echinachea, Licorice, Selenium and others
Infections	A, B1, B5, **B6, C**	Zinc		Garlic poultice with essential oils, Boost immune system
Kidney Stones	A, B6	Magnesium		
Memory	Choline			Ginko, Gotu kola, Siberian Ginseng
Menopause		Calcium	Tryptophan	Black Cohosh, Don Quai, Hops Foenugreek, Ginseng, Licorice
Metabolism	B2, B5, B6,			
Multiple Sclerosis / Myelin Sheath	B5, B6, B12	Chromium, Copper	Choline, Histidine, Serine, Valine	
Muscle Cramps/ Spasms	A, B2, B3, B5, B6, D, E	Calcium, Magnesium, Sodium	Isoleucine	Kava, Lavender
Nails	B2	Calcium, Zinc	Methionine	
Nerve Disorders	B1, B3, B5, B6, B12, Choline, D, Inositol, PABA	Calcium, Phosphorus, Potassium	Alanine, Glutamine, Isoleucine, Taurine, Tryptophan	Indian Ginseng, Lavender, Ligustrum, Oats, Shizandra, Skullcap, Valerian
Neurotransmitters	B6, C, Choline	Sodium/ Potassium cellular exchange	Phenylalanine, Tryptophan	
PMS	B6, E	Magnesium		

PROBLEM	VITAMINS	MINERALS	AMINO ACIDS	HERBS
Radiation Damage			Aspartic Acid, Histidine	
Shingles	B6, B12, B complex, C, E	Zinc	Lysine	Combine equal amounts of tincture of Oatstraw, St. John's Wort & Skullcap take 1 tsp. four times per day. Olive Leaf Extract, Pau d'arco Topically: Licorice
Skin	B2, B5, B6, B12, D, Folic Acid, Inositol, PABA	Copper, Selenium, Zinc	Methionine	Chamomile, Evening Primrose Oil, Licorice root, Milk Thistle, Pau d-arco, Sarsaparilla
Sleep / Insomnia	Choline, Inositol	Calcium, Magnesium	Tryptophan	Chamomile, Gotu Kola, Hops Passionflower, Skullcap, Valerian
Stress	B6	Magnesium	Arginine, Threonine	California Poppy, Chamomile, Ginseng, Siberian ginseng, Skullcap, Valerian
Teeth	C, D	Calcium, Phosphorus, Zinc	Threonine	
Urinary Tract	C			Blueberry, Cats claw, Cranberry, Garlic, Nasturtium, Rose hips, Uva ursi

> > < <

This table © 2001 by Carolyn Gorman in *Less-Toxic Alternatives, Revised Edition* - May not be reprinted without author's written permission.

Part III: Less-Toxic Alternatives

For allergic and environmentally aware individuals

The following less-toxic alternative products have proven safe for most people. Items marked less-toxic may not be tolerated by all - any item should be tested before use, especially if you are sensitive to any of the components. Please realize that the marketplace changes rapidly and we cannot guarantee that all products and suppliers are available at any one time. Please notify us if you find some listings are out-of-date.

Special note: Items marked with this symbol ᵒ may not be tolerated by all.

> < <

Air Handling

Indoor Air Quality

We breathe 10,000 to 20,000 liters of air each day. Anthony Cortez of Tufts University says there are 1 million molecules of chemicals in one breath of air.

Your climate control system can give you control of the humidity, temperature, purity, and allergenic content of the air in your home.

Central systems are ideal. When window air conditioning units are used, they must have proper filtration and be cleaned regularly. Electric space heaters must be carefully selected, placed, and maintained in order to provide a healthy alternative.

> < <

Your Climate Control System

The type of air handling system and its location are of major importance. Space heaters, wood stoves and fireplaces can be a source of contamination. Gas and oil systems must be properly placed and monitored regularly to prevent chemical exposure.

<u>YOU SHOULD AVOID</u>

Climate control systems that may increase indoor air contamination and expose
occupants to natural gas, methyl mercaptan and gas combustion by-products
Fuel-fired furnaces in attic or basement (not specially constructed)
Fuel-fired furnaces or heaters in living area, especially near sleeping area
Fuel-fired furnaces vented through unlined brick chimneys

Gas floor and wall furnaces
Direct oil forced-air furnaces can expose one to fumes (tank should be outside)
Plastic or fiberglass ductwork
Unvented gas heaters
Wood stoves and fireplaces
Radiators that contain diethylaminoethanol as a rust inhibitor

LESS-TOXIC ALTERNATIVES

Ceramic Radiant Heaters: Allergy Alternative, The Living Source, Nirvana
    Safe Haven (steel cabinet), Radiant Heater Corp.
Closed system energy-efficient, electric-start gas furnace[a] (optimal protection
    if placed in a sealed room in the attic or basement. This necessitates fresh
    air intake and combusted air exhaust to outside. When in the basement, a
    door opening only outside offers the best protection.)
Copper pipes in floor (with proper power source)
Delonghi sealed radiator-type portable heaters
Electric baseboard heaters (water filled or regular)
Electric forced-air heat (with proper power source in attic or basement)
Fuel-fired furnace (6 ft. from house or in sealed room in basement – vented
    outside)[a]
Heat pumps (with motor and insulation outside air stream)
Heat recovery ventilators need at least 1 air exchange per hour
Metal ductwork with insulation and vapor barrier on the outside
Portable Convection Heater (metal construction): Lifekind Products
Radiators[a] (with proper power source)
Solar systems: Real Goods
Three-stage fuel-fired (gas or oil) furnace that uses a water boiler to heat air or
    supply radiator heat
A carbon monoxide monitor should be put near furnace if it is in living area

> > < <

Heat / AC Filtration Systems

YOU SHOULD AVOID
All oil or Hexachlorophene impregnated filters
Filters containing glues if you are sensitive to adhesives

LESS-TOXIC ALTERNATIVES
Activated charcoal filters for chemicals: The Living Source
    (Note: heat and humidity can decrease carbon absorption efficiency)
Electrostatic filters (98% efficient at 3 microns – filters particulates including
    dust, pollen and mold): AEHF, Allermed, Dust Free (Allerx), Environ-
    mentally Sound Products, The Living Source, E. L. Foust (Ultra Filter)
Magnatron Electrostatic Permanent Filter: Allergy Relief Shop
Permatron – Space-Gard Filters: National Allergy Supply
Potassium Permanganate filters formaldehyde

VENT OUTLET FILTERS (after the ductwork)
AEHF
Cheesecloth layered on air ducts
Charcoal filter material: Allergy Relief Shop
Final Filter" – 3-stage filter for floor, wall and ceiling vents (activated carbon,
    microbe shield and passive electrostatic filtration): Dasun
WINDOW UNIT AC FILTERS: The Living Source

> > < <

Filter Efficiency

The following table shows the different levels of efficiency of various filtration systems (particulates include pollen, mold and bacteria):

Type of Filter (use only as directed)	Dust	Particulate
Standard AC Filters		
Fine open cell foam & textile denier non-woven fibers	30%	0%
Thin paper-like mat of glass & cellulose fibers	35%	0%
Glass fiber, multi-ply cellulose, &/or wool felt	40%	10%
Mats:		
5-10mm fibers, 6-12 mm thick	60%	25%
3-5mm fibers, 6-20 mm thick	80%	40%
1-4mm fibers (various fiber & glass mix)	90%	55%
0.5-2mm fibers (usually glass)	98%	90%
Charcoal Filters	90%	89.3%
Electronic Air Filter Systems	98%	95%
Electrostatic Filters (at 5.0 microns)	100%	98%
Space-Gard Filters (at 1.0 micron)	100%	98%
Untreated HEPA Filters (at 0.3 micron)	100%	99.99%
(High Efficiency Particulate Accumulator)		
Barrier cloth (at 0.1 micron)	100%	100%

NOTE: 1 inch equals 25,400 microns

> > < <

Air Purifications Systems

YOU SHOULD AVOID
Purifiers that contain glue, painted surfaces or construction materials that can
    contaminate the environment

LESS-TOXIC ALTERNATIVES
Portable and whole house systems with metal cabinets and components,
    minimal glue and less-toxic filtration media

PORTABLE OR SINGLE ROOM AIR PURIFIERS
Aireox Air Purifiers: Abundant Earth, Aireox, Dasun, The Living Source,
    NEEDS, Nirvana Safe Haven
Air Quality Systems (AQS): The Living Source

AllerAir Air Solutions (Steel housing – 5 filters): Allergy Relief Shop, NEEDS, Nirvana Safe Haven

Allermed: Allermed, Allergy Relief Shop

Amaircare: National Allergy Supply

Austin Air Purifiers (Steel housing)[a]: AEHF, Absolute Environmental's, Allergy Relief Shop, Allergy Relief Store, Priorities, NEEDS, Nirvana Safe Haven

Care 2000 (Stainless steel housing/UV light): NEEDS, Nirvana Safe Haven

C-90A 4 stage electronic air cleaner (2 stage ionizer, particulate collector plates[a] and activated carbon - housing won't emit gas): Friedrich AC Co.

Dust Free: Allerx

Enviracare[a]

Foust Air Purifiers: E.L. Foust, The Living Source

Foust Desktop Air Purifiers: E.L Foust, The Living Source

Lifekind Products 3-stage (Carbon, HEPA and VOC filter)

Other portable air purifiers: Allergy Alternative, Mountain Energy Supply

UV-C CELLS TO INSTALL IN H/AC SYSTEMS
Dust Free Nomad & Triad

WHOLE HOUSE SYSTEMS
Allermed

Amaircare Whole House Systems: Natural Solutions, Pure n Natural

Honeywell Air Exchanger

Lifebreath Clean Air Furnace: Nutech Energy Systems

Pure Air Systems: Allergy Relief Shop

SunPure UV Air Purifier

HEAT RECOVERY VENTILATORS
BossAire, Inc.

Lifebreath (Whole House HRV & ERV): Nutech Energy Systems

TherMax Energy Recycling Ventilators: Kooltronic, Inc.

AUTO AIR PURIFIERS
Aireox Car Air Purifier: Aireox, Dasun, The Living Source, NEEDS

Auto/RV Air Cleaner: Allerx

Foust Auto Air: AEHF, E.L. Foust, Gazoontite, The Living Source

Portable Hepa Auto Filter: Lifekind Products

Sanuvox Next Generation Air Purifier: The Living Source

PERSONAL AIR PURIFIERS & IONIZERS
AEHF, The Living Source, NEEDS, Priorities, Pure n Natural, Real Goods

OZONATORS (Eliminates volatile hydrocarbons)
Use only as directed – run 2-4 hours, then air 8 hours before entering room

AEHF, The Living Source (Sonozaire), NEEDS (Kleen-Air King)

ZEOLITE (A natural mineral that helps remove toxic gas and odors)
Powder and breather bags: Absolute Environmental's, Dasun, Earth Friendly Products, Nirvana Safe Haven, Real Goods

> > < <

Air Duct Cleaning
YOUR DUCT WORK IS YOUR AIR LINE

YOU SHOULD AVOID
Most chemicals used to clean or seal duct, and toxic mold inhibitors

LESS-TOXIC ALTERNATIVES
Vacuum and brush ducts or have professionally cleaned

Absolute Environmental's Allergy Store

National Air Duct Cleaners Association

Texas Power Vac Inc.

Some local heating/AC firms perform this service, but carefully check their procedures and any chemicals they use.

Arrange to be away from the premises during cleaning and for at least an additional 4-8 hours for chemically sensitive or 1 hour for those who are more tolerant of chemical exposure.

If contaminated ductwork is flex-duct instead of metal, it may have to be completely replaced.

FOR MOLD IN DUCTS
AFM Safety Clean[□] and AFM X-158 Sealant[□]: Allergy Relief Shop, Allerx, The Living Source, NEEDS

Hydrogen peroxide

Oxine[□]

Ozonator – Eliminates volatile hydrocarbons *(use only as directed)*: AEHF, The Living Source, NEEDS

Zephiran (Benzalkonium) Chloride 17%[□] *(use only as directed)* – 1 part to 10 parts water: Abrams Royal Pharmacy *(prescription required)*

> > < <

Humidity Regulators & Gauges

YOU SHOULD AVOID
Equipment containing glue, painted surfaces or construction materials that contaminate. Be careful of mold growth and microbial contamination. Avoid ultrasonic systems.

LESS-TOXIC ALTERNATIVES
Maintain proper temperature/humidity ratio (70/50%) to keep mold and dust mite growth at a minimum.

Use only distilled water in humidifiers, and clean units daily with Borax – avoid mold and microbial contamination.

Sunlight and circulating air aid in humidity regulation.

Relative humidity and temperature gauges are available from many local sources plus Allergy Relief Shop, Allergy Relief Store, National Allergy Supply, Real Goods

HUMIDIFIERS

AprilAire attached metal steam humidifier: Research Products
Cool mist portable humidifiers□
Metal steam humidifier: E.L. Foust
Portable steam humidifiers□
Real Goods
Slant/Fin GF-350 Humidifier (Ultraviolet Technology): Natural Solutions, Pure
   n Natural

DEHUMIDIFIERS

Calcium Chloride Crystals – Damp Rid Moisture Absorber Tray: local
   supermarkets, The Living Source
Closet Dehumidifier□: Allergy Relief Store
Dehumidifiers (clean daily with Borax): Air Technology Systems, Humidex,
   Nirvana Safe Haven (steel cabinet), Real Goods (steel cabinet), and White
   Westinghouse (steel cabinet with hose connection)
Industrial and commercial dehumidifiers: Desert Aire

> > < <

Breathing Aids

Filtration Masks

YOU SHOULD AVOID
Masks containing polyester, plastic, rubber or other elements to which you
   may be sensitive

LESS-TOXIC ALTERNATIVES
Cotton or Silk Masks with Charcoal Filters*: AEHF, Allergy Relief Shop,
   Allerx, Dixie Peterson (retail & wholesale), The Living Source
Eco Rap (All cotton, bandana style, adjustable chin strap and nose clip –
   replaceable activated carbon filters): Dasun Co.
Handkerchiefs with charcoal filter insert: The Living Source
HEPA Mask or Charcoal Mask: Allergy-Asthma Technology
Industrial type silicon with charcoal/HEPA filters: Gempler
3M Chemical/Pollen Masks□ : The Living Source
*Coconut charcoal is standard, but wood and bituminous charcoal are also
   available from some sources. Plain all-cotton or all-silk masks may be
   used if charcoal is a problem.

> > < <

Respiratory & Oxygen Supplies

YOU SHOULD AVOID
Plastic tubing and rubber or plastic masks

Less-Toxic Alternatives

LESS-TOXIC ALTERNATIVES
Ceramic masks: AEHF, Allergy Relief Shop, The Living Source
E Cylinder oxygen tank, regulator and cart: AEHF, The Living Source
Glass & metal humidifier bottle: AEHF, The Living Source
Stainless steel tubing: AEHF
Tygon tubing: AEHF, Allergy Relief Shop, The Living Source
Denim carrying case: The Living Source
The following resources provide supplies for those suffering from asthma and other respiratory problems (a prescription may be required). Products vary between suppliers, but may include peak flow meters, oxygen equipment, compressors, nebulizers, and supplies: AEHF, The Living Source, National Allergy Supply

> > < <

Building & Home Improvement

It is important for your home to be a haven from contaminated outside air. This makes for relaxation and rejuvenation.

To preserve the integrity of your home, products should be chosen that are low in formaldehyde, petrochemicals, volatile hydrocarbons and tung oil.

The wise builder or home handyman chooses products low in formaldehyde and fungicides. Solid wood and plywood are substitutes for forbidden particleboard.

Less toxic paints, sealers and wood finishing products are acceptable alternatives to products containing petrochemicals, and tung oil. The use of natural fibers and products contributes to improved air quality in your home.

> > < <

Cabinets

YOU SHOULD AVOID
Commercial brands that may contain aldehydes, cellulose, urethane, hydrocarbons, and polyvinyl chloride
Do not use particleboard and avoid plywood if possible

LESS-TOXIC ALTERNATIVES

METAL CABINETS for kitchen, bath, etc.
St. Charles Blue Steel and Glass Cabinets
Designs by Droste

WOOD CABINETS
Use solid poplar, white oak or other selected hardwoods
Plywood is not recommended. If you must use it – use interior grade (exterior is too resinous), air for at least six weeks (preferably 3 months), then seal with a less-toxic wood sealer.

> > < <

Carpeting & Rugs

Enjoy the warmth of natural fiber carpets with select backing

YOU SHOULD AVOID

Excess glue, 4-PC (Phenylcyclohexene), synthetic latex backing, foam pads, styrene butadiene, formaldehyde, and chlorinated hydrocarbons

LESS-TOXIC ALTERNATIVES

Choose carefully: synthetic jute or cloth backings, continuous filament, Berber, and pads of felt, jute or rag

Bio-Floor wool & hemp carpet (100% natural and untreated): Earth Weave

Cotton rugs/carpet: Dellinger, GAIAM, Harmony, Heart of Vermont (cotton fiber 9x12 rugs), Janice's (cotton rag rugs, bath rug and seatcover), White Lotus (rugs)

Earth Weave Carpet Mills

Hemp rug: Earth Weave, Real Goods

Jute rugs/carpet: Earth Weave, Real Goods

Karastan-Bigelow Carpets are tolerated by some[a]: Peerless Imported Rugs

Natural fiber area rugs/carpets: Peerless Imported Rugs, Natures Carpet (chemical free for the chemically sensitive)

Nylon carpet with no added stain resistant chemicals: Sutherland Mill – Collins & Aikman

Sisal rugs[a]: Hendricksen Naturlich Flooring

Wool rugs/carpet: Carousel Carpet Mills, Chambers, Helios (woven), Hendricksen Naturlich Flooring, Nirvana Safe Haven (untreated/undyed), Sinan Co. (untreated, undyed, natural latex[a] backing)

Wool yarn plus fleece on linen rugs: Heart of Vermont

PADS

Felt pads: Hendricksen Naturlich Flooring

Jute pads: Hendricksen Naturlich Flooring, Sinan Co. (jute with horsehair[a] or camel hair[a])

Wool &jute pads: Earth Weave

WHEN DEALING WITH EXISTING CARPETS

If you are unable to remove carpeting that is producing environmental sensitivities and have followed the recommended procedures for carpet cleaning, then cover the floor with Thermoply Storm-Bracing.

Seal seams and baseboards edges with Polyken tape: AEHF, The Living Source

Barrier cloth can also be used to cover carpet.

See section on Upholstery & Carpet Cleaners for additional alternatives for care of existing carpets

> > < <

Flooring

YOU SHOULD AVOID

Due to formaldehyde content, avoid synthetic, stain-resistant wall-to-wall carpet, solid vinyl tiles with wax finishes and particleboard sub-flooring. Be careful to avoid hardwood strip filler containing toluene.

LESS-TOXIC ALTERNATIVES

STONE: cement, ceramic tile, marble, slate, terra cotta, terrazzo brick - set with C-Cure Grout, Portland Cement Thin Set, Laticrete, Permabond 902 (non-modified), or Custom Blend Thin Set (no additives)

Euro Marble & Granite

WOOD: Test all wood before construction begins. Solid aspen, beech, birch, maple, oak, poplar, and teak should be considered first. Floors should be solid wood. Hardwood floors with baked-on finish must be carefully selected. Sub-flooring should be solid wood, exterior grade plywood, or formaldehyde-free plywood. Redwood can be used outside. (*See Paint Section for less-toxic wood finishes*)

Junckers hardwood flooring

Mannington finished wood plank flooring

Medite II, Medex, and Medite FR formaldehyde-free fiberboard[a]: SierraPine

Trinity Floor Co.

Untreated white and red oak: Superior Floor Covering

PARQUET TILES: ¼" oak can be nailed. Other parquet must be applied with water-soluble adhesive. Tile wood strips should be stapled together, not glued.

VINYL: (products should be tested first)[a]

Duravinyl (brittle composite with a no-wax surface): American Biltrite

Plain battleship linoleum from natural raw material: Forbo Industries

CORK TILE & ADHESIVES

Bioshield (Eco Design), Hendricksen Naturlich, Natural Cork, Trinity Floor

> > < <

Insulation, Vapor Barriers & Walls

YOU SHOULD AVOID

Too much, too little, or improperly placed insulation. If the home is not properly insulated, outside humidity and temperature will penetrate the walls and affect the inside climate. However, if the house is too tight, windows will sweat, and the humidity produced inside the house can cause mold growth. Therefore a proper balance must be achieved, and adequate ventilation must be provided.

Blown-in insulation may be hazardous to some. If blown insulation is installed, you should remain away from home until the house can be thoroughly cleaned. Avoid the use of fiberglass insulation that has urea extended phenol-formaldehyde binder.

Fiberglass may be more carcinogenic than asbestos, according to a 1995 report from researchers at the Occupational Safety and Health Administration and the National Institute for Environmental Health. In 13 studies, lung cancer was significantly higher in rats exposed to glass wool than in those who were not. Besides exposure at home, over 13 million Americans are exposed to fiberglass at their jobs, according to Victims of Fiberglass, a California based non-profit corporation.

LESS-TOXIC ALTERNATIVES

VAPOR BARRIERS

Vapor barriers are used on the outside of the house under siding or brick veneer in warm, humid climates to prevent outside humidity from entering the home. In very cold climates, insulation is placed behind the inside wall. Vapor barriers may also be used on the ground in crawl spaces. Caution must be taken to allow the house to breathe, or inside humidity will rise above acceptable levels and cause mold growth.

Dennyfoil (aluminum) Vapor Barrier: Denny Wholesale, The Living Source
K-Shield Radiant Vapor Barrier & Radiant Barrier Ultra: AEHF
Radiant Barrier (aluminum quilted with a thread)
Stainless steel foil and tape: Alpine Industries
Super R Radiant Barrier – perforated for attic: Forbo Industries, Real Goods
Thermo-Ply Sheating: Simplex Products
86001 Vapor Barrier (no plastic or foil – liquid can be brushed, rolled or sprayed – will seal plywood or particleboard against outgassing / resists mold and mildew): Palmer Industries, Inc.

INSULATION

Should be foil backed
Cotton insulation
Air Krete$^{\circ}$: Palmer Industries, Inc.
InsulSafe Owens Corning$^{\circ}$: yellow, pink, white
Icynene insulation system: Icynene Inc.
Manville Unbonded B-Fiber
Microcell (foam)$^{\circ}$ reflective insulation
Volcanic Stone Cementitous Foam

WALLS

Sheetrock (aged at least 6 weeks – preferably 3 months)
    U.S. Gypsum or Georgia Pacific (formaldehyde free is available)
Plaster
Porcelain Panels – Architectural porcelain enamel on metal or hardboard
    Baked enamel on glass or steel: American Porcelain
    Porcelain on aluminum: Mapes Industries

116

SIDING
Brick, Wood (hard), Metal

> > < <

Lighting

YOU SHOULD AVOID
Halogen bulbs burn at a high temperature. They are made with quartz, thereby filtering radiation. However, they can emit damaging ultraviolet light causing sunburn, increased risk for cataracts, and skin cancer. If you have unshielded halogen bulbs, ask your supplier to replace them with a double envelope – glass-shield type.

LESS-TOXIC ALTERNATIVES
Chromalux full spectrum incandescent light bulbs: Allergy Relief Shop, American Environmental Products, NEEDS

Full spectrum incandescent bulbs/lights and fluorescent tubes and bulbs: American Environmental Products (Light-A-Lux, E-Bulb, Sad-Lite), Natural Lifestyle, The SunBox Co., Tomorrow's World

Full spectrum fluorescent lamps: American Environmental Products (Glad Lite desk lamp), Vita-Lite Plus (table lamp)

Full spectrum light boxes: American Environmental Products (Sad-Lite, Sun-A-Lux), Healthy Environments (Sad-Lite), The SunBox Co.

Full spectrum tubular skylight: Abundant Earth

Ott-Lite full-spectrum light bulbs, fluorescent light bulbs, tubes and task lamps: Allergy Relief Shop, GAIAM, Harmony, The Living Source, NEEDS, Real Goods, Tomorrow's World, Whole Foods

Ott-Lite full-spectrum Portable Light Box: Allergy Relief Shop, GAIAM, Harmony, NEEDS, Real Goods, Whole Foods

Ott-Lite full-spectrum Therapy Lamp (to treat SAD Syndrome): Allergy Relief Shop, GAIAM (Happy Light), Harmony (Happy Light), The Living Source, NEEDS (Ott Sun-A-Lux), Pure n Natural (Biolite), Real Goods (Happy Light), Tomorrow's World (Happy Light)

Solar powered lights, lanterns and flashlights: GAIAM, Harmony, Real Goods, Tomorrow's World, Whole Foods

> > < <

Mastics, Caulks, Grouts, etc.

YOU SHOULD AVOID
Mastics and caulks if they contain petrochemical solvents such as xylene and toluene, and glycol ethers. Petroleum and rubber-based grouts and grouts fortified with mold retardants.

LESS-TOXIC ALTERNATIVES

CAULKS & SEALERS
100% Clear Silicon Caulk°
AFM caulks & sealers°: The Living Source, NEEDS
Dap Kwik Seal Tub & Tile Caulk°
GE Silicon Sealer°
Phenoseal line of caulks and sealers°: AEHF, Gloucester Co.

GROUTS
AFM Safecoat grouts and sealers: AEHF, Allergy Relief Shop, The Living
    Source, NEEDS, Nirvana Safe Haven
AR Grout: C-Cure
Custom Blend° (without additives)
Hydroment by Bostick (use polymer free)
Laticrete (cement, sand and pigment – additive free)
Marble dust and cement
Sinan Co. (not for showers or tubs)
Texrite
Portland Cement (no fungicides)
    For joints 1/8 inch or less - 1 part each sand and cement
    For joints up to ½ inch - 2 parts sand and 1 part cement
    For joints over ½ inch - 3 parts sand and 1 part cement

GROUT SEALER
Sodium Silicate
AFM Safecoat Hard Seal (for all grouts): AEHF, Allergy Relief Shop, The
    Living Source, NEEDS, Nirvana Safe Haven

MASONRY OR CONCRETE SEALER
AFM Concrete & Driveway Sealer°: AEHF, Allergy Relief Shop, The Living
    Source, NEEDS
Sinan Co.
Sodium Silicate: Humco Labs (for distributor), Trinity Ceramic Supply
Thoroseal°
Xypex Concrete Waterproofing
9400 Masonry Waterproofing (breathable, solvent-free – impregnates and seals):
    Palmer Industries, Inc.

PAVING SEALERS
AFM Safecoat Paver Seal°: Allergy Relief Shop, The Living Source, NEEDS

SHEETROCK SEALER / JOINT COMPOUNDS
BIN° (contains alcohol)
Murco Joint Compound
Sodium Silicate: Humco Labs (for distributor), Trinity Ceramic Supply

MASTICS FOR PARQUET
AFM Safecoat 3-in-1 Adhesive°: AEHF, Allergy Relief Shop, The Living
    Source, NEEDS

Almighty Adhesive[□]: Allergy Relief Shop
Elmers Glue

MASTICS FOR VINYL

AFM Safecoat 3-in-1 Adhesive[□]: AEHF, Allergy Relief Shop, The Living Source, NEEDS
Almighty Adhesive[□]: Allergy Relief Shop
Elmer's Glue[□]
Self Adhesive Vinyl[□]

> > < <

Paints, Finishes & Sealants

Colors are happy and beautiful, and bring joy to life. Most of us like colors surrounding us inside our homes, on the walls, floors, etc. Paint on the walls can be uplifting, yet paint must not contain chemicals that create health problems.

YOU SHOULD AVOID

Paint products that contain hexane, pentanes and petroleum distillates, volatile hydrocarbons, formaldehyde, kerosene, alcohols, cadmium, ammonia, aluminum, coal tar, dioxane, titanium, zirconium and lead.
Paint strippers that contain methylene chloride and toluene.

LESS-TOXIC ALTERNATIVES

PAINTS, FINISHES, ETC.[□]

AFM Safecoat paints, finishes, sealants, adhesives, etc. (needs to be applied under dry conditions – thin coats, if second coat is needed, paint must be allowed to dry 2-3 days between coats): AEHF, Allergy Relief Shop, The Living Source, NEEDS, Nirvana Safe Haven, RH of Texas
Auro Paint[□]: Sinan Co.
Anchor Paint
Benjamin Moore[□] - EcoSpec Pristine
BioShield[□] Paint, Finishes & Sealers: Eco Design
Dupont Lucite[□]
EnviroSafe[□] (water base Paint)
Glidden 2000[□]
Casein Milk Paint: Eco Design
Livos products
Miller Paint (interior and exterior)
Murco
Milk Paint: Old-Fashioned Milk Paint Co.
Add 2-3 Tbsps. baking soda to each gallon of paint to inhibit odor (may affect bonding quality of paint), or wash the newly painted surface with a baking soda solution after the paint has dried.
Use latex paint without additional biocides or fungicides.

Paint only on dry days – apply thin coat – if second coat is necessary, wait 7-10 days to apply.

PAINT STRIPPERS & THINNERS

AFM SafeChoice Liftoff & Paint Removers[a]: The Living Source, NEEDS, Nirvana Safe Haven

Auro[a]: Sinan Co.

BioShield Natural Citrus Thinner[a]: Eco Design

CitraSolv[a]: GAIAM, Harmony, Real Goods, Whole Foods

Health Masters[a]

Livos

3M Safest Stripper[a]

Trisodium Phosphate (1 lb. trisodium phosphate to 1 gallon hot water) – brush on, let stand for 30 minutes, then rinse off. Stubborn areas may have to be brushed with a steel brush.

Homemade stripper[a] – boil equal parts linseed oil, turpentine, and vinegar[a]

Some surfaces will be safer sanded instead of stripped, but be careful of sanding if the possibility of lead paint exists.

WOOD TREATMENTS

AFM Safecoat: AEHF, Allergy Relief Shop, The Living Source, NEEDS, Nirvana Safe Haven

Aqualac Waterborne Lacquer: Trinity Coatings Co.

Auro Wax (plant derived oil sealant for wood): Sinan Co.

Bioshield Wax – penetrating oil and wax: Eco Design

Livos

Penetrating oil for floors: Sinan Co.

HOMEMADE FORMULAS:

    #1: 3 parts olive oil with 1 part lemon juice
    #2: 1 part linseed oil with 1 part vinegar[a]
    #3: Boil 1 qt. beer, 1 Tbsp. sugar and 2 Tbsp. beeswax, cool, buff.
    #4: Boil 6 Tbsp. beeswax, 3 cups Linseed Oil (food grade), cool, buff.
    #5: Almond oil and lemon juice - Let set 1 hour and buff.

Do not use excess oil. Oil with lemon juice or vinegar can become rancid. Buff weekly with soap and water, thoroughly clean every 3 months.

WOOD STAIN

AFM Safecoat Durostain[a]: AEHF, Allergy Relief Shop, The Living Source, NEEDS, Nirvana Safe Haven

Health Masters

Livos

Organic Nuts: Hammons Products Co. (To make stain – boil shells until the desired color is reached, apply with paint brush, let sit until desired darkness, then wipe off – can repeat for darker finish.)

Weather-Bos

Less-Toxic Alternatives

WOOD SEALANT

AFM Safecoat sealers[a]: AEHF, Allergy Relief Shop, The Living Source, NEEDS, Nirvana Safe Haven

Aquafabulon: Nigra Enterprises

Aqualac Waterborne Lacquer: Trinity Coatings Co.

Crystal Aire & Crystal Shield: Pace Chemical Industries, Nirvana Safe Haven

Hydroline and Hydrolite (water-based urethanes): Basic Coatings, Inc.

Livos

9400W – Wood water-proofing (breathable, solvent free – impregnates and seals): Palmer Industries, Inc.

DECK PREPARATION

AFM Safecoat sealers[a]: AEHF, Allergy Relief Shop, The Living Source, NEEDS, Nirvana Safe Haven

Deck Prep & Waterproofing - Nisus Corp

Weather-Bos[a]

BRUSH CLEANER

Boil vinegar[a], simmer brushes a few minutes, then remove, and wash in tolerated detergent and water.

Livos

SPRAYERS

Hudson Deck Sprayer (hand pump-up pressure sprayer for use with sealants etc.): Allergy Relief Shop

> > < <

Roofing & Roof Ventilation

YOU SHOULD AVOID

Asphalt roof coatings and particleboard underlayment.

Carefully select roofing material in accordance with sensitivities. If EMF sensitive, avoid metal; if sensitive to terpenes, avoid cedar.

LESS-TOXIC ALTERNATIVES

Substitute K-Shield Foil Radiant Vapor Barrier for petroleum-laden felt used under composition shingles.

Solid wood strips are preferred for roofing underlayment. Exterior grade plywood may be acceptable for some, but the underside of the plywood may require a sealer.

Turbines or attic ventilation is important for chemical reduction.

Tile, Metal, Slate or Concrete

Wood shingles (check local ordinances, flame-retardant treatment may be required)

Thermoflex reflective roof and wall covering

Weather-Bos Roof Formulas

ROOFING SEALERS
AFM Safecoat Dyno Flex and Dynoseal□: Allergy Relief Shop, The Living Source, NEEDS, Nirvana Safe Haven

ROOF VENTILATION
Solar Attic Fan: Real Goods, Tomorrow's World

> > < <

Saunas

YOU SHOULD AVOID
Health club saunas may use undesirable chemicals for cleaning, other occupants may wear irritating colognes, and diligence may not be given to keeping down mold.

LESS-TOXIC ALTERNATIVES
Home saunas: AEHF, Heavenly Heat Saunas, Radiant Heater Corp.
Cedar pre-built & cedar kits: The Sauna Warehouse□
Portable (metal frame with organic cotton inside): Fred Nelson
Kit for a glass & stainless steel sauna: Fred Nelson
Grandpa Fred's Very Mild Sauna Soap (vegetable oil base): Fred Nelson
Hemp Sauna Accessories: Real Goods
Teak spa-style mat (teak wood and leather): Chambers

> > < <

Swimming Pool & Spa Water Filtration
(See also Food and Water section for household water filters)

LESS-TOXIC ALTERNATIVES
Copper & Zinc Ion Exchange Filter: EcoDesign
Swimming Pool & Spa Purification
Baquacil and Bromine (alternatives to Chlorine)□
Diatomateous Earth
Ozonator
Vision Purifiers (flow-through catalyst-activated treatment process) Dickson Bros.
Solar Pool Purifier – Floatron: Real Goods
Electrode filtration: Eco Smarte
Natural Water Environments
Zodiac Pool Care Inc.

Swim For Your Health ~ Keep Pools Refreshing & Stimulating

> > < <

Wallpaper & Wallpaper Paste

YOU SHOULD AVOID
Vinyl-coated wallpaper and cloth-textured wallpaper
Mold inhibitors and insecticide in paste – nothing is both safe and mold-proof or insect-proof
It is best if you can avoid wallpaper entirely

LESS-TOXIC ALTERNATIVES

WALLPAPER
Aluminum Wallpaper

WALLPAPER PASTE
Borax or Boric Acid: use 1 Tbsp. to a quart of starch to make anti-mold & anti-insect paste.
Golden Harvest Wheat Paste
Metylan

WALLPAPER CLEANER
Borax (Dissolve ¼ cup in 1 gallon hot water, stir to blend, saturate a sponge with solution and use it to wash walls. - Use with care; if left wet on walls, it could remove the wallpaper.)
Washing Soda and water

> > < <

CONSULTATION SERVICES: There are various resources that will help you with your building, remodeling, and home improvement problems. *(See section on Building Consultation in Resources Directory for more information.)*

> > < <

Children's Special Needs

Today's actions will determine tomorrow's world. We must make wise choices to insure a bright future for our children who are our responsibility, our legacy and our hope for tomorrow. The importance of healthy decisions takes on a new dimension when viewed through the lives of the future.

Children are more susceptible to chemical exposure than are adults. Relative to their weight, a child's body surface is three times greater than that of an adult, thus they absorb more chemicals from skin contact per pound of body weight than an adult.

Children have a higher metabolic rate than adults, and small children breathe twice as much air as an adult per body weight. They also have lower levels of specific chemical detoxification enzymes that affect their ability to metabolize and eliminate chemicals.

Children eat more fruits, vegetables and juices than adults. This exposes them to a greater health risk from pesticides used in growing produce.

Hormones found in food exposes them to the unnatural effect of hormones during important growth years.

Children's cells divide more rapidly than adults. During the first two years of life, the nerves are being created with a myelin sheath. The brain continues to grow throughout childhood. Therefore, exposure to neuro-toxins can have damaging neurological effects.

Children also tend to put objects into their mouths, and they spend more time playing in the dirt and on the floor of their home. This can expose them to lead and other contaminants in dirt and enhance the effect of pesticides used in the home.

Making correct choices is never more important than in decisions affecting children. Careful selection must be made in the use of household cleaners, building materials, pest control, and especially in items used in a child's study, play and sleep areas. Pure water and less chemically contaminated food are essential to their health. A new dimension of stewardship is required to protect their world.

Many of these items have been dealt with in other areas of this book, but a few of the specialized items that affect only children are listed on the following pages. It is also important to consider the computers, reading boxes, etc. that are listed in the Office & Workplace Section, because most children today start using computers at an early age.

> > < <

Baby Items

YOU SHOULD AVOID
Toxic chemicals in bedding, clothing, and disposable diapers. Not only are many of these chemicals harmful to the child, disposable diapers pose a serious threat to our environment because they do not thoroughly decompose. Chlorine bleach, dioxin and pesticides used in fabrics also pose a threat to both our children and the environment.

LESS-TOXIC ALTERNATIVES

BEDDING FOR BABIES
Bassinets, baby bunks & cribs: Abundant Earth, Eco Baby, Lifekind Products, NEEDS, Real Goods, White Lotus

Cotton blankets: A Happy Planet, Abundant Earth, B.Coole Designs, Crown Mattress, Eco Baby, Ecosport, Ethical Shopper, GAIAM, Harmony, Heart of Vermont, JAMS, Janice's, Lifekind Products, Mama Moon, Real Goods, Tomorrow's World

Cotton crib sheets: A Happy Planet, Abundant Earth, Eco Baby, Ecosport, Ethical Shopper, JAMS, Janice's, Lifekind Products, Mother Harts Infant Sheets, Organic Cotton Alternatives, White Lotus

Cotton quilt (handquilted): Ethical Shopper, Honeysuckle Dreams

Cotton or wool comforters: A Happy Planet, Abundant Earth, Tomorrow's World

Crib mattresses, bumpers & pads: Chemically Sensitive Living, Crown City Mattress, Janice's, Lifekind Products, Nirvana Safe Haven, Organic Cotton Alternatives (crib futon & bumpers), Real Goods, Tomorrow's World, White Lotus

Silk/flannel blanket & pillow: The Baby Lane

Wool blankets: Lifekind Products, Mama Moon

Wool Puddle Pad: Tomorrow's World, White Lotus

Wool & cotton bunting: Mama Moon

CAR SEAT COVERS
Wool: Mama Moon

CLOTHING FOR BABIES & TODDLERS
A Happy Planet, Alternative Baby, Alternative Undies, B.Coole Designs, Chemically Sensitive Living, Diamond Organic, Earthlings, Eco Baby (clothing and shoes), Ecosport, Ethical Shopper, Feeling Goods, GAIAM, Green Babies, Green iDeals, Green Marketplace, Harmony, Island Hemp Wear, JAMS, Lifekind Products, Oskri Organics, Real Goods, Whole Foods

DIAPERS
A Happy Planet, Alternative Baby, Alternative Undies, B.Coole Designs, The Baby Lane, Born to Love, Chemically Sensitive Living, Earthwise Basics, Eco Baby, Ethical Shopper, The Living Source, Mama Moon, The Nurtured Baby, Organic Bebé, Oskri Organics

DIAPER BAGS
Alternative Baby (Hemp/Cotton)

DIAPER COVERS, SOAKERS, WRAPS & TRAINING PANTS
Wool and/or cotton: The Baby Lane, Born to Love, Earthwise Basics, Eco Baby, Organic Bebé (wool)

Diaper Doublers: Alternative Baby, Organic Bebé

FURNITURE FOR THE NURSERY
WOOD: Abundant Earth, Eco Baby, Golden Furniture Maker, Organic Bebé (high chair), Real Goods (crib), White Lotus

GIFT BASKETS: EcoExpress

ORGANIC BABY FOOD
Diamond Organic

Earth's Best Baby Food: Frankferd Farms, Organic Bebé, and many grocery and health food stores)

Organic Provisions

PERSONAL CARE PRODUCTS FOR BABIES
Aubrey Organics baby shampoo, lotion and soap: Environmentally Sound Products

Baby's First Wipes: The Living Source
California Baby Products: Organic Bebé
Country Affair Goat Milk Soap: Alternative Baby
Country Comfort baby powder, oil and cream: Environmentally Sound Products
Natural Products Store Baby Shampoo
Simmons Natural Body Care baby products

SLINGS
Alternative Baby (organic cotton or hemp), The Baby Lane, Eco Baby, Ethical Shopper, Mama Moon (hemp and cotton)

WIPES, WASHCLOTHS, TOWELS, BIBS, ETC. FOR BABIES
A Happy Planet, Alternative Baby, Eco Baby, Ethical Shopper, GAIAM, Harmony, JAMS, Mama Moon, Whole Foods

NOTE: www.borntolove.com gives a vast list of baby and children's needs (including cloth diapering resources) by state & name – some are organic, others are just 100% cotton.

> > < <

Toys & Dolls

LESS-TOXIC ALTERNATIVES
Dream Dough (non-toxic food product): JAMS
Gift Crate: EcoExpress
Hemp Balls: A Happy Planet
Kid's Hold It All Bag (cotton): Janice's
Natural fiber and wood toys produced without toxic chemicals: The Baby Lane, Childsake, Earthwise Basics, Eco Baby, Heart of Vermont, JAMS (wood puzzles), Nova Natural, Whimsicality
Non-toxic Roy-Toy Wood Building Logs: Vermont Country Store
Organic dolls, stuffed animals, puppets etc.: Abundant Earth, Alternative Baby, B.Coole Designs The Baby Lane, Childsake, Earthwise Basics, Eco Baby, Ethical Shopper, Fair Trade Naturals, Feeling Goods, Green Babies, Honeysuckle Dreams, JAMS, Janice's, Lifekind Products, Mama Moons, Oskri Organics, Real Goods, Whimsicality

~ ~ ~ ~ ~ ~

Chewing Gum

Children can make their own less toxic chewing gum with the Chewing Gum Kit from Verve. The kit uses chicle gum base (harvested by Central American chicleros from rain forest trees), powdered sugar, corn syrup, flavor packets, pan, instructions, and the story of chicle.

> > < <

Art Supplies

YOU SHOULD AVOID
Children love to be creative, but commercial art supplies often contain dyes, chemicals and additives that are dangerous to children.

LESS-TOXIC ALTERNATIVES

CRAYONS, CHALK, FINGERPAINT, PENCILS, ETC.
Beeswax Crayons in Wooden Box, Modeling Beeswax & Colored Pencils: The Baby Lane

Nova Natural Toys & Crafts has a complete line of less-toxic supplies

Stockmar Beeswax and Prang Soybean Crayons: Childsake

Stockmar Modeling Beeswax: Childsake

Prang Soybean Crayons: Childsake

Homemade Fingerpaint
1 cup flour, 1 cup water, 1 ½ tsps. salt and food coloring

Directions: Mix ingredients well in a small bowl or cup

Homemade Eggshell Sidewalk Chalk
6 eggshells (thoroughly washed), 1 tsp. very hot tap water, 1 tsp. flour

Directions: Grind eggshells into fine powder. Mix with flour and water to form a paste. Roll into a stick shape, and wrap with a paper towel. Let dry (about 3 days). For sidewalk art (not for blackboards)

Homemade Sidewalk Paint
¼ cup cornstarch, ¼ cup water, 6-8 drops food coloring

Directions: Mix cornstarch and water. Add food coloring and stir.

GLUE
Elmer's Carpenter Wood Glue

Elmer's white or yellow glue

Sanford Elephant Glue

Homemade Paper Paste
1/3 cup flour, 2 Tbsps. Sugar, 1 cup water, ¼ tsp. oil of cinnamon

Directions: Mix flour and sugar in saucepan. Add water and stir until smooth. Cook over low heat until clear, stirring constantly. Remove from heat, and add oil of cinnamon.

Homemade Waterproof or Glass Glue
2 packets unflavored gelatin, 2 Tbsps. Cold water, 3 Tbsps. Skimmed milk, Several drops oil of cloves (optional)

Directions: Sprinkle gelatin over cold water, and set aside to soften. Heat milk to boiling, and stir in softened gelatin mixture. Add oil of cloves as a preservative if glue is to be kept for over a day. Store in a jar. Set jar in hot water to soften for use.

PLAY DOUGH & BUBBLES

Children love to play with play dough and blow bubbles, but commercial brands often contain dyes and additives that are dangerous to children. The following are less-toxic alternatives:

Homemade Non-Edible Play Dough (Do not eat)
2 cups water, 1 cup salt, 2 Tbsps. oil, safe food coloring as desired, 4 tsps. cream of tartar, 2 cups flour

Directions: Heat the water on low heat in a large 6-8 quart pan. Add salt and simmer until completely dissolved. Add oil and food coloring for desired color. Mix the flour and cream of tartar, then add to water, stirring constantly with a wooden spoon. Don't worry about lumps, they will work out when the dough cools. Store in refrigerator

Homemade Cornstarch & Salt Play Dough (Do not eat)
2 cups salt, 2/3 cups water, 1 cup cornstarch, ½ cup additional water

Directions: Mix salt and 2/3 cup water in pan and cook on medium for 4-5 minutes. Turn off heat. Mix cornstarch and ½ cup cold water in bowl. Stir into cooked mixture, and cook on medium until mixture is thick. Cool thoroughly before use.

Homemade Oatmeal Play Dough (Do not eat)
1 cup flour, 1 cup water 2 cups oatmeal

Directions: Mix ingredients together thoroughly and knead until smooth. This is not supposed to be edible, but will not hurt children if they eat it.

Homemade Edible Play Dough
2 cups smooth peanut butter, 2 cups rolled oats, 2 cups dried milk, 2/3 cups honey. Optional ingredients: safe food coloring, Rice Krispies, coconut, chocolate chips, red hots

Directions: Mix ingredients until thoroughly combined. Have children wash hands before using and work on waxed paper. Store leftover dough in airtight container.

Homemade Bubbles
1/3 cup safe dish soap or baby shampoo, 1 ¼ cups water, 2 tsp. sugar, Safe food coloring as desired, 2 Tbsps. glycerine (optional – makes more durable bubbles)

Directions: Combine ingredients and pour into unbreakable bottle. Can use spoons with holes in them, straws, wire bent into a circle and covered with string, etc. to make bubble blowers.

> > < <

Cleaning Agents
Bathroom Cleaners

YOU SHOULD AVOID

Commercial cleaners may contain chlorine, glycol ether, hydrocarbons and other volatile toxic chemicals. Toilet bowl cleaner frequently contains sodium bisulfate, which forms sulfuric acid in water, but similar products may also contain equally dangerous hydrochloric or phosphoric acid.

LESS-TOXIC ALTERNATIVES

AFM Safety Clean[a] & Super Clean[a]: AEHF, Allergy Relief Shop, The Living Source, NEEDS

Bioshield Soap Cleaner and Toilet Bowl Cleaner: Eco Design

Bon Ami: AEHF

Borax (2 Tbsps.) plus ½ cup low suds detergent and ¼ cup calcium carbonate make a good bathtub cleaner (Store in a jar or old salt shaker) sprinkle on area and rub with cloth, rinse with clear water.

Earth Friendly Shower Kleaner

EarthRite products: NEEDS

Ecover[a]: AEHF

Enviro-Magic Tile Tub & Grout Cleaner: AEHF

GoldenKaire Cleansing Solution (cleans, purifies, and deodorizes): Dasun

Home Soap: Life Tree, Environmentally Sound Products

HomeFree Multi Cleaner[a]: Allergy-Asthma Tech.

Hydrogen Peroxide (germicide) and cream of tartar paste make a good cleaner for sinks and bathtubs

Natural Line Basin, Tub & Tile Cleaner: Real Earth

Nature Clean Tub & Tile Cleaners & Toilet Bowl Cleaner: AEHF, The Living Source

Nature Clean Kitchen & Bath Spray Cleaner: AEHF, The Living Source

Planet: Planet Products

Ring Eraser (pumice stone with handle for cleaning toilets): Vermont Country Store

Sol-U-Guard disinfects

Zephiran (Benzalkonium) Chloride 17%[a] (*use only as directed*) – 1 part to 10 parts water: Abrams Royal Pharmacy (*prescription required*)

¼ cup baking soda and ½ cup white vinegar[a] mixed with warm water to clean tub and tile

TOILET BOWL CLEANERS

Borax (1 Tbsp.) plus hot water

Denture cleaning tablets[a]

Descale It Toilet Bowl Cleaner: AEHF

Earth Friendly Toilet Bowl Cleaner

Paste of borax and lemon juice, or vinegar[a] and baking soda

Nature Clean Toilet Bowl Cleaner: AEHF, The Living Source

LIME & SCALE REMOVERS

Borax (in waterless toilet bowl)

Mix 2 parts ammonia, 1 part vinegar[a], and a little baking soda (in waterless toilet bowl)

DeScale It Lime-Eater[a]: AEHF

Vinegar[a] strips lime deposits from sinks and showers

> > < <

Dishwashing Compounds

YOU SHOULD AVOID

Commercial powders, granules and liquids may contain perfume, formaldehyde, hydrocarbons, petroleum surfactants and arsenic.

LESS-TOXIC ALTERNATIVES

Allen's Naturally Dishwashing Liquid & Automatic Dishwasher Powder: Allergy Relief Shop, Janice's, NEEDS

Ambio-Clean: Rainman Int.

Amway Dish Drops[a]

Biofa Dishwashing Liquid

Bioshield: Eco Design

Castile Soap (contains no petroleum): Environmentally Sound Products

Dishmate: Earth Friendly Products

Dr. Bronner's Soap: The Living Source

EarthRite (contains little, if any petroleum): NEEDS, some grocery stores

Ecover[a]: AEHF

Electra-Sol Automatic Dishwashing Detergent[a]

Granny's Old-fashioned E-Z Maid: AEHF, Allergy Relief Shop, The Living Source, NEEDS

HomeFree Dishwashing Liquid[a]: Allergy-Asthma Tech.

Natural Line Hand Dishwashing Detergent: Real Earth

Nature Clean Automatic Dishwashing Powder, Liquid & Cleaning Lotion: AEHF, The Living Source

Neo-Life Automatic Dishwashing Powder: The Living Source

Neo-Life LDC (formerly Yellow) or Green: The Living Source

Palmolive Liquid Automatic Dishwasher Detergent

Premium Dishwashing Liquid with Aloe Vera and Calendula and Automatic Dishwashing Detergent: Life Tree, Environmentally Sound Products

Rain Fresh Automatic Dishwasher Powder: The Living Source

Seventh Generation: GAIAM, Harmony, Real Goods, Whole Foods

Shaklee Basic D[a]

Sunlight Powder Automatic Dishwasher Detergent

Washing Soda (Sodium Carbonate) – Arm & Hammer

Combine 1 part Borax to 1 part washing soda; mix, then label as dishwasher compound. Add ¼ cup to dishwasher per load.

Use vinegar[n] to remove stains in either glass or metal coffeepots
Combine liquid soap and vinegar[n] to remove grease.

> > < <

Disinfectants & Germ Removers

YOU SHOULD AVOID
Phenolated products, chlorinated products, or products containing alcohols
and formaldehyde.

LESS-TOXIC ALTERNATIVES
AFM Safety Clean: AEHF, Allergy Relief Shop, The Living Source, NEEDS
Australian Tea Tree Oil – from Melaleuca tree (mix 2 tsp. in 2 cups of water
and spray area): Desert Essence, Arizona Health Foods
Borax
GoldenKaire Cleansing Solution: Dasun
Hydrogen Peroxide
Purasol[n]
Spectracidal Disinfectant Agent[n]: Apothe-Cure *(compounding pharmacy)*
(broad micro-flora spectrum killer for all forms of disease-producing mold,
bacteria, viruses and protozoa – use instead of isopropyl alcohol)
Sol-U-Guard
Zephiran (Benzalkonium) Chloride 17%[n] *(use only as directed)* – 1 part to 10
parts water: Abrams Royal Pharmacy *(prescription required)*

> > < <

Drain Cleaners

YOU SHOULD AVOID
Commercial caustic granule and liquid cleaners that may contain volatile toxic
chemicals such as 1,1,1-Trichlorethane.

LESS-TOXIC ALTERNATIVES
Actina Waste Conditioner: The Living Source
BioFree Drain Cleaner
Drain Care (enzymes): Allergy Relief Shop
Earth Enzymes Drain Cleaner: Earth Friendly Products
Greasemate: Earth Friendly Products
Nature's Key Drain Opener & Plumbing Cleaner (enzymes): Dasun
Nature's Clean Septic Treat (reactivates bacteria): Dasun
Natural Line Enzyme Stain & Odor Treatment: Real Earth
Organics Drain Opener: AEHF
Pango Pressure Gun
Trisodium phosphate
Home Remedies:
Clean drains weekly to kill all mold - Keep drains closed when not in use

Baker's Yeast – Pour 1 packet of baker's yeast down the drain, let it stand for 20 to 30 minutes. Then pour a quart of warm/hot water down the drain. Run tap water to ensure that the drain is clear.

Baking soda and water – Pour ½ cup baking soda the down drain and follow with 3 cups boiling water – let it bubble and gurgle for a while before rinsing with hot water.

Baking soda (1 cup) and vinegar⁰ (½ cup) – Pour soda in drain first, add vinegar and cover tightly until fizzing stops, repeat as needed. Flush with hot water.

Baking soda (½ cup), vinegar (1 cup) and boiling water (2 pints) – Cover and let set for a few minutes or overnight – then rinse with hot water

Baking soda (¾ cup) and salt (¾ cup) followed by 1 pint boiling water. Let set overnight then flush with water

Epsom salts used weekly in drains

Plunger followed by baking soda treatment

Washing Soda – Pour 3 Tbsps. washing soda down the drainpipes once a week to prevent problems.)

Weekly prevention: mix baking soda (2 oz.), salt (1 oz.) and cream of tartar (1 oz.). Pour down drain, followed by 1 gallon boiling water then 1 gallon cold water.

FOR GREASE IN TRAPS

Mix 1 cup salt, 1 cup baking soda, and ¼ cup cream of tartar. Put ¼ cup in drain every week. Add 2 cups boiling water, leave 5 minutes then rinse with cold water.

Nature's Key Drain Opener & Plumbing Cleaner: Dasun

FOR GARBAGE DISPOSALS

Deodorize with baking soda or citrus peels

All-Natural NOC Concentrate: Dasun

Eat your food off sparkling dishes, washed over germ-free drains and cooked in chemically less-contaminated ovens.

> > < <

Dry Cleaning

YOU SHOULD AVOID

Commercial dry cleaners use dry cleaning fluid that contains toxic chemicals such as 1,1,1-Trichlorethane, Tetrachlorethylene, Trichloroethylene and Naphthalene.

LESS-TOXIC ALTERNATIVES⁰

Wet cleaning is a water alternative for 70% of the articles labeled "Dry Clean Only."

A new type of dry cleaning equipment utilizes odorless non-chlorinated hydrocarbon fluid: Prestige-Exceptional Fabricare, Our Cleaner World

If these processes are not available in your area or by mail, select a dry cleaner that cleans in a location separate from the storage facility. To prevent unnecessary exposure, dry cleaners should frequently change filters and cleaning solution.

Sweater Fresh[n]: Natural Lifestyle

IF YOU MUST WEAR DRY-CLEANED CLOTHES

If your clothes have any smell when they are returned from the dry cleaner, return them and have the residue removed.

Hang freshly cleaned clothes outside or in the garage to air. Never store in a bedroom closet near sleeping quarters. Dry cleaning fluid has a half-life of 40 days.

> > < <

Floor Cleaners & Polishes

YOU SHOULD AVOID

Commercial cleaning fluids that contains toxic chemicals.

LESS-TOXIC ALTERNATIVES

To clean vinyl/linoleum floors, combine 1 cup white vinegar[n] with 2 gallons water.

AFM SuperClean: AEHF, Allergy Relief Shop, The Living Source, NEEDS

Bioshield Soap Cleaner, Floor Soap & Floor Milk: Eco Design

Earth Friendly Products

Ecover's Floor Soap (for wood floors)

Home Soap: Life Tree, Environmentally Sound Products

Livos waxes

Orange Glo: Appel Co.

Nature Clean Floor Cleaner: AEHF, The Living Source

Neolife Green

Planet: Planet Products

> > < <

Furniture Polish & Cleaner

YOU SHOULD AVOID

Scratch covers and oils containing ammonia, fragrance, glycols, nitrobenzenes and petroleum distillates.

LESS-TOXIC ALTERNATIVES

Almond oil

Beeswax (natural)

Bioshield Wood & Furniture Polish: Eco Design

Dryaden Furniture Polish: Livos

Dust Bunny (electrostatic dust cloth – needs no chemical treatment[n]: Allerx

Earth Friendly Furniture Polish: AEHF

Enviro-Magic Lemon Oil Furniture Polish & Treatment: AEHF, The Living Source

Glanos Liquid Wax: Livos

Murphy's Oil Soap[a]

Natural Line Furniture Polish: Real Earth Environmental

Olive Oil: mix 3 parts olive oil and 1 part white vinegar[a], or mix 1 part lemon juice and 2 parts olive or vegetable oil

Orange Plus: Earth Friendly Product

Raw Linseed Oil (Food Grade): mix 1/8 cup linseed oil, 1/8 cup vinegar[a] and ¼ cup lemon juice

Salt: As a grease cleaner, apply salt to absorb grease.

Tea: Use a cloth dipped in cool tea to dust furniture

Vinegar[a]: Use 1 cup vinegar[a] with 1 gallon of warm water.

Homemade Furniture Polish

Boil a tea bag in ¾ cup water. Let set at least 1 hour. Remove tea bag. Add ½ cup olive oil, 1 Tbsp. vanilla and 2 Tbsps. lemon juice. Put in a small bottle and shake well before using. Rub with a soft cloth until tackiness disappears.

Scratch Remover

Use lemon juice and salad oil. Rub with a soft cloth.

Water Stain/Spot Remover

Toothpaste

Lemon juice

Salt and vinegar mixture

10 drops lemon oil with 2 cups vodka. Immediately rub and dry.

Coffee Cup Stain Remover

Moist salt

Allow your furniture to breathe too!

> > < <

General Household Cleaners

YOU SHOULD AVOID

Sprays and liquids that may contain hydrocarbons such as benzene and terpenes such as pine oil.

LESS-TOXIC ALTERNATIVES

AFM SafeChoice products[a] (Safety Clean, Super Clean, X-158): AEHF, Allergy Relief Shop, The Living Source, NEEDS, Nirvana Safe Haven

Allen's Naturally All-Purpose Cleaner[a]: Allergy Relief Shop, Janice's, NEEDS

Amway LOC[a]

Ambio-Clean (a special blend of natural amino acids, vegetable oil and water which dilutes with water – can be used for various cleaning tasks): Rainman Int.

Aubrey Organics Earth Aware & Liquid Sparkle: AEHF, NEEDS

Baking Soda

Biofa Household Cleaner
Bioshield Soap Cleaner: Eco Design
Bon Ami Cleaning Product: AEHF, The Living Source
Borax
Citra-Solv (contains d-limonene)[a] : Environmentally Sound Products
Citrus Shine Total Home Cleaner: Mia Rose Products
Dr. Bronner's Peppermint Castile Soap: Arizona Health Foods, The Living Source
EarthRite products: NEEDS
Earth Wise Fresh Mint
Enviro-Magic Mildew Stain Away, Super Cleaner & Supra Citra: AEHF
GoldenKaire Cleansing Solution: Dasun
Home Soap Household Cleaner: Life Tree, Environmentally Sound Products
HomeFree Multi Cleaner[a]: Allergy-Asthma Tech.
Planet: Planet Products
Mela Magic (concrete cleaner)
Murphy's Oil Soap
Natural Chemistry All Purpose Cleaner[a]: Allergy Relief Shop
Natural Line All Purpose Cleaner: Real Earth
Nature Clean Kitchen and Bath Spray: AEHF, The Living Source
Neo-Life Super 10 (formerly Rugged Red): The Living Source
Orange Plus: Earth Friendly Products
Organics All-Purpose Cleaner, Degreaser & Stain Remover: AEHF
Shaklee Basic H[a]
Trisodium Phosphate
Washing Soda
Zephiran (Benzalkonium) Chloride 17%[a] (*use only as directed*) – 1 part to 10 parts water: Abrams Royal Pharmacy (*prescription required*)
Mix 2 parts ammonia, 1 part vinegar[a] and a little baking soda in water
Mix 3 Tbsp. dry mustard and water into a paste. Apply to area and let set until dry (removes perfume)
Mix ¼ cup baking soda, ¼ cup washing soda and water – make paste. Apply to area, let dry (removes petroleum-based products)
Mix 1 tsp. liquid soap with 1 tsp. borax and 1 squeeze of lemon in 1 quarter of warm water

> > < <

Laundry

BLEACHES
YOU SHOULD AVOID
Laundry bleaches that contain chlorine and fragrances
LESS-TOXIC ALTERNATIVES
Borateem Bleach[a]

Borax-20 Mule Team
Chlorox 2[a]
Hydrogen peroxide (use ½ cup to washer)
Itteki Natural replacement for chlorine bleach: The Living Source
Lemon juice - put ¼ cup in rise cycle then hang in the sun to dry – the sun and
    lemon juice together act as a natural bleach
Miracle White[a]
Mrs. Stewart's Bluing[a] (mineral dye derived from iron) will help brighten
    white laundry
Nature Clean Non-Chlorine Power & Liquid Laundry Bleach: AEHF, The
    Living Source
Seventh Generation: GAIAM, Harmony, Real Goods, Whole Foods
Snowy[a]
Sodium Hexametaphosphate (¼ to 1 cup per 5 gallons of water): The Living
    Source / or unscented Calgon – 1/8 cup per load
Sodium Percarbonate (hydrogen peroxide and sodium carbonate): AEHF
The Brightener: Allerx

> > < <

DETERGENTS
YOU SHOULD AVOID
Powders and liquids that may contain perfume, formaldehyde, phenol, alcohols,
    naphthalene and other chemicals.
LESS-TOXIC ALTERNATIVES
Allen's Naturally Biodegradable Liquid Laundry Detergent: Allergy Relief
    Shop, Janice's, NEEDS
Ambio-Clean: Rainman Int.
Amway SA8[a]
Arm & Hammer Detergent[a] (use only as directed)
Awalan wool and silk wash: Sinan Corp.
Baking Soda
BioShield Powder and Liquid Laundry Soap: Eco Design
Borax
Ceramic laundry discs: Allergy Relief Shop, The Living Source
Earth Smart Laundry Cleaning Discs
EarthRite products: NEEDS
Ecos Laundry Detergent: Earth Friendly Products
Ecosave Magnetic Washball: Allergy Relief Shop
Ecover Natural Delicate Wash (for wool, silk and all natural fabrics): AEHF
Granny's Old Fashioned[a] Laundry Liquid & Power Plus (use only as directed):
    AEHF, Allergy Relief Shop, The Living Source, NEEDS
Heart of Vermont Laundry Soap: Heart of Vermont
HomeFree Liquid Laundry Detergent[a]: Allergy-Asthma Tech.
Premium Laundry Liquid: Life Tree, Environmentally Sound Products
Natural Line Laundry Detergent/Softener: Real Earth Environmental

Less-Toxic Alternatives

Nature Clean laundry products: AEHF, The Living Source
Neo-Life G-1 Powder (non-petroleum – low phosphate): AEHF, The Living Source
Shaklee Basic H
San-O-Zon (mineral compound)
Seventh Generation: GAIAM, Harmony, Real Goods, Whole Foods
Snowflake Laundry Soap
SuperGlobe: Dixie Peterson
T-Wave Natural Laundry Cleaning Discs: Natural Lifestyle
Vinegar
Wood clothes dryers (save your money and your clothes):

> > < <

FABRIC SOFTENERS & ANTISTATIC
YOU SHOULD AVOID
Most commercial strips and papers as they may contain perfume and
  hydrocarbons.
LESS-TOXIC ALTERNATIVES
½ cup apple cider vinegar
¼ to ½ cup baking soda in rinse water (softener and deodorizer)
Bounce Free
Dryer Fresh: Natural Lifestyle
Nature Clean Fabric Softener: AEHF, The Living Source

> > < <

PRE-WASHES & STAIN REMOVERS
YOU SHOULD AVOID
Sprays, liquids and aerosols that may contain chlorine, formaldehyde, toluene,
  benzene or tetrachloroethylene.
LESS-TOXIC ALTERNATIVES
All natural N.O.C. Concentrate – odor and stain remover: Dasun
Allen's Naturally Fabric Softener: Allergy Relief Shop, NEEDS
Baking Soda
Borax
Club Soda
The B.O.S.S. – odor and stain remover: Dasun
Enviro-Magic Super Spot Remover & Magic One-Spray: AEHF
Flora Bright (natural papaya enzyme bleach): Natural Lifestyle
Granny's Old Fashioned Soil Away: Allergy Relief Shop, The Living Source,
  NEEDS
Hydrogen Peroxide
  (care must be exercised to avoid damage to colored garments)
Lemon Juice (may use together with sea salt)
Nature Clean Laundry Stain Remover: AEHF, The Living Source
Nature's Key Spot & Stain Remover: Dasun

Neo-Life Super 10 (Formerly Rugged Red): The Living Source
Planet: Planet Products
Salt
Stain & Odor Remover: Earth Friendly Products

SPECIAL STAIN REMOVAL
Blood
Soak in cold water.
Bleach with ¼ cup Borax and 2 cups water, then wash with an acceptable
   detergent.
Hydrogen peroxide will also bubble blood out of clothing. If the spot is on a
   colored garment, be aware that peroxide may also remove the color.
The B.O.S.S. (odor & stain remover): Dasun
Granny's Old Fashioned Soil Away: Allergy Relief Shop, NEEDS
Nature's Key Spot & Stain Remover: Dasun
Chewing gum and adhesives: CitraSolv – GAIAM, Harmony, Real Goods,
   Whole Foods

Crayon
Granny's Old Fashioned Soil Away: Allergy Relief Shop, NEEDS

Fresh fruit or vegetable stain
Boiling water

Grease stains
Borax and water (cover stain, rub in and wipe off – then rinse well)

Ink spots
1 Tbsp. cream of tartar and 1 Tbsp. lemon juice with cold water
Granny's Old Fashioned Soil Away: Allergy Relief Shop, NEEDS

Oil stains
Rub white chalk or talcum power into stain before laundering
Eucalyptus oil (put on cloth and rub affected area – allow to soak in before
   laundering)

Perspiration
Sponge with white vinegar⁵ or lemon juice, or apply a solution of two aspirins
   and water.

Rust stains
A mixture of lemon juice and salt and place in sunlight
Enviro-Magic Rust-Away III: AEHF

Scorch marks: Grated onion

Tar stains
Eucalyptus oil (put on cloth and run affected area – allow to soak in before
   laundering)

Wine stains: Salt or club soda

> > < <

Metal Cleaners

Brighten your brass, shine your silver, caress your copper with natural cleaners, and the metal in your life will really be gold.

YOU SHOULD AVOID

Most commercial cleaners contain ammonia, ethanol, fragrances, paraffin, petroleum distillates, and sulphur compounds.

LESS-TOXIC ALTERNATIVES

ALUMINUM CLEANERS

2 Tbsps. cream of tartar and 1 quart hot water

Lemon juice on a cloth, then rinse with warm water

Note: Keep washing soda (sodium carbonate) away from aluminum as it may attack the surface of the metal.

BRASS & BRONZE CLEANERS

Toothpaste

Dampen table salt with vinegar[n] or lemon juice. Rub. Brass will look brighter and need less polishing if rubbed with olive oil after each polishing.

2 tsps. salt and 1 Tbsp. flour plus enough vinegar[n] to make a paste – put salt and flour in a small bowl, then add vinegar. Rub on with sponge, let dry, then rinse in hot water. If any discoloration remains, use toothpaste.

1 Tbsp. salt and 2 Tbsp. flour plus enough water to make a paste. Cover object. Allow to dry and buff with soft cloth.

Clean and polish with Worcestershire sauce

Sour milk or yogurt (coat object, allow to dry, rinse and buff with soft cloth)

After cleaning, rub with olive oil to increase brightness

COPPER CLEANERS

If copper is tarnished, boil in water, 1 tsp. salt and 1 cup white vinegar[n] for several hours. Wash in hot soapy water, rinse, then dry.

Use lemon juice or vinegar and salt

Sour milk or yogurt (coat object, allow to dry, rinse and buff with soft cloth)

CHROME / CHROMIUM CLEANERS

Lemon peel (rub, rinse and polish with a soft cloth)

Pure undiluted apple cider vinegar[n] (apply with a soft cloth, and polish with a paper towel)

Whiting (calcium carbonate) is available at paint stores. Apply with a damp cloth. Dry with a soft cloth.

GOLD CLEANERS

Wash in warm, soapy water. Dry with a cloth, then polish with a chamois.

JEWELRY CLEANERS

(For metal and hard stone jewelry - not recommended for pearls)

Denture tablets[n] in water - let set 15 minutes

Toothpaste on old toothbrush - scrub jewelry

SILVER CLEANERS

Electrolyte method: 1 tsp. cream of tartar or baking soda in 1-2 pints of water. Use an aluminum pan or a pan with a piece of aluminum foil in it. Boil 2 to 3 minutes, making sure the water covers the silver. Remove the silver, rinse, dry and buff.

Salt removes tarnish caused by contact with eggs

Soapy solution of baking soda and water (rub, rinse and dry)

Whiting (on a soft cloth)

Toothpaste

STAINLESS STEEL POLISH

Earth Friendly Stainless Steel & Metal Cleaner

Mineral Oil

> > < <

Mold Inhibitors

YOU SHOULD AVOID

Commercial sprays that may contain chlorine, formaldehyde hydrocarbons, or biocides

LESS-TOXIC ALTERNATIVES

AFM Safety Clean° and X-158° Mold Retardant: AEHF, Allergy Relief Shop, Allerx, The Living Source, NEEDS

Australian Tea Tree Oil – from Melaleuca Tree (mix 2 tsp. in 2 cups of water and spray area): Desert Essence, Arizona Health Foods

Baking soda and enough water to make a paste. Apply with stiff brush.

Borax is a natural bleach and anti-mold agent. After drying areas, sprinkle a small amount in the moldy places to retard the mold growth.

Borax & baking soda placed in appropriate areas helps absorb moisture.

Borax (1 tsp. plus 3 Tbsps. vinegar° or lemon juice)

Citracidal (20 drops to 1 quart water)

Full spectrum florescent light (UV source) – leave on at least 4 hours per day in any room without windows

Garden sulfur kills mold on stones

Keep areas well lighted, dry and increase air circulation.

Leave a light on in closets to reduce mold

Lemon Juice (full strength)

Lemon Juice plus salt

Mold Rid (calcium chloride crystals) moisture absorber tray – use only as directed. Helps reduce humidity and mold growth.

Ozonator (use only as directed): AEHF
   (Run 2-4 hrs., then air 8 hrs. before entering room)

Paramycocidin (mix 10 drops in 2 cups of water and spray area)

Purasol

Sol-U-Guard – Melaleuca Oil: Mela Magic

UV Lights: National BioLite, Tsoralite, Dermalight, International Lite

Vinegar[a] (full strength)

Vinegar[a] and salt – equal parts

Washing soda – sprinkled in appropriate places

Zeolite: AEHF, Absolute Environmental's, Dasun, Real Goods

Zephiran (Benzalkonium) Chloride 17%[a] - general germicide/fungicide (*use only as directed*) – 1 part to 10 parts water: Abrams Royal Pharmacy (*prescription required*)

For shoes: rotate your shoes, put baking soda in them, sun and air them to remove moisture

For mold on books – microwave 30-60 seconds – use caution

Rub each page with baking soda

> > < <

Oven & Barbecue Cleaners

YOU SHOULD AVOID

Commercial sprays, jellies and pastes due to propellants, detergents, glycol ethers, and lye.

LESS-TOXIC ALTERNATIVES

Aluminum foil or disposable foil oven liner (do not allow to touch food)

Amway LOC[a] (in very hot water)

Baking Soda and Salt (blended together)

Baking Soda and Steel Wool

Baking Soda and water paste – spread over greasy areas and leave for 3 minutes – then wash off with hot water and a cloth

Borax (2 tsps.) and liquid soap (2 Tbsp.) mixed with warm water

Nature Clean Non-Toxic Oven & Barbecue Cleaner: AEHF, The Living Source, Frank Ross

Neolife Super 10 (Formerly Rugged Red) - in very hot water

Salt – sprinkle on warm spills (will make later removal easier)

Self-cleaning oven (turn on and leave)

Note: Do not use abrasive cleaners on self-cleaning ovens as it can damage the coating.

Washing Soda in warm water

> > < <

Room Air Fresheners

YOU SHOULD AVOID

Aerosols and stick-ups that may contain alcohols, glycols, perfumes, petroleum distillates, hydrocarbons, paradichlorobenzene and quaternary ammonium compounds

LESS-TOXIC ALTERNATIVES
Activated Charcoal Blanket: Nirvana Safe Haven
Adzorbstar: The Living Source
Air Filters *(see Heating / Air Conditioning Filters)*
All Natural NOC Concentrate (removes bacterial based odors): Dasun
Australian Tea Tree Oil: Desert Essence, Arizona Health Foods
    (Mix 2 tsps. in 2 cups of water and spray area)
Baking Soda
Bathroom exhaust fans, ceiling fans and other electric fans help circulate the
    air, but they must be kept clean.
Borax is a natural deodorant
The B.O.S.S. – odor and stain remover: Dasun
Charcoal
Cider vinegar[a] will remove pet odors
Circulating air helps freshen any room
Citrus Air Fresheners[a]: Environmentally Sound Products
Electric fan (blow air out of a musty room)
Enviro-Dynamics Odor Trap: AEHF
GoldenKaire Cleansing Solution: Dasun
Grated orange or lemon rind (place in a small saucer)
Hygenaire (fan circulates solution of grapefruit seed extract & vegetable
    glycerin)
Natural Chemistry Smells and Stains: Allergy Relief Shop
Natural Line Enzyme Stain & Odor Treatment: Real Earth
Odorbusters: The Living Source
Orange Plus: Earth Friendly Products
Rose petals
Simmering scents: cinnamon, citrus, cloves, eucalyptus[a], herbs, spices (be
    careful of added fragrances)
Smells-B-Gone for pet and other odors: The Living Source
Strike a match in the bathroom to remove odors – avoid inhaling smoke
UniFresh: Earth Friendly Products
Vanilla extract (place 1 or 2 Tbsp. in a small bowl)

ODOR ABSORBERS
Apple – cut into pieces (use in small area)
Bac-azap: Nisus Corp.
Baking Soda
Bread – several slices in open container (use in small area)
CarraFree™ Odor eliminator: Mom's Aloe Store
Charcoal
Enviro-Dynamics Odor Trap: AEHF
Lemon
Ozonator (use only as directed – eliminates volatile hydrocarbons): AEHF
    (Run 2-4 hours, then air 8 hrs. before entering room)
Auto Ionizer[a]: Real Goods
Vanilla extract (place 1 or 2 Tbsp. in small bowl absorbs paint odors)

Zeolite (a natural mineral which removes toxic air gases and odors from the environment) – powder and breather bags: AEHF, Absolute Environmental's, Dasun, Real Goods

> > < <

Scouring Powder

YOU SHOULD AVOID
Commercial cleansers and powders, cleaning pads and sponges containing chlorine and volatile organic hydrocarbons

LESS-TOXIC ALTERNATIVES
Baking Soda (for coffee and tea stains)
Bon Ami Enviro-Dynamics Odor Trap: AEHF
Borax
Dr. Bronner's peppermint castile soap plus baking soda
Calcium carbonate (¼ cup) plus borax (2 Tbsps.)
Ecover Cream Cleaner
Sodasan – vegetable soap and pumice stone
Washing Soda
Mix hydrogen peroxide and cream of tartar (tub and sink cleaner)[□]
Mix 12 parts baking soda, 7 parts powdered soap and 81 parts pumice[□]
Mix 9 parts calcium carbonate and 1 part trisodium phosphate.[□]
Mix borax and ½ cup safe, low suds detergent and ¼ cup calcium carbonate (tub cleaner)[□]
Powders may not be suitable for all surfaces due to abrasiveness.

FOR HEAVY SCOURING
Use any of the following with a tolerated scouring powder.
   Plain copper or stainless steel coils and balls
   Plain steel wool
   Stainless steel scrubber

Properly label all mixtures

> > < <

Upholstery & Carpet Cleaners

YOU SHOULD AVOID
Sprays and spot removers that contain volatile hydrocarbons
Commercial carpet cleaning and shampooing solutions may contain aromatic, aliphatic and chlorinated hydrocarbons, petroleum distillates and sodium salts of fatty alcohol sulfates.
Avoid any applications that will not dry within 12 hours.
Pesticides, herbicides, insecticides, fertilizer, etc. can remain in carpet for long periods of time because they are not subject to the decomposition of rain, sun and air movement.

Carpet can also harbor lead and asbestos from outside. So leave the shoes you
wear outside the home.

LESS-TOXIC ALTERNATIVES

CARPET STEAM CLEANERS & SHAMPOOS

AFM SafeChoice Carpet Shampoo: AEHF, Allergy Relief Shop, The Living
Source, NEEDS

AFM Super Clean: The Living Source

Allerpet (to remove pet dander): Absolute Environmental's

Granny's Old Fashioned Karpet Kleen: Allergy Relief Shop, NEEDS

Home Soap: Life Tree, Environmentally Sound Products

Lifekind Products Steam (Cleaning) Machine

Nature Clean Carpet & Upholstery Cleaner: The Living Source

Natural Chemistry Smells and Stains: Allergy Relief Shop

Neo-Life Green or Super 10: The Living Source

Orange Glo: Appel Co.,

Steam clean with Perrier or Club Soda

See next page for dust mite removal and page 200 for flea and tick removal

CARPET STAIN REMOVERS

For A Wide Variety of Stains

All Natural N.O.C. Concentrate – odor and stain remover: Dasun

The B.O.S.S. (odor & stain remover): Dasun

Granny's Old Fashioned Soil Away: Allergy Relief Shop, NEEDS

Nature's Key Spot & Stain Remover: Dasun

Blood

Soak in cold water.

Bleach with ¼ cup Borax and 2 cups water, then wash with an acceptable
detergent.

Grass

Rub with glycerin. Allow to sit one hour. Wash.

Grease spots

Cover the grease spot with baking soda. After one hour, vacuum the area
thoroughly.

OR sprinkle Fuller's Earth on the spot. It absorbs the grease like a sponge in
15 minutes to 2 hours. Be careful with colors; they may lighten if exposed
too long.

OR use borax on a damp cloth

Ink

Cream of tartar and drops of lemon juice. Rub, then brush off powder. Sponge
with warm water. Repeat if needed.

Mold

Soak in vinegar[a], then rinse in a baking soda and water solution. Rinse with
water only, absorb, and quickly dry with a heater or fan.

Tea: Use boiling water.

Urine
Sponge the area with baking soda and water. Rinse with warm water, then shampoo carpet as usual.

Sponge vinegar[n] onto carpet and absorb excess moisture

Wine stains: Club soda

CARPET SEALANTS
AFM SafeChoice Carpet Guard & Lock Out: AEHF, Allergy Relief Shop, The Living Source, NEEDS

CARPET ODOR ABSORBERS
Borax or baking soda (sprinkle dry on carpet – do not walk on carpet after application – vacuum with HEPA or water filter)

Ozonator (use only as directed – run 2-4 hours, then air 8 hours before entering room) – Eliminates volatile hydrocarbons: AEHF, NEEDS

CLEANING SERVICES
Texas Power Vac (Carpet and Air Duct Cleaning)

DUST MITE CONTROL
Allersearch X-MITE & ADS[n]: Allergy Relief Store, Allerx

Dr. Bronner's Liquid Eucalyptus Soap (kills dust mites)

Ecology Works Dust Mite Control[n]: Allergy Relief Shop

Steam clean with tannic acid to remove dust mites ($\frac{1}{2}$-$\frac{3}{4}$ tsp. in 2 quarts water): Abrams Royal Pharmacy

> > < <

Vacuum Cleaners

IS YOUR VACUUM YOUR FRIEND?
Do you clean it regularly?
Do you displace mites and mite feces regularly?
or Do you capture and destroy the Mighty Mite?
A good vacuum with a HEPA filter
removes particulates from floor, air and furnishings

YOU SHOULD AVOID
Cleaners that do not eliminate dust and dust mites.

LESS-TOXIC ALTERNATIVES
Amway – distributor

Euroclean (HEPA): Gazoontite

Filter Queen

Galaxie Central Vacuum System

Miele: Absolute Environmental's, Sinan Corp.

Nilfisk (with HEPA filter): Nilfisk, Allergy Relief Store, The Living Source, National Allergy Supply, Natural Solutions Environmental, Nigra Enterprises, Real Goods

Phantom (HEPA)

Rainbow (water trap system): various local distributors

Thermax (water trap with 2nd stage disposable electrostatic filter): Allergy Relief Shop, and various local distributors

Vita-Vac Vacuum Cleaner (14-layer cellulose bag plus activated charcoal and HEPA filters): Vita-Mix Corp.

> > < <

VACUUM BAGS/FILTERS

YOU SHOULD AVOID

The use of standard bag systems is not generally recommended.

LESS-TOXIC ALTERNATIVES

If it is necessary to use standard bag systems, we recommend the use of specially prepared paper bags and vinyl or rubber lined outer bags.

Micro Clean vacuum bags and filters (may be used with various vacuum types)[a]: Allergy Control Products, Allergy Relief Store, Priorities

Thermax bags and filters: Allergy Relief Shop

> > < <

Window Cleaners

YOU SHOULD AVOID

Commercial products which may contain ammonia, butyl cellosolve, alcohol, naphtha, glycol ethers

LESS-TOXIC ALTERNATIVES

AFM SafeChoice Glass Cleaner: AEHF, Allergy Relief Shop, The Living Source, Nirvana Safe Haven

Allen's Naturally Non-Toxic Glass Cleaner: Allergy Relief Shop, Janice's, NEEDS

Baking soda

Bioshield Glass Cleaner: Eco Design

Bon Ami Cake Soap

Earth Friendly Window Cleaner

HomeFree Window Cleaner[a]: Allergy-Asthma Tech.

Mix 2 Tbsps. borax or baking soda in three cups of water.

Mix ¼ cup vinegar[a] or lemon juice to a quart of water

Mix 1 tsp. Sodium Hexametaphosphate (unscented Calgon) and 1 drop liquid soap in warm water in a spray bottle

Natural Chemistry Glass Cleaner: Allergy Relief Shop

Nature Clean Window and Glass Cleaner: AEHF, The Living Source

Organica Window and Glass Cleaner: AEHF

Zephiran (Benzalkonium) Chloride 17%[a] (use only as directed) – 1 part to 10 parts water: Abrams Royal Pharmacy (prescription required)

> > < <

Special Cleanups

Certain cleaning projects require special procedures for the environmentally sensitive and health conscious. The following suggestions are for those special situations. *See also Special Stain Removal and Carpet Stain Removers.*

EuroSteam is a portable, hot, dry steam cleaner and sanitizer for all types of cleaning and disinfecting situations on all surfaces even penetrating cracks and crevices. It is chemical free, and will safely remove mold and mildew, wax buildup, adhesive residue, dried-on food, pesticides, oil and even burned-on grease plus everyday dirt and grime.

ADHESIVE

For removing adhesive labels/decals – soak in white vinegar[□]
CitraSolv: GAIAM, Harmony, Real Goods, Whole Foods

CRAWL SPACES

For cleaning up pesticides and mold in vent spaces under the house: Remove contaminated soil if possible; then cover the ground with 6 mm. black plastic; then 3 inches sand or gravel or 1 to 2 inches Portland cement; then sprinkle with water to form crust.
Use circulating air (may use push-pull fans) and ultraviolet light
For odor problems in crawl space use Bac-Azap[□]: Nisus Corp
Zephiran (Benzalkonium) Chloride 17%[□] *(use only as directed)* – 1 part to 10 parts water: Abrams Royal Pharmacy *(prescription required)*
Water must not be allowed to stand under house. Use gutter, drains or terracing to deflect water from house.

MOLDS

Borax & Vinegar: Use 1 tsp. borax and 3 Tbsp. vinegar[□] or lemon juice.
Enviro-Magic Mildew Stain Away: AEHF
Grapefruit seed extract
Ozonator (use only as directed – run 2-4 hours, then air 8 hours before entering room) – Eliminates volatile hydrocarbons: AEHF, NEEDS
Seal concrete walls in basement with a safe concrete sealer, and use dehumidifiers to prevent mold growth
Zephiran (Benzalkonium) Chloride 17%[□] *(use only as directed)* – 1 part to 10 parts water: Abrams Royal Pharmacy *(prescription required)*
If there is extensive water damage, remove and discard damaged sheetrock, wood, ceiling tiles, etc. which may contain mold.
Mold exposure can cause disease, allergies and can be life threatening. Identify mold. Expert removal may be required.
(See also Mold Inhibitors above)

OILS

Make paste of ¼ cup washing soda and ¼ cup baking soda. Let dry, then remove.
AFM Super Clean: AEHF, Allergy Relief Shop, The Living Source, NEEDS

CitraSolv: GAIAM, Harmony, Real Goods, Whole Foods
Mela Magic
Nature's Key Spot & Stain Remover: Dasun
Pure Solvent: Healthy Kleaner, Greenspan
Trisodium Phosphate

PERFUME

AFM Super Clean: AEHF, Allergy Relief Shop, The Living Source, NEEDS
Mustard paste – Mix enough water with 3 tsp. of dry mustard to form a paste.
    Rub on and allow to dry, then wash off with water.

PESTICIDES

Chlorox$^\square$ and water
Ozonator (use only as directed – run 2-4 hours, then air 8 hours before entering
    room) – Eliminates volatile hydrocarbons: AEHF, NEEDS
Soap and water
Discard item if it cannot be cleaned or has had direct pesticide contact.
See also instructions above for cleaning crawl spaces.

PORCELAIN STAINS

Baking soda

REFRIGERATORS & FREEZERS

Place an open container of baking soda in the refrigerator/freezer wash with
    baking soda in warm water when defrosting or cleaning unit.
Zeolite Refresh-A-Frig: Dasun, Earth Friendly Products, Real Goods

SKUNK ODOR

Bac-A-Zap$^\square$: Nisus Corp.
Saturate person, pet or material that has been sprayed with ordinary tomato
    juice; wash and repeat if necessary.

Household cleaning can add luster to your home.
Careful selection can add luster to your blood cells.

> > < <

Clothing & Accessories

Clothing

YOU SHOULD AVOID

Clothes that may contain formaldehyde designated as permanent press, crease
    resistant and flame retardant; chlorine bleach; or azo or aniline dyes that
    may affect anemia or a decrease in peripheral oxygen supply.
Fabrics treated with polyethylene glycol (PEG) increase wearer comfort by
    absorbing heat under cold temperatures and releasing heat in warm
    temperatures. Non-wrinkle cottons are being developed by treating the
    fabric with quaternary ammonium salts of triethanolamine derivatives.

Less-Toxic Alternatives

Although these three chemicals are not highly toxic, they can cause contact dermatitis in sensitive individuals. (Hank Becker & Bruce Kinzel in Agricultural Research, Jan.-Feb. 1991.)

Exposure to certain dyes and chemicals in fabrics can result in rashes, itching and asthma. If more naturally colored fibers were used, many toxic chemicals associated with the dying process would not be needed including sodium dichromate, pyridine, ethyl acetate, methanol, acetone, cyclohexanone, chlorinated hydrocarbons, formaldehyde, and pine oil. This would reduce exposure of workers to toxic chemical and provide healthier, more comfortable clothing.

LESS-TOXIC ALTERNATIVES
AEHF (organic cotton socks, t-shirts, shorts for adults)
A Happy Planet (men, women, children and infants – organic cotton and hemp)
Alternative Undies (men's & women's underwear – organic cotton, silk and hemp)
B.Coole Designs (all ages)
Bauer, Eddie
Blue Canoe (women's underwear and casual wear – organic cotton)
Canary Fashions
Decent Exposures (cotton undergarments for women and children)
Deva Lifewear (men's and women's green and organic cotton, wool and silk clothing, undergarments)
Diamond Organics (organic cotton for women and babies)
Earthlings (organic cotton clothing for children and infants)
Earth Speaks
Eco-Baby (infants to adults)
Eco-Organics (hemp and organic cotton clothing for men and women)
Ecosport (men, women, unisex and baby clothes)
Ethical Shopper (infants to adults)
Fair Trade Naturals
Feeling Goods (infants to adults)
GAIAM
Grass Roots Natural Goods
Green Babies (infants and young children)
Green iDeals
Green Marketplace (adults, children and babies)
Greenpeace (adults, children and babies)
Harmony
Heart of Vermont
Island Hemp Wear (hemp and organic cotton clothing for children and adults)
James River Traders
JAMS (children's organic clothing)
Janice's (men's and women's underwear, socks, sleepwear, casual wear)
Land's End

Maggie's Organic Products (available from Ethical Shopper)
My Favorite Planet
Natural Lifestyle (organic cotton underwear, socks, casual wear)
Organic Threads
Oskri Organics (adults and babies)
Patagonia (sportswear for all ages – outdoor wear)
Real Goods (organic cotton)
Royal Silks
SOS from Texas (organic cotton sportswear / t-shirts)
Thai Silk
Thirteen Mile Lamb & Wool
Tomorrow's World
Under the Canopy (Organic cotton, wool, hemp women's clothing)
Vermont Country Store (natural fabric clothing for adults)
Whole Foods
WinterSilks (clothing, undergarments for men and women)
Costumes/Period Clothing: B.Coole Designs

WASHING METHOD FOR NEW CLOTHES

All clothes must be washed prior to being worn to remove the contaminants of the manufacturing process. Any or all of the following methods can be used or repeated.

#1: Put 1 cup powdered milk in washer. Fill with water and agitate a few minutes to dissolve milk. Add clothing. Soak 2-3 hours. Spin.

#2: Put ½ to 1 cup AFM Super Clean (AEHF & The Living Source) in washer. Fill and agitate a few minutes to blend. Add clothes. Soak over night. Spin.

#3: Put 1 cup vinegar[n] or ¼ cup sodium hexametaphosphate (The Living Source) in water. Fill and agitate to blend. Add clothes. Soak 12-24 hours. Spin. Then rinse with ¼ cup baking soda.

THE WASH OF LAST RESORT

If soaking your clothes for several days in white vinegar[n] or overnight in water with a box full of powdered milk does not achieve desired results, you can try this method. It will remove natural cotton oil odor and certain organophosphate pesticide residues, but not herbicides. Do colored clothes one color at a time.

Put a drop of water on new cotton clothing – if it beads up or doesn't soak right in immediately, return it because it has too much formaldehyde and chemical finish which is not water soluble. Even this method will not work. If the water soaked in, proceed.

• Add 2 cups chlorine bleach to a full, agitating washer with your clothes in it. (Warning: it is best to have someone who is not environmentally sensitive do this for you or hold your breath and run outside – be sure to pause a moment before you inhale because the bleach fumes have clung to the clothes you're wearing.)

Less-Toxic Alternatives

- Do a full wash cycle, but do not remove from washer. Be sure they have rinsed thoroughly in plain water. If your washer has a second rinse cycle, use it; or manually set if for a second rinse. You must rinse out all the bleach before proceeding to the next step because bleach and ammonia would combine to make a deadly chlorine gas.
- Neutralize the residual bleach by doing a full wash cycle with 1 cup clear ammonia (with no perfume) or "sudsy ammonia" (which contains a surfactant). Add this after the washer is full and agitating.
- Do a full wash cycle, but do not remove from washer. Now do a third wash cycle with one pound of baking soda. After this cycle is completed you can remove clothes from washer.
- Dry well, then dry an additional 30-50 minutes at high heat to remove residual ammonia. Heat is critical at this step.
- Wash and dry repeatedly (2 to 8 times) until you can tolerate the clothing. This is hard on clothes, but it is only done once. After a couple of washings you can usually wash them with your other clothes.

NOTE: This washing method also works for natural silks, which are all fumigated by law, but will often turn them gold in color. It is not reliable for previously perfumed or fabric softened clothes.

PRESSURE COOKER METHOD:
This recently discovered method was reported to Share, Care and Prayer:

Clothes of certain materials can be cooked in a pressure cooker at a temperature in excess of 300 degrees. This allows chemicals whose boiling points exceed those of water to volatilize and escape to outside air. This should be done outside to avoid contamination of indoor air.

Your clothes should protect and reflect your beauty.

> > < <

Miscellaneous Accessories

LESS-TOXIC ALTERNATIVES
Backpack, Bookbags, Travel Bags: A Happy Planet, Eco-Organics, Grass Roots Natural Goods
Belts: B.Coole Designs, Deva Lifewear
Canvas & Hemp Bags: B.Coole Designs, Grass Roots Natural Goods
Fanny Pack: Feeling Goods
Gloves: AEHF, B.Coole Designs, Ethical Shopper, Janice's, Vermont Country Store (white cotton gloves for men and women)
Handkerchiefs: The Living Source, Real Goods, Thai Silk
Hats & Hair Accessories: B.Coole Designs, Deva Lifewear, Ethical Shopper (men, women and children), Grass Roots Natural Goods
Luggage: cotton, hemp or leather: Grass Roots Natural Goods
Purses: Deva Lifewear, Ethical Shopper, Thai Silk, Under the Canopy
Silk & Cotton Scarves: B.Coole Designs, Thai Silk, Under the Canopy

Silk Neckties: Thai Silk
Wallets: A Happy Planet, Eco-Organics, Ethical Shopper, Grass Roots Natural
  Goods

> > < <

Shoes, Boots, etc.

YOU SHOULD AVOID
Most commercial shoes, boots, purses and luggage contain acrylic, vinyl
  chloride, formaldehyde and/or hexane in glues and tanning process.

LESS-TOXIC ALTERNATIVES
Shoes need to be individually selected. Due to construction, any may be
  intolerable to the very sensitive.
Shoes: Cordwainers, Grass Roots Natural Goods, Heart of Vermont, Janice's
  (slippers), Swedish Clogs, Inc., Under the Canopy (only some of their
  shoes are non-toxic)
Hemp Shoestrings: Island Hemp Wear

> > < <

SHOE & LEATHER CARE

YOU SHOULD AVOID
All synthetic, odoriferous polish preparations which may contain 1,1,1-
  Trichloroethane

LESS-TOXIC ALTERNATIVES
Olive, herbal, lanolin or nut-derived oil (use with chamois, then shine)
Rotate shoes regularly to give them a chance to air
Sprinkle baking soda in shoes to keep them fresh and odor free
Odor Eliminator for Shoes: The Living Source

WATERPROOFING
Pecard leather waterproofing products: Pecard Chemical Co.

LEATHER CLEANERS / POLISH
¾ cup vinegar" + ¼ cup food grade Linseed Oil – rub in leather
¼ cup lanolin + ¼ cup food grade Linseed Oil – blend & rub in
Saddle Soap or mild soap
Zeolite Boot & Foot Powder: Absolute Environmental's

> > < <

Food & Water

What we eat and drink dictates what we are.
Choices to be made require thoughtful consideration.

Food Contamination

Food can contain more than vitamins and minerals.
Less-chemically contaminated food, cooked with bottled or filtered water,
in glass, iron, or steel utensils on an electric cooktop
is the recommended procedure for proper health maintenance.

YOU SHOULD AVOID

Hormone and antibiotic fed beef that can interfere with your own hormones
and immunity.

Arsenic in chicken feed.

Pesticide sprayed fruits and vegetables that are neurogenic and carcinogenic
such as DDT and Dioxin.

Foreign produce may contain chlorinated hydrocarbons which are fat stored.
(DDT, an insecticide still used in food production in some foreign countries,
enhances the effect of estrogen on the body, thereby increasing cancer
risk.)

Seafoods that may contain surprise ingredients such as heavy metals

Phenol lined cans and welded seam cans (seam is flat with a thin, dark, sharply
defined line along the joint. Soldered seams are crimped with a smear of
silver-grey metal on the outside of the seam and have lower lead levels.
Cans with plastic lacquer inner coating leach a toxic compound (bisphenol-
A) into foods and liquids – it is an estrogenic compound, and it disrupts
hormonal activity.

LESS-TOXIC ALTERNATIVES

Organically grown foods are available at many health food and specialty stores
and on the internet (see Organic Food Sources in Resources Directory).

FRUIT & VEGETABLE WASH

Allen's Naturally Fruit & Veggie Wash: Allergy Relief Shop, Janice's, NEEDS
Clean Greens: Allergy Relief Shop
Earth Friendly Fruit & Veggie Wash
Edcor
Fit²: local grocery stores
Grapefruit Seed Extract
Hydrogen Peroxide

ALUMINUM-FREE BAKING POWDER

Mix 3 parts baking soda to 3 parts rice, corn, potato or arrowroot flour, and 2
parts cream of tartar. If using the mixture immediately, you can eliminate
the starch and mix ¼ tsp. of baking soda to ½ tsp. cream of tartar.
Rumford Baking Powder

CONCENTRATED LIQUID SWEETENER
Boil 8 cups organic juice until reduced to two cups. Cool and freeze. To use, warm a knife under hot water and cut out the amount of frozen juice needed, returning remainder to freezer.

> > < <

Food Preparation
Food preparation can cook more than your goose.
It can add significant pollutants to kitchen air.

YOU SHOULD AVOID
Charcoal grills, gas cooktops, gas grills, halogen cooking surfaces. Avoid cooking with wood chips – smoking meats with Mesquite wood introduces the most polycyclic aromatic hydrocarbons (carcinogenic) into the food.

Cooking utensils can add more than heat and palatability to foods. Avoid plastic or Teflon-coated cooking utensils, plastic storage containers (not safe in microwave) and aluminum pots/pans

Also avoid other sources of aluminum: Antacids (see alternatives below), baking powder, bleached flour, city water supplies, antiperspirants and deodorants, processed cheese, table salt, soft drink cans. Aluminum is also frequently used in strengthening materials used in dental crowns. Aluminum has an affinity for the brain and parathyroid.

Antacid Alternatives: Tums, Riopan and Tri-Salts.

LESS-TOXIC ALTERNATIVES
Champion Juicer: The Living Source
Cotton coffee filters: Environmentally Sound Products, Tomorrow's World
Hemp coffee filters: A Happy Planet, Grass Roots Natural Goods
Stainless Steel Dish Drain: Natural Lifestyle
Stainless steel kitchenware: Diamond Organic, Natural Lifestyle, also available in many local stores
Stainless steel toaster
Vita Mix food processors: Vita-Mix Corp.
Wood dish rack: Real Goods
Wood utensils: Diamond Organic, many local stores
Exhaust ventilation (through the roof or to the outdoors)

COOKING APPLIANCES
Corning Ware Cooktops
Electric cooktops and grills
GE Induction Cooktops
JennAir
Sun Oven: Abundant Earth, Real Goods, Tomorrow's World
Solar Cooker: Real Goods

COOKING UTENSILS
Baked enamel or porcelain

Cast iron

Corning Ware

Corning Visions Cookware (available direct from the factory with non-stick coating)

NEOVA Waterless Cookware (stainless steel): Vita-Mix Corp.

Stainless steel cookware/bakeware: Natural Lifestyle, local stores

REFRIGERATORS & FREEZERS

Sun Frost refrigerators and freezers: Abundant Earth, Sun Frost

Vestfrost Refrigerator and Freezer (CFC free): Tomorrow's World

Whirlpool (CFC free)

A NOTE ABOUT FOOD PREPARATION: It is best to steam, stir-fry, microwave (preserves the most nutrients), bake, broil (flame above does not introduce polycyclic aromatic hydrocarbons), or fry in an acceptable oil (olive and canola have the lowest trans-fatty acids) - this is best for meats.

WARNING: PLASTIC & MICROWAVES DON'T MIX: Never thaw frozen meat product in its original packaging, such as foam trays and plastic wraps. Styrene and PVC (i.e.: margarine tubs, cottage cheese cartons, whipped topping bowls) should never be used for cooking in a microwave. They are not heat-stable and can melt or warp, thereby allowing harmful chemicals to migrate into foods. Likewise, plastic wrap should never directly touch food in a microwave.

> > < <

Food Storage

It is important where and in what you store food.

YOU SHOULD AVOID

Aluminum foil, plastic food wraps, plastic icebox dishes, plastic sandwich bags, waxed paper

LESS-TOXIC ALTERNATIVES

Cellulose bags (derived from cell walls of plants): Allergy Relief Shop, Environmentally Sound Products, Janice's, The Living Source, Natural Lifestyle, NEEDS

Cellophane (wood derived cellulose)

Cheesecloth (100% organic cotton): Natural Lifestyle

Cotton muslin re-usable lunch bag: Eco-Bags

Glass jars

Mesh, cotton canvas, string, hemp and muslin produce and shopping bags: Abundant Earth, The Cloth Bag Co., Eco-Bags, Eco-Organics, Ethical Shopper, Environmentally Sound Products, Janice's, The Living Source, Tomorrow's World

Organic Cotton Vegetable Crisper Bag: Janice's

Stainless Steel or Glass Vacuum Bottles: A.K. Das, Natural Lifestyle, The Thermos Co.

Vacuum bottles should be periodically cleaned with baking soda and warm water or vinegar and water. Let sit 15 minutes, then wash in warm water and a tolerated detergent.

Wood toothpicks: Diamond Brand Inc., Marquis Dental Mfg.

Do not be a toxic chemical dump!

> > < <

Drinking Water Filtration

YOU SHOULD AVOID

Unfiltered tap water and well water that may contain contaminants and various chemicals.

LESS-TOXIC ALTERNATIVES

Filtered water – provided the filter housing is metal, preferably stainless steel, and filtration media is compressed activated charcoal, charcoal with ceramic, or reverse osmosis with charcoal. Use no silver or plastic in filtration media.

Cold water filtration structure matrix: Pure Water Place

Doulton steel case – ceramic/activated carbon filters: AEHF, Naturally Pure Products, NEEDS

First Need – Activated Charcoal Portable Unit for Campers

Garden hose filter: Abundant Earth, Lifekind Products, The Living Source, Tomorrow's World

Glass-bottled spring water (check the location of the spring)

Gravity Water Filter (ceramic and charcoal filters): Lifekind Products

Icemaker Filters: Abundant Earth, The Living Source

Mariner Stainless Steel Travel Water Filter

Portable/travel filters: AEHF

Portable reverse osmosis filter: Tomorrow's World

Pure 'n Simple: Dasun

Reverse Osmosis plus Charcoal Filter: AEHF, Allergy Relief Shop, Dasun

Reverse Osmosis: Naturally Pure Products

Shower Filters: Abundant Earth, AEHF, Allergy Relief Shop, Dasun, Environmentally Sound Products, E. L. Foust, Lifekind Products, The Living Source, Naturally Pure Products, NEEDS, Pure n Natural, Tomorrow's World

Stainless Steel Charcoal Water Purifiers: AEHF (Aqua Clear), Culligan, Cuno, Everpure, Nontoxic Environments, RH of Texas, Pure Water Place (Structure Matrix)

Stainless Steel Carbon Block (.09 micron): Multi-Pure - Natural Lifestyle

Travel Water Filter: Abundant Earth, Allergy Relief Shop, The Living Source

Water Distiller: AEHF, Scientific Glass, Nigra Enterprises

WaterSense: Dasun

Whole-house filtration systems: AEHF, Allergy Relief Shop
Water purifiers (several types): Nirvana Safe Haven
(Combination systems can also be created by AEHF)
See Water in Part II for a comparison between water filtration systems.
Be selective with your liquid source.

> > < <

Household Goods

The beds in which you sleep, the clothing you wear on your body,
and the materials with which you work
all contribute to your general state of health!
Choose wisely and travel the less-toxic road.
Prevent cellular damage.

> > < <

Mattresses & Intersprings

YOU SHOULD AVOID
All featherbeds, foam mattresses, waterbeds, and most conventional mattresses.

LESS-TOXIC ALTERNATIVES
Organically grown materials that do not include chemical flame-retardants and pesticides – these usually require a physician's prescription. Choose your mattress carefully – no item is tolerated by everyone. If possible, mattresses should be washable. All components should be washed prior to mattress creation.

COTTON MATTRESS & BOX SPRING SETS
A Happy Planet, Abundant Earth, Allergy Relief Shop, Chemically Sensitive Living, Furnature, Janice's, NEEDS

COTTON/WOOL[□] INNERSPRING & BOX SPRING SETS
A Happy Planet, Chemically Sensitive Living, Crown Mattress, Heart of Vermont, Lifekind Products, NEEDS, Tomorrow's World

COTTON MATTRESSES / FUTONS
Abundant Earth, Allergy Relief Shop, Chemically Sensitive Living, Crown City Mattress, Heart of Vermont, Lifekind Products, Nirvana Safe Haven, Organic Cotton Alternatives, Superior Mattress, Tomorrow's World, White Lotus, Palmer Bedding[□] (cotton and canvas / not organic but chemical free)

COTTON EXERCISE/YOGA MAT
GAIAM, Harmony, Janice's, Lifekind Products, Organic Cotton Alternatives, Tomorrow's World, White Lotus (Stowaway)

NATURAL MATTRESSES
Hemp: Tomorrow's World   Wool: Heart of Vermont

WOOL□ MATTRESS TOPPER
White Lotus

METAL SPRINGS WITH COTTON BLANKETS OR PADS
Capitol City Springs

METAL BED FRAMES
Chambers, Garnet Hill, Land's End

WOOD BED FRAMES
Chambers, Eco Baby, Garnet Hill, Heart of Vermont, Land's End, Nirvana
Safe Haven, Tomorrow's World, White Lotus

> > < <

Pillows

YOU SHOULD AVOID
All feather and foam pillows.

LESS-TOXIC ALTERNATIVES

NATURAL COTTON AND / OR WOOL□
Abundant Earth, AEHF, A Happy Planet, Allergy Relief Shop, Allergy Relief
Stores, Chemically Sensitive Living, Eco Baby, Gazoontite, Healthy
Environments, Heart of Vermont, Janice's, K.B. Cotton Pillows, Lifekind
Products, The Living Source, NEEDS, Priorities, Shepherd's Dream,
Tomorrow's World, White Lotus

COTTON SOFA / THROW PILLOWS
Chemically Sensitive Living, Fair Trade Naturals, Grass Roots Natural Goods
(hemp), Honeysuckle Dreams, Janice's

COTTON EYE PILLOWS□
Abundant Earth, Honeysuckle Dreams

ORTHOPEDIC PILLOWS / NECK PILLOWS
Abundant Earth, Janice's, NEEDS, Shepherd's Dream (wool)

> > < <

Sheets, Blankets, etc.

YOU SHOULD AVOID
All formaldehyde and petrochemicals in treated fabrics
Possible EMF exposure in electric blankets

LESS-TOXIC ALTERNATIVES
Most of us spend about a third of our life in bed; therefore our beds and
bedrooms should be the healthiest place possible – a sanctuary that is free

of chemicals; a place to heal, recuperate and sleep in peace. For better health, we should consider replacing synthetic fibers with organic fibers that have not been treated with pesticides or chemicals.

Wool[a] is naturally flame-retardant and can absorb large amounts of moisture under all sleeping conditions. Scientists have found that, compared to polyester comforters, the heart rate under wool-filled comforters was significantly lower 100% of the time.

For those allergic to wool, organic cotton is the next best choice, and it is usually somewhat cheaper than wool.

COTTON SHEETS & PILLOWCASES

A Happy Planet, Abundant Earth, AEHF, Allergy-Asthma Tech. (Simple: chemical free 100% cotton), Allergy Relief Shop, Chemically Sensitive Living, Coyuchi Inc., Eco Baby (all sizes), Fieldcrest Cannon, GAIAM, Gazoontite, Grass Roots Natural Goods, Harmony, Janice's, J. P. Stevens, Lifekind Products, The Living Source, Natural Lifestyle, Nirvana Safe Haven, Priorities, Real Goods, Tomorrow's World, Wamsutta Pacific

COTTON FLANNEL SHEETS

A Happy Planet, Abundant Earth, Eddie Bauer, Chambers, Heart of Vermont, Lifekind Products

COTTON KNIT (JERSEY) SHEETS & PILLOWCASES

A Happy Planet, Abundant Earth, Feeling Goods, Harmony, Janice's, Tomorrow's World

BARRIER CLOTH SHEETS

Eco Baby, Janice's

SILK SHEETS & PILLOWCASES

Gazoontite

BLANKETS

COTTON OR WOOL[a]: A Happy Planet, Abundant Earth, AEHF, Allergy Relief Shop, B.Coole Designs, Eco Baby, GAIAM, Gazoontite, Harmony, Heart of Vermont, Janice's, Lifekind Products, The Living Source, Oskri Organics, Real Goods, Shepherd's Dream / SILK[a]: Chambers, Garnet Hill

COTTON OR WOOL[a] COMFORTERS, QUILTS & SPREADS

A Happy Planet, Chemically Sensitive Living, Eco Baby, GAIAM, Gazoontite, Harmony, Heart of Vermont, Janice's, Lifekind Products, NEEDS, Nirvana Safe Haven, Shepherd's Dream, Tomorrow's World

COTTON &/OR WOOL[a] FUTON COVERS

Abundant Earth, Heart of Vermont

COTTON DUVET & COMFORTER COVERS

A Happy Planet, Abundant Earth, Allergy Relief Shop, Coyuchi Inc., Lifekind Products

SLEEPING BAGS / SLEEPSACKS
Janice's, The Natural Bedroom

ACTIVATED CHARCOAL BLANKET
Nirvana Safe Haven (absorbs odors and chemical fumes)

For Baby Bedding see Baby Needs Section.

> > < <

Mattress Cases, Covers & Pads

YOU SHOULD AVOID
Plastic and vinyl coverings

LESS-TOXIC ALTERNATIVES
Barrier cloth (to control dust and dust mites), cotton or wool mattress pads.

MATTRESS, BOXSPRING & PILLOW COVERS/CASES
AEHF, A Happy Planet, Allerx, Chemically Sensitive Living (barrier cloth), Eco Baby, GAIAM, Harmony, Heart of Vermont, Janice's, Lifekind Products, The Living Source, NEEDS

MATTRESS PADS
COTTON OR WOOL[□]: AEHF, A Happy Planet, Allergy Relief Shop, Eco Baby, GAIAM, Harmony, Heart of Vermont, Lifekind Products, Nirvana Safe Haven, Shepherd's Dream, Tomorrow's World; SILK[□]: Chambers

WOOL[□] MATTRESS TOPPERS
A Happy Planet, Eco Baby, GAIAM, Harmony, Lifekind Products, Nirvana Safe Haven, Tomorrow's World, White Lotus

BARRIER CLOTH FABRIC
(By the Yard) AEHF, Heart of Vermont, Janice's, Natural Guard, The Living Source (SafBarrier)

> > < <

Bathroom & Kitchen Linens & Supplies

YOU SHOULD AVOID
Plastic and vinyl shower curtains; dyes in linens; and dyes, perfumes and skin conditioners in facial and toilet tissues.

LESS-TOXIC ALTERNATIVES

BATH ACCESSORIES
Chambers (Metal and Glass), GAIAM, Harmony, Simmons Natural Body Care (Bamboo Soap Rack and Sisal-Ramie Soap Sack)

BATH BRUSHES & SCRUBBERS
Simmons Natural Body Care (Natural Bristle Brushes)

BATH SPONGES / LOOFAHS (Natural Sponges)
Allergy Relief Shop, Eco Organics, GAIAM, Harmony, Simmons Natural Body Care, Whole Foods

BATH TOWELS & WASH CLOTHS
COTTON: AEHF, A Happy Planet, Allergy Relief Shop, Chemically Sensitive Living, Eco Baby, Fair Trade Naturals, Feeling Goods, GAIAM, Gazoontite, Harmony, Heart of Vermont, Janice's, Lifekind Products, The Natural Bedroom, Oskri Organics, Priorities, Simmons Natural Body Care (washcloths), Tomorrow's World

SHOWER CAPS – BARRIER CLOTH
Janice's, The Living Source

SHOWER CURTAINS
COTTON: Abundant Earth, Abundant Earth, AEHF, Allergy Relief Shop, Environmentally Sound Products, GAIAM, Harmony, Heart of Vermont, Janice's, Lifekind Products, NEEDS, NOPE (White or Natural), and Tomorrow's World
HEMP: Abundant Earth, Feeling Goods, Grass Roots Natural Goods, Real Goods, Tomorrow's World
Brass shower roller rings: GAIAM, Harmony

FACIAL & TOILET TISSUES
Dye and perfume-free products
Seventh Generation: GAIAM, Harmony, Real Goods, Whole Foods

KITCHEN LINENS
Organic cotton kitchen towels, dishcloths, napkins, potholders, aprons, etc.: Fair Trade Naturals, Janice's, Lifekind Products, The Living Source
Natural hemp kitchen towels, napkins, and potholders: A Happy Planet, Abundant Earth, GAIAM, Harmony
Natural hemp placemats and tablecloth: A Happy Planet, Grass Roots Natural Goods

> > < <

Curtains & Draperies

YOU SHOULD AVOID
Heavy fabrics that must be dry-cleaned or are vinyl backed.

LESS-TOXIC ALTERNATIVES
All curtains and blinds must be washed, dusted or aired regularly to prevent dust accumulation.
Mini-blinds
Washable cotton curtains: Fair Trade Naturals

> > < <

Furniture

YOU SHOULD AVOID
Overstuffed furniture, furniture with particleboard or plywood, toxic stains and varnishes, lead-based or petroleum-based paints.

LESS-TOXIC ALTERNATIVES

PURE WOOD FURNITURE
Abundant Earth, Eagle Cabinets & Construction, Eco Baby (infant to adult), Feeling Goods, Golden Furniture Maker, Heart of Vermont, Ilami Furniture Gallery, Land's End, Nirvana Safe Haven (Pacific Rim unfinished maple), White Lotus (Pacific Rim, Norka, and Vermont Mission)

CEDAR OUTDOOR FURNITURE
Lifekind Products (unfinished)

METAL, GLASS & MARBLE FURNITURE
Land's End, San Miguel de Allende, Inc.

NATURAL COTTON OR HEMP FURNITURE SLIPCOVERS
Fair Trade Naturals, GAIAM, Harmony, Tomorrow's World

HEMP HAMMOCK
Abundant Earth

UPHOLSTERED FURNITURE
Organic cotton on maple frames with steel innersprings – no synthetic foams, polys or formaldehyde: Furnature
Less-toxic replacement cushions for existing furniture: Furnature

NOTE ABOUT PIANO CARE: Ask piano tuner to avoid cleaning your piano with naphtha, and avoid pesticide application on felt pads. Lacquer is also toxic. Dust piano with a clean cloth or a less-toxic furniture polish. Avoid replacing felts with new ones until absolutely necessary.

> > < <

Fabrics & Sewing Supplies

YOU SHOULD AVOID
Commercial fabrics in draperies and upholstery that can contain formaldehyde in Scotchguard or wrinkle-resistant treatment
Synthetic fabrics used in clothing and household goods
Cotton contaminated with pesticides, etc. including the following Methyl Parathion, Trifluralin, Cyanazine, Tribufos (DEF or Folex), Dioxin, and heavy metals such as chromium and copper

LESS-TOXIC ALTERNATIVES
BARRIER CLOTH: (see page 160)
FABRIC DYES: Allegro Natural Dyes

NATURALLY GROWN COLORED, ORGANIC COTTON
Fox Fiber

NATURALLY TANNED LEATHERS
Bison Specialties (Brain Tanned Hides / Vegetable Tanned Soles)

ORGANIC COTTON or WOOL[a]
Cotton Plus, Crocodile Tiers (curtains, fabrics, linens, etc.), Eco Baby, Ecosport, Heart of Vermont (cotton and wool[a]), Janice's, The Living Source (cotton), Thirteen Mile Lamb & Wool

ORGANIC COTTON OR WOOL[a] BATTING
Heart of Vermont (both), The Living Source (cotton)

SEWING NOTIONS: Janice's

WOOL YARN
Thirteen Mile Lamb & Wool

> > < <

Home Safety

LESS-TOXIC ALTERNATIVES

SAFETY MONITORS (Carbon Monoxide, EMF, Smoke)
Carbon Monoxide Monitor/Detector (if you heat your home or water with gas): Allergy Relief Shop, Environmentally Sound Products, Real Goods

Carbon Monoxide Monitor Tester (checks monitor's efficiency): Environmentally Sound Products

Carbon Monoxide Test Kit – Heads Up: Abundant Earth, AEHF

Cellular Phone Sensor (Detects RF radiation & EMF): Allergy Relief Shop

Christmas Tree Fire Alarm: Environmentally Sound Products

Electro Sensor (EMF) – Sonic Technology: AEHF, Environmentally Sound Products

EMF Meter and Tri-Field Meter

EMF Regulator: Quantum Life (transforms electrical fields into a soothing, coherent wave): NEEDS

Gaussmeter (rental – detects ELF): Magshield

Microwave Oven Test Kit – Heads Up: AEHF, Allergy Relief Shop

Portable Solar Panel: Real Goods, Tomorrows World

Safe Digital ELF/VLF Meter (EMF)

Solar Smoke Alarm: Real Goods

Suncatcher Solar Chargers: PowerQuest, Real Goods
(See additional test kits in Resources Section)

FIRE SAFETY
Use baking soda and/or a lid to smother kitchen grease fires

Fire Cap Fire Extinguishers: Allergy Relief Shop

Planned escape route: family should decide in advance, practice, and post a planned route of escape and an outside meeting place in case of fire,

OTHER SAFETY PRECAUTIONS

All medications should be stored out of the reach of children.

All chemical products should be stored out of the living area and out of children's reach.

> > < <

Miscellaneous Household Goods

AUTO BATTERY CORROSION REMOVER
Baking soda and water

AUTO SEAT COVERS
Abundant Earth (Hemp)

EMERGENCY MEDICAL BRACELETS
Medic Alert

GIFT BASKETS
EcoExpress

HEALTH SIGNS (About Chemical Sensitivity)
Dixie Peterson, The Living Source

HEATING PAD & HOT WATER BOTTLE COVERS
Barrier Cloth: The Living Source

IRONING BOARD COVERS & PADS
Barrier cloth or cotton muslin: The Living Source

RUSTY BOLT/NUT REMOVER
Carbonated beverage - especially colas

STORAGE & LAUNDRY AIDS
Cotton Accessory/Shoe Holder: Janice's
Cotton Gift Bags: Abundant Earth
Delicate fabric bags: Janice's
Ironing Board Covers & Pads (Barrier cloth): Janice's, The Living Source
Laundry Bags/Pouches: Janice's, Real Goods
Tabletop ironing board: Janice's
Wood Laundry Racks: Real Goods

UNTREATED COTTON TENTS
Denver Tent Co.
Blue Star Tents
(These must be washed and aired)

> > < <

Office & Workplace
Computers

YOU SHOULD AVOID
Excessive exposure to glare and electromagnetic radiation. Many people are
sensitive to non-ionizing electromagnet radiation emitted by computers.
There is some evidence that the plastic cases also emit harmful chemical
emissions – particularly new computers when temperatures increase after
prolonged usage.

LESS-TOXIC ALTERNATIVES
COMPUTERS
Monorail Model 7245 Personal Computer[a] (Screen is a color LCD - liquid
crystal display – virtually no radiation emitted), and there is virtually no
smell from out-gassed models. It uses very little power, and generates
very little heat.)
Apple Computer has a solar power pack for its Powerbook[a]

ANTI-GLARE/ANTI-RADIATION FILTERS
These screens serve to decrease extremely low frequency of electrical fields –
not magnetic fields
3-M Anti-glare/Radiation Filters (reduces glare and blocks 99.9% ELF/VLF
emissions): Micro Warehouse
Kensington Anti-Radiation Filters: Micro Warehouse
NoRad Radiation Blocking Shield (also eliminates static electricity, glare and
reflections)

COMPUTER SHIELDS
Image Guard (copper/nickel steel screen): Magshield
Magnetic shielding alloy sheets: Magshield
Silver Lining Net (EMF shield fabric)

STEEL COMPUTER CABINETS
Computers can be placed in stainless steel cabinets and vented outside or to an
air purifier to reduce chemical contaminants:
Stainless Steel Cabinets: Allermed
Galvanized Steel Computer & TV enclosures: The Safe Reading & Computer
Box Co. (Fred Nelson)

ELECTROMAGNETIC METER/TESTING
An electromagnetic meter can be used to check for magnetic, electronic, or
radio/microwaves and electromagnetic hot spots.

KEYBOARDS, ETC.
EMX keyboard neutralizes coherent EMF
Keyboards should be placed 18" from monitor
Organic Wrist Wrest: Abundant Earth

Correction Fluid

YOU SHOULD AVOID
Polyacrylate binder, light petroleum naphtha, toluene, and trichloroethylene

LESS-TOXIC ALTERNATIVES
Water based correction fluid: Opti Light

> > < <

Glues

YOU SHOULD AVOID
Super-stick glues, airplane glues, epoxy glues, rubber cement - may contain toluene which is a CNS depressant

LESS-TOXIC ALTERNATIVES
Elmer's Carpenter Wood Glue, White Glue or Yellow Glue
Sanford Elephant Glue

> > < <

Lubricants

YOU SHOULD AVOID
All petroleum-based machine oils.

LESS-TOXIC ALTERNATIVES
EZ-1 Synthetic Lubricant^a: Allergy Relief Shop
Graphite (check with the manufacturer before using it)
Light Mineral Oil, medicinal grade (may be purchased from a pharmacy)
Plain Castor Oil or Jojoba Oil (use on hinges, doors, latches, etc.)
Motors requiring no lubrication are preferred.
Pure Silicon Oil

> > < <

Office Furnishings & Furniture

YOU SHOULD AVOID
Particleboard, plastics, polyurethane, toxic glues, stain resistant materials, and wall partitions which trap pollutants.

LESS-TOXIC ALTERNATIVES
Handcrafted solid black cherry wood: White Lotus
Solid wood furniture (water-based finishes preferred)
Metal or glass and metal furniture
Chairs of metal or solid wood with natural cloth cushions

> > < <

Papers

YOU SHOULD AVOID
Chlorine bleached papers

LESS-TOXIC ALTERNATIVES
Banana and coffee papers (recycled without chemicals): Costa Rica Natural
Chlorine-free papers (must be specifically requested): Atlantic Recycled Paper
    Co., GreenLine Paper Co., Quill, Real Recycled
Hemp paper, envelopes, notepapers, cards: A Happy Planet
Hemp & cereal straw paper: Tree-Free ECO Paper
Organic cotton, hemp and coffee bean papers: Green Field Paper Co.

> > < <

Reading Boxes & Bags

YOU SHOULD AVOID
Petrochemical exposure

LESS-TOXIC ALTERNATIVES
Reading boxes: Allermed, The Living Source, The Safe Reading & Computer
    Box Co. (Fred Nelson)
Cellulose reading bags: AEHF, The Living Source

> > < <

Miscellaneous Office & Workplace Supplies

YOU SHOULD AVOID
Toxic chemicals in the workplace, and telephones with pesticide in receiver,
    plastics

LESS-TOXIC ALTERNATIVES
GIFT BASKETS: EcoExpress
HEMP STRING: A Happy Planet
METAL PENS & PENCILS
SILK BUSINESS CARD CASE: Ethical Shopper
SOLAR WATCH: Real Goods
WOOD WRITING INSTRUMENTS (PENS): Goodkind Pen Co.

> > < <

Personal Care Products

Many alternative products are available from the various mail order or
internet resources listed later in this book and/or from local health food stores.
Some are items that you can prepare yourself.

Antiperspirants & Deodorants

YOU SHOULD AVOID
Sticks, sprays, aerosols and roll-ons that may contain aluminum, zirconium, ammonia, ethanol, formaldehyde and fragrances.

LESS-TOXIC ALTERNATIVES
Alvera Aloe Deodorant (Texas Best Unlimited L.P.): AEHF, The Living Source
Baking soda or borax (pat under the arm)
Clearly Fresh & Natural (Jason Natural Cosmetics): AEHF
Deodorant Stone/Crystal: Environmentally Sound Products, Real Goods, Simmons Natural Body Care
Desert Essence Deodorant: Desert Essence, AEHF, Arizona Health Foods
Gillette Sport Stick Deodorant[a]
Home Health herbal Magic Deodorant: Allergy Relief Shop
Kiss My Face Active Enzyme: AEHF, NEEDS
Kiss My Face Liquid Rock/Crystal: AEHF, NEEDS
Lavalin Underarm Deodorant Cream: The Living Source
LeCrystal Stone, Roll-On, Spray or Stick: Allergy Relief Shop, Janice's, The Living Source
Lichten Natural Deodorant: The Living Source
Mill Creek Roll-On Herbal
Naturally Fresh Deodorant: AEHF
Nature de France Deodorant: NEEDS
Real Purity: Chemically Sensitive Living, The Living Source
Right Guard Roll-On (unscented)[a]
Simple Anti-Perspirant: AEHF, Allergy Relief Shop, The Living Source, NEEDS
Tom's Herbal Roll-On (unscented): NEEDS, Organic Bebé
> *Check the health food store for many of the above products.*

FOOT DEODORANTS
LeCrystal Foot Deodorant Spray: Allergy Relief Shop
Naturally Fresh Foot Spray: AEHF
> *Uncover your true scent.*

> < <

Antiseptics & Antibacterials

YOU SHOULD AVOID
Iodine (if allergic to it), and isopropyl alcohol (can be especially irritating to sensitive skin and babies or small children)

LESS-TOXIC ALTERNATIVES
Australian Tea Tree Oil from Melaleuca Tree: Desert Essence, Arizona Health Foods
Blue Cypress Germ Zapping Hand Cleaner – Aubrey: AEHF

Grapefruit Seed Extract
Home Health Antibacterial Liquid Soap°: Allergy Relief Shop
Hydrogen Peroxide
Nature's Gate Antiseptic Liquid Soap: AEHF
Orange Plus Waterless Handcleaning Towels: Earth Friendly Products
Zephiran (Benzalkonium) Chloride 17%° *(use only as directed)* – 1 part to 10
    parts water: Abrams Royal Pharmacy *(prescription required)*
Zephiran (Benzalkonium) Chloride wipes and towelettes° (use instead of alcohol
    wipes) AEHF, The Living Source
Zinc Oxide

> > < <

Bath, Hand & Face Soaps

YOU SHOULD AVOID
Commercial bars/liquids containing high amounts of perfume, fatty alcohols,
    and deodorants.
Note: Determine whether the soap has a glycerin or coconut oil base, and if
    you are allergic to these substances. This will definitely affect your
    sensitivity response to it.

LESS-TOXIC ALTERNATIVES
Aubrey Organics soaps: AEHF, Arizona Health Foods, NEEDS
Aveeno-Bar (Oatmeal)
Baby oil will help remove paint or grease from hands
Dr. Bronner's Magic Soap: The Living Source
Castile soap (glycerin): Environmentally Sound Products
Clearly Natural Glycerin Soap: AEHF, Clearly Natural, eNutrition, The Living
    Source
Clinique
Conti Castile (Purpose)
Dionis Goat Milk soaps°: Allergy Relief Shop
Granny's Old-fashioned Body Satin: AEHF, Allergy Relief Shop, The Living
    Source, NEEDS
Green tea contains polyphenols which are natural antioxidants, and aids in
    preventing cellular damage
Hemp & Essential Oil soaps°: Eco-Organics
Herbal soaps: Auromere
Ivory°
Kiss My Face soaps: AEHF, Arizona Health Foods, Chemically Sensitive
    Living, Janice's, The Living Source, NEEDS
Mineral Bath salts: Eco-Organics
Natural Glycerin Soaps: Terressentials
Natural Loofa with glycerine soap: Clearly Natural
Nature's Bounty Goat Milk Soap – plain bars (25% whole goat milk – for oily
    skin) and oatmeal bars (45% whole goat milk that provides more moisture
    for dry skin): The Living Source

Nature Clean Pure Soaps (bar and liquid): AEHF, The Living Source
Nature's Gate soaps: AEHF
Neolife Green Personal Care Cleaner: The Living Source
Neutragena (unscented)
Olive Oil Bar Soap: Janice's
Olive oil base natural bar soaps: Environmentally Sound Products
Palma Christi Bar Soap°: Allergy Relief Shop
Psoriasil Medicated Scalp and Body Wash°: Allergy Relief Shop
Pure New England Face Soap
    (Vegetable, almond oil, Vitamin E, Aloe Vera)
Rainforest Aloe Vera & Copaiba (no coconut oil)
Reviva Seaweed Soap (pure vegetable-based seaweed): Reviva Labs
Santa Fe Cactus Bar Soap°: Allergy Relief Shop
Simmons Pure Soap: Simmons Natural Body Care
Simple soaps and cleansers (bar and liquid): AEHF, Allergy Relief Shop,
    Janice's, The Living Source, NEEDS
Sirena (coconut oil based): AEHF
Soap Critters (natural glycerine soap for children): Clearly Natural,
    Drugstore.com
Tom's Natural soaps: AEHF, NEEDS
Ultra Botanicals (MSM) Facial Wash: The Living Source
                 ~ Caress your skin ~
                    > > < <

Cosmetics

YOU SHOULD AVOID

Avoid skin care products which contain propylene glycol and sodium lauryl
    sulfate. These are definite skin irritants. Avoid petroleum-derived products,
    such as mineral oil. These adhere to the surface of the skin to form a
    barrier, preventing moisture absorption. Glycerin actually draws moisture
    from the surface of the skin and is to be considered for use in a conditioner
    only if it is the 4th or 5th ingredient preceded by vegetable-based oil. Never
    use a moisturizer that contains isopropyl muristate and di- or tri-
    ethanolamine. These form cancer-causing nitrosamines.

Cosmetics whose ingredients include fragrance.   It is impossible to know
    which of over 200 ingredients this means. Some cause headaches, dizziness,
    rash, hyperpigmentation, violent coughing, vomiting, skin irritations, and
    more.

Petrolatum (particularly in lip care products) can produce photosensitivity and
    promote sun damage, drying and chapping.

Mascara may contain quaternium 15 and thimerosol.

Liquids, powders, cakes and sticks may contain any of the previously listed
    allergens, chemicals, coal tar dyes, drying agents, irritants, microbial growth
    inhibitors, and preservatives.

LESS-TOXIC ALTERNATIVES[12]

Cosmetics should nourish the skin, contain emollients and humectants, and be non-irritating and non-drying. Be sure all cosmetics are labeled fragrance free. Add to your beauty, not your sensitivities.

Allercreme

Almay

Aubrey Organics (contains coconut oils): Arizona Health Foods, Natural Lifestyle, NEEDS

Aziza

Bare Essentials

Bath and Beauty Works

Clinique

Earth Science Beta Ginseng cleansers, cremes, etc.

Ecco Bella Mascara and Vitamin E Lip Smoother: Ecco Bella, NEEDS

Indian Earth

Jojoba: The Living Source

Naturade: NEEDS

Organic cotton balls, swabs & cosmetic rounds: Abundant Earth, AEHF, Allergy Relief Shop, GAIAM, Grass Roots Natural Goods, Harmony, JAMS, The Living Source, Natural Lifestyle, Organic Essentials

Paul Pender: Chemically Sensitive Living, Natural Lifestyle, NEEDS

Rachel Perry

Real Purity (line of cosmetics): Chemically Sensitive Living, The Living Source

Simple Eye Makeup remover and cleansers: The Living Source

Homemade Skin Toner

Combine ½ cup lemon juice, 1 cup distilled water and 2/3 cup witch hazel in a bottle. Shake well before applying with a clean cotton ball.

Homemade Bath Salts

Combine 1 part sea salt, 2 parts baking soda and 3 parts Epsom salts. Shake well before using.

Homemade Foaming Bath Oil

Blend together 1 cup oil, ½ cup safe liquid soap, 1 Tbsp. vanilla and ¼ cup honey (optional). Shake well before using ¼ cup per bath.

IMPORTANT NUTRIENTS

Almond Oil, Beeswax, Coconut Oil, Collagen, Lanolin, Linoletic Acid, Fruit Oils, Tea Tree Oil, Vitamins E (Tocopherol) & C (minimize moisture loss)

IMPORTANT SKIN PROTECTANTS

Allantoin, Cocoa Butter, Humectants (maintain moisture balance)

Aloe Vera Gel & Collagen Amino Acid

Moisturizers: Chamomile and Oatmeal

> > < <

Dental Care
Toothpaste, Toothbrushes & Mouthwash

Brush and clean your teeth and breath.
Don't kill them with 'als, 'ols, and 'zyls.

YOU SHOULD AVOID

Most tooth cleaners as they can contain ammonia, benzyl alcohol, ethanol, formaldehyde, glycols and flavors. Toothpaste and mouthwashes may have dyes including blue #1 (possible carcinogen).

Toothbrushes with plastic handles and bristles

LESS-TOXIC ALTERNATIVES[□]

AMNI Mouthwashes: The Living Source

Baking Soda or baking soda (2 parts) to 1 part salt (mix in a blender to form a fine powder)

Breath Buddies (World Organic – for bad breath): The Living Source

Calendula Mint Free: Janice's

Desert Essence Tea Tree Toothpaste: Desert Essence, Chemically Sensitive Living, NEEDS

Enzymatic Therapy Oral Basics Mouthwash: The Living Source

GoldenKaire Cleansing Solution (toothbrush cleaner): Dasun

Herbal Toothpaste: Auromere

Homemade Herbal Toothpaste: 1 tsp. dried Irish moss (red algae), 1 cup water, 1 tsp. salt, 1 tsp. soda and a few drops of chlorophyll - soak moss 15 minutes in spring water, bring to a boil, boil 15 minutes. Strain gel through cheesecloth. Mix salt and soda, and add to gel. Add chlorophyll.

Homemade Mouthwash: Australian Tea Tree Oil: Desert Essence, Arizona Health Foods

Put 4-5 drops per cup of water. Make only a few days supply each time.

Homeodent Toothpaste: Allergy Relief Shop

Lemon Homeodent Toothpaste (Boiron-Borneman Inc.): AEHF

Natural Dentist Toothpaste: Allergy Relief Shop

Natural Dentist Mouth & Gum Therapy: Allergy Relief Shop

Nature de France Toothpaste

Nature's Gate: Janice's

OraRinse, OraPatch & OraBan: Mom's Aloe Store

Peelu Chewing Gum: The Living Source

Peelu Dental Fibers: AEHF

Peelu Toothpaste & Mouthwash: AEHF, The Living Source, Simmons Natural Body Care

Real Purity Natural Toothpaste: Chemically Sensitive Living, The Living Source

Salt 'N Soda Natural Toothpowder: Allergy Relief Shop

Sensodyne Toothpaste

Thursday Plantation Tea Tree Dental Floss
Thursday Plantation Tea Tree Toothpaste: NEEDS
Tom's Natural Flossing Ribbon: AEHF, NEEDS
Tom's Natural Toothpaste: AEHF, Chemically Sensitive Living, Eco-Organics, NEEDS, Organic Bebé
Viadent
Weleda Herbal Toothpaste
Wood and natural bristle toothbrushes: Heart of Vermont, Janice's
Note: Toothbrushes or toothbrush heads should be replaced once a month to prevent viruses (such as herpes) and bacterial problems.

> > < <

Hair Care

The average head has 150,000 hairs. Hair can certainly add beauty to our being, yet we don't always treat it with respect. Harsh shampoo, alcohol, dyes, bleaches and soaps can cause it to choke. Care should be exercised in your choice of hair care products.

YOUR HAIR REFLECTS YOUR HEALTH

Hair can be a reflection of an individual's overall health. Dull/brittle hair can be a result of salty, chlorinated or sudsy water; swimming; over-shampooing; chlorine; sun damage; or too much heat in hair drying.

Hair loss can be due to mistreatment of hair; but it can also be the result of chemical exposure, stress/tension, thyroid disease, heredity, excess salt, white sugar, decreased iron, hair dyes, dryers, dandruff, oral contraceptives, lack of B vitamins, or malnutrition.

VITAMINS WHICH HELP YOUR HAIR

Vitamins which nourish and build the health of your hair include: vitamin A, fatty acids (Omega 3 and 6), vitamin E, choline, and B vitamins. Dull hair is often a result of a vitamin A deficiency.

COMBS & BRUSHES
YOU SHOULD AVOID
Plastic handles and bristles

LESS-TOXIC ALTERNATIVES
Wood and natural bristles: AEHF, Allergy Relief Shop, GAIAM, Harmony, Heart of Vermont, Janice's, Natural Lifestyles, Simmons Natural Body Care

SHAMPOOS AND CONDITIONERS
YOU SHOULD AVOID
Most commercial brands contain many harmful chemicals used as emollients (moisturizing agents), emulsifiers (used to thoroughly blend non-mixable liquids), humectants (hold in moisture), and surfactants (wetting agents permitting water to spread out and penetrate easily).

These harmful chemicals include:

- Fragrance,
- Ethanol (drying to the hair and a central nervous system depressant that can affect heart rate, blood pressure and respiration)
- Formaldehyde (mucous membrane and heart irritant)
- Nitrosamines (carcinogens)
- Sodium lauryl sulfate (can be an eye irritant)
- Sodium trideceth sulfate
- PEG-150 distearate
- Coal tar (carcinogenic)
- Quaternium-15
- Polyquaternium-10 or quaternium ammonia compound (eye irritants and may cause dermatitis and damage hair)
- TEA (triethanolamine)
- DEA (diethanolamine) nitosating agents
- PVP/VA Copolymer (a petroleum-derived chemical) is used in hairsprays, wavesets, and other cosmetics. Its particles may contribute to foreign bodies in the lungs.
- Stearalkonium chloride (used in hair conditioners and creams) causes allergic reactions. These not only damage your hair but also your health.

LESS-TOXIC ALTERNATIVES[a]

AFM SafeChoice Head & Body Shampoo: AEHF, The Living Source, NEEDS, Simmons Natural Body Care

AFM Satin Touch Shampoo: Allergy Relief Shop, Environmentally Sound Products, The Living Source, NEEDS

Aubrey Organics shampoos: AEHF, Arizona Health Foods, Environmentally Sound Products, Natural Lifestyle, NEEDS

Aubrey Organics B5 Design Gel: AEHF, Arizona Health Foods, NEEDS

BioLand hair products: Fair Trade Naturals

Giovanni Shampoo and Conditioner: Simmons Natural Body Care

Granny's Gently Yours & Rich'N Radiant shampoos: AEHF, Allergy Relief Shop, The Living Source NEEDS

Granny's Old-Fashioned Soft & Silky Conditioner: AEHF, Allergy Relief Shop, The Living Source

Hemp & Essential Oil Shampoos and Conditioners[a]: Eco-Organics

Home Health Everclean Anti-Dandruff Shampoo & Chamomile Shampoo[a]: Allergy Relief Shop

J.R. Liggett's Old Fashioned Bar Shampoo: Simmons Natural Body Care

Kiss My face Olive & Aloe Shampoo: AEHF, Arizona Health Foods

Lemon juice – will rinse out excess shampoo

Magick Botanicals shampoos & conditioners[a]: Allergy Relief Shop, Living naturally, NEEDS, Simmons Natural Body Care

Mayonnaise – a good conditioner

Mill Creek Shampoo & Conditioner: AEHF, NEEDS

Natural Products Store Baby Shampoo
Nature Clean Herbal Shampoo & Organic Conditioner: AEHF, The Living
    Source
Nature's Bounty shampoos (no coconut oil): The Living Source
Nature's Gate Tea-Tree Oil Shampoo & Conditioner: The Living Source
Neo-Life Green: The Living Source
Patricia Allison (glycerine base): Allergy Relief Shop, The Living Source
Rainforest (has sodium laurel sulfate)
Rose Petal Shampoo
Santa Fe Shampoo & Bath Gel: [n]: Allergy Relief Shop
Ski Kai Shampoo (free of coconut and alcohol)
Simple Gentle Shampoo: AEHF, Allergy Relief Shop, NEEDS
Simple Gentle Conditioner: Allergy Relief Shop, The Living Source, NEEDS
Terressentials herbal shampoo
Tom's Shampoo – almond oil and aloe vera (has glycerol and sodium laurel
    sulfate): Eco-Organics, Ethical Shopper, NEEDS
Ultra Botanicals (MSM Shampoo & Conditioner): The Living Source
Unicure Natural shampoo and conditioner[n]: Allergy Relief Shop

Homemade Hot Oil Treatment
Shake together ½ cup olive oil and ½ cup boiling water in a pint jar until
the oil forms in tiny droplets. Massage into hair and cover for 15-20
minutes, then shampoo as normal.
Note: Be sure to condition the ends and not necessarily the roots.

For Gum in Hair
Use peanut butter or vegetable oil followed by a tolerated shampoo

HAIRSPRAYS & WAVESETS
YOU SHOULD AVOID
PVC/VA Copolymer, a petroleum-derived chemical used in hair sprays,
    wavesets and other cosmetics can cause toxic lung reactions.

LESS-TOXIC ALTERNATIVES[n]
Aubrey Organics Natural Mist Hair Spray (alcohol/scented)[n]: AEHF, Arizona
    Health Foods, Natural Lifestyle, NEEDS
Aloegen Natural Super Hold Hair Spray (alcohol)[n]: AEHF
Magick Botanicals Styling Gells and Hairspray [n]: Allergy Relief Shop,
    Chemically Sensitive Living, NEEDS, Simmons Natural Body Care
Mill Creek Hair Spray (alcohol/herbal fragrance)[n]: AEHF, NEEDS
Naturade Aloe Vera 80 (no alcohol or fragrance): AEHF, NEEDS
Real Purity Natural Styling Gel: Chemically Sensitive Living, The Living
Source
Source Hair Spray & Setting Lotion: The Living Source

Homemade Hair Spray
2 cups boiling water, 1 tsp. Knox gelatin, & 1 Tbsp. vinegar[n]
Mix together and strain through coffee filter. Put in sprayer bottle.

HAIR DYES
YOU SHOULD AVOID
Hair dyes can irritate the skin and have been known to cause cancer of the
  breast, bladder, ovaries, uterus, cervix and lungs; non-Hodgkins lymphoma
  (according to an American Journal of Public Health Nebraska Study); and
  leukemia. Ammonia and hydrogen peroxide can be skin irritants and
  sensitizers.
Dyes also contain p-phenylenediamine (skin irritant). Dark hair dyes are the
  most potent. Synthetic colors are believed to be cancer-causing agents.

LESS-TOXIC ALTERNATIVES[a]
Chemically Sensitive Living,
Lagona: Green Marketplace
Natural Henna (available from health food stores)
Paul Pender
Herbal tint: Whole Foods Markets
Vegetable based hair dyes (health food stores)
Vita Wave hair coloring products[a]: Allergy Relief Shop, Natural Lifestyle,
  NEEDS

HEAD LICE TREATMENTS
YOU SHOULD AVOID
Commercial preparations which may contain Lindane

LESS-TOXIC ALTERNATIVES
Innomed Lice Comb, A-200 Shampoo[a] & A-200 Lice Control Spray[a]: Hogil
  Pharmaceutical
Lifekind Organic Lice Shampoo: Lifekind Products
Medicomb (available from pharmacies) – use after delousing
Neolife Green to shampoo, followed by coconut oil rinse and comb out with a
  special fine-tooth nit comb.
Not Nice to Lice Shampoo[a] and Nit Comb: Biocontrol Network
Homemade preparation: Mix enough garlic, nettle and tea tree oils (3:3:1) to
  coat child's hair, cover with a towel and leave overnight, then shampoo
  with garlic shampoo or Neolife.
Essential oil treatment: combine 2 oz. vegetable oil; 20 drops tea tree essential
  oil; and 10 drops each essential oil of rosemary, lavender and lemon. Apply
  to dry hair and cover with shower cap or plastic bag. Wrap with a towel
  and leave for one hour, then shampoo and rinse hair several times to help
  cut the oil. May have to repeat treatment for several weeks to eliminate
  any new lice that may be hatching.
Tea tree oil and hot (131°F) water. Shampoo and comb 2 times the first week,
  1 time per week the second week and 1 time per week the 3rd week.

Treatment Notes
If possible, use a lice killing shampoo listed above. Ordinary shampoos have
  no effect on lice.

Less-Toxic Alternatives

Comb hair with a special lice comb immediately after shampooing. This is essential as lice eggs or nits are "cemented" to the hair shaft and must be physically removed before they hatch and re-infest the scalp.

Repeat shampooing and combing after seven to ten days. Unless you do, you could experience re-infestation.

Examine all other family members for lice and nits (eggs), and treat if present.

You must soak all combs, brushes and hair accessories in <u>very</u> <u>hot</u> water.

Wash clothing, towels, bedding and draperies in <u>very</u> <u>hot</u> water, and do not share these with others in the family until the problem is totally gone.

Dry clean non-washable items or store in air-tight bags for 30 days.

Vacuum (and steam if possible) furniture, carpets and mattresses thoroughly.

PERMANENT WAVES

YOU SHOULD AVOID

Commercial perms containing ammonia; dyes; fragrances; crotonic acids (skin irritant); ammonium thioglycolate (can cause severe burns, blistering and hemorrhaging under the skin); formaldehyde (skin irritant); ammonium carbonate (can cause dermatitis); DEA (diethanolamine) or TEA (triethanolamine) can cause cancer, eye problems, dryness of hair and skin; polyvinyl pyirolidone (may lead to lung irritation); mineral oil (clogs pores) or glycols

LESS-TOXIC ALTERNATIVES

Ask your hairdresser about ammonia and formaldehyde-free perms.

Creative Curl by Redkin□

Giovanni□

Ogilvie□

Thermo Perm Naturally by Helene Curtis□

Vita Wave Perms: Allergy Relief Shop, The Living Source, Natural Lifestyle, NEEDS

Wellaperm□ – available from health food stores

Curl your hair – not your toes.

> > < <

Men's Shaving & Hair Care Needs

YOU SHOULD AVOID

Bleaches, fragrances and preservatives

LESS-TOXIC ALTERNATIVES

Aloe Vera & Unscented shaving soaps: Simmons Natural Body Care

CarraDerm™ Moisturizing Cream□: Mom's Skin Care

Colgate Shaving Soap & brush instead of shaving cream in cans

East of the Sun Shaving Mug and Brush: Simmons Natural Body Care

Kiss My Face Natural Moisture Shave: AEHF, The Living Source, NEEDS

Lagona: Green Marketplace

Moonflower Herbals Hair Oil: Simmons Natural Body Care

My Brother's Keeper

Nat'l. Lifestyle Suppliers

Paul Pender (shaving cream & aftershave)

Real Purity Hypo Allergenic Shave Cream: Chemically Sensitive Living, The Living Source

Simple Soothing Shave Gel: AEHF, The Living Source, NEEDS

Tom's Shaving Cream: NEEDS

Witch hazel (use as aftershave)

> > < <

Nail Care

Nails are a substructure of epidermis composed mainly of keratin. They reflect your health. They grow 1/500th to 1/20th of an inch per week. These conditions can indicate a correlating nutrient deficiency:

- Brittleness – iron, vitamin A or calcium deficiency; thyroid or kidney dysfunction
- Chip, peel, crack or break – general nutritional deficiency, insufficient protein or hydrochloric acid.
- Horizontal & vertical lines/ridges – fatty acid or vitamin B deficiency
- Horizontal lines – physical or psychological stress
- Splitting – poor digestion
- Spoon-shaped – iron deficiency, B12 deficiency
- Vertical lines – poor health or kidney disorder
- White spots – zinc deficiency

YOU SHOULD AVOID

Nail polish containing toluene, acrylics and nail lacquers, and adhesives for artificial nails. Artificial nails can breed bacteria and result in serious nail infections.

LESS-TOXIC ALTERNATIVES[a]

Delore Nail Treatment from Natural Oils (in health food stores)

Estee Lauder – Finish Nail Lacquer (in drug stores)

European Secrets Nail Enamel (in beauty salons)

Nail Brush (wooden handle/natural bristles): Simmons Natural Body Care

Revlon Strong Wear (toluene and formaldehyde free)

> > < <

Perfumes

YOU SHOULD AVOID

Commercial fragrances consist of a combination of natural essential oils, aroma chemicals and solvents in a base of alcohol.

These harmful chemicals include acetone (CNS depressant) aldehydes (dermatitis/carcinogenic); alcohol (CNS depressant); ammonia; propylene glycol (an immuno-toxic chemical); formaldehyde (mucous membrane irritant); musk ambreette (can cause central and peripheral nervous system damage); phenols; toluene (very toxic - can produce headaches, nausea, narcosis); glaxolide; hedione; phenyl ether; vertofix; benzyl acetate; cyclohexanol (can depress central nervous system, inhibit motor activity, cause flaccidity, spasm and death); linalool (can affect motor and muscular functions, cause depression and respiratory disturbances); benzyl salicylate, linalyl acetate; citronella; methylione gamma; hexyl cinnamic aldehyde; arryl salicylate; iso bomylacetate; benzophenones (can cause hives); ethanol; and orris root (a sensitizer).

Toluene-laced fragrances are also being used in furniture wax, tires, plastic garbage bags, inks, hair gel, hairspray, kitty litter and many other commercial products.

LESS-TOXIC ALTERNATIVES[o]

Eastern Star Creme Perfumes[o]: Simmons Natural Body Care

Eden Botanicals Aromatic Resins[o]: Simmons Natural Body Care

Pure essential oils: Aroma Vera, Inc., Aura Cacia, Leydet Arromatics, Original Swiss Aromatics, Simmons Natural Body Care

Natural homemade essential oils from herbs, flowers and the sun

- Put a large amount of fresh flower or herbs in a large glass jar and cover with distilled water. Seal top and place in direct sunlight. When an oil forms on top, skim it off, and save it in a small jar. Repeat as needed. Save oil in airtight bottles.
- Put water in bottom of double boiler. Put 1 cup sunflower or almond oil on top, and heat until warm. Pack top with very fresh fragrant flowers or herbs, cover tightly and heat on very low for 2 hours. Squeeze oil from leaves and replace with fresh ones. Repeat until desired fragrance is reached; strain and place in airtight bottles.

Perfume Remover

Mix enough water with 3 tsp. of dry mustard to form a paste. Rub on and allow to dry, then wash off with water.

> > < <

Skin Care

Your skin is the body's largest vital organ – covering an area of approximately 19 square feet, and weighing about 7 pounds. It is the first line of defense to prevent invasion into the body by germs, bacteria, etc. Its main functions are to regulate body temperature through sweat glands, detoxify organs of poison, respire by absorbing oxygen and expiring carbon monoxide, absorb nutrients, and manufacture vitamin D. It also contains sense receptors for pain and tactile sensory stimulation.

The skin has two clearly defined layers, the epidermis and dermis, which require care and feeding. It must be cleansed of dirt and dry skin cells, and stimulated to increase circulation and the functioning of hormones and oil-producing glands in order to remove an estimated 1/3 of the body's toxins.

Soothe and beautify the real you from the inside out, from head to toe. Your skin must be nourished in order to function properly. Oils can be applied to soften and moisturize it. Vitamins A, C, E, and B, and essential amino acids need to be abundant in the diet or supplemented to insure skin health.

Skin can reflect sensitivities and poor dietary habits (eczema, rashes, acne or dermatitis). It must be protected from sunburn, artificial fabrics and dyes or irritation can occur. Know your body's needs, sensitivities and limitations, so your skin can serve you well.

> > < <

MOISTURIZERS

YOU SHOULD AVOID
Commercial brands that may contain ammonia, colors, perfume and ethanol.

LESS-TOXIC ALTERNATIVES
All types of skin needs adequate vitamins and minerals that can usually be found in organic moisturizers and cleansers.

Alba Botanica Very Emollient Body Lotion: The Living Source

AloeCeuticals™ Snow and Sun™ Lip (SPF 15), Sunburn Spray & Sports Gel (for burns): Mom's Aloe Shop

Aloe Vera (use from the plant)

Aubrey Organics: AEHF, Arizona Health Foods, Environmentally Sound Products, Natural Lifestyle, NEEDS

Autumn Harp Unpetroleum Lip Balm: Allergy Relief Shop, Environmentally Sound Products

Bee Pollen Skin Nutrition Cream: The Living Source

Camocare Gold (intense facial therapy)

CarraDerm™ Moisturizing Cream[n]: Mom's Skin Care

Carrot Oil

Earth Science Bet Ginseng lotions and cremes

Elizabeth Van Buren Unscented Lotion: Simmons Natural Body Care

Enzymatic Therapy (formulas for cold sores, fever blisters, psoriasis, worts, moles and liver spots): The Living Source

Eucerin

Granny's Old-fashioned Moisture Guard / Lotion: AEHF, Allergy Relief Shop. The Living Source, NEEDS

Kiss My Face Aloe Moisturizer: AEHF, Arizona Health Foods, NEEDS

Hemp & Essential Oil Moisturizer[n]: Eco-Organics

Herbal Aloe Force Topical Gel: The Living Source

Horsetail Extract

Hyaluronic acid

Lagona: Green Marketplace

Lansinoah For Healthy Feet & Lansinoah Soothe & Heal: AEHF

Linseed Oil

Magick Botanicals moisturizers and lotion[a]: Allergy Relief Shop, NEEDS
Margarite Zinc Cream: The Living Source
Naturade moisturizers: NEEDS
Nature's Bounty Moisturizing Cream: The Living Source
Nature's Gate Moisturizing Lotion: The Living Source
Patricia Allison Vita Balm: Allergy Relief Shop
Patricia Allison Petal hand & body balm: Allergy Relief Shop, Living Source
Primrose Oil
Shea Butter
Simple Products moisturizers, bath and shower creams and gels: AEHF, NEEDS
Simmons Lip Balm: Simmons Natural Body Care
Simple cleansing products[a] – Deep Down Facial Mask, Skin Toner, Active Cleansing Lotion, Gentle Cleansing Scrub & Refreshing Facial Wash, Gel: AEHF, The Living Source, NEEDS
Simple Eye Zone Benefits Cream: AEHF, The Living Source, NEEDS
Simple Extra Gentle Eye Makeup Remover: AEHF, The Living Source, NEEDS
Simple moisturizing cremes, oils, lotions, etc.: Allergy Relief Shop, The Living Source, NEEDS
Simple Nourishing Night Cream: AEHF, The Living Source, NEEDS
Ski Kai: Whole Foods
Terressentials
Ultra Botanicals moisturizers: The Living Source
Wheat Germ Oil
Vitamin E Oil

Homemade Moisturizing Lotion

- 2 ounces Aquaphor (a salve-like mixture that makes the oil and water mix – available at drug counters)
- 7 ounces of edible oil (i.e. Safflower, Sesame, Sunflower – do not use cottonseed, corn, soybean, or peanut oil)
- Chlorine Free Water (Spring or Distilled) 7 ounces

Mix on low speed in your blender or by stirring until you have a pleasing consistency. Label the mixture as a moisturizing lotion. Apply a generous coat of moisturizer to skin as needed.

Skin toners can include extract of chamomile, aloe vera, calendula or rose.

If you have oily skin, consider a conditioner with witch hazel.

> > < <

SUNSCREENS & SUNBLOCKS

It is essential to protect your skin from the damaging rays of the sun. Excessive sun exposure can damage skin, giving it a leathery appearance. It also causes basal cell carcinoma (skin cancer). The SPF number equals the estimated time in the sun without burning.

YOU SHOULD AVOID
Commercial brands that may contain mineral oil, dyes, fragrances and petrochemicals

LESS-TOXIC ALTERNATIVES[a]
Alexandra Avery (with PABA and sesame oil)
Alba Botanica Sun Screen-Daily Shade SPF 16 Lotion: The Living Source
Aubrey Organics Sun Shade 15 & Ultra 15 & Rosa Mosquerta Sun Protection Herbal Butter – SPF 15: AEHF, Arizona Health Foods, NEEDS
Aubrey Organics Titania – SPF 25: AEHF, NEEDS
Bullfrog[a] (no PABA, fragrance) – SPF to 36
Clinique Special Defense Sun Block[a] (no PABA or fragrance) – SPF 25
Cocoa butter
Ecological Formulas Oxy-Screen Anti-Oxidant Sunscreen SPF 15: The Living Source
Light colors reflect heat, dark colors absorb heat.
Lily of the Desert Skinsaver Sunblock (Aloe Vera, no PABA) – SPF 40
Logona Sunscreen for Children – SPF 27
Naturade Aloe Vera 80 – Kids Sunblock (PABA, fragrance free) – SPF 30: The Living Source
Natural Lifestyle, Green Tea Sun Block for Children – SPF 25 (UVA & UVB protection): AEHF, NEEDS
Pro Tec Sun Screen SPF 30+: The Living Source
Rachel Perry Tanning
Real Purity Sunscreen SPF 15: The Living Source
Simmons Natural Body Care SPF 15 Sunblock
Wysong Sun Block: Ecco Bella
Wear hats that provide shade for face, long sleeves and leg covers to protect your skin from damaging rays.

Homemade fragrance-free sunblock:
16 ounces of oil (almond, olive, rice, or whatever you tolerate), 2 oz. of beeswax, 3 heaping Tbsps. of USP grade Titanium Dioxide or Zinc Oxide (take care NOT to inhale these powders)

Directions: Heat oil in kettle, then drop in a few beeswax chunks. Test consistency by dripping a puddle on foil and allowing to cool (freezer will speed cooling). Add more wax for firming, more oil if it's too hard. The amount of titanium dioxide or zinc oxide you add determines the opacity (whiteness). Should be stored in refrigerator and small containers used on outings. The oil and beeswax make a good hand and skin lotion, and a firmer version is good for dry lips (can be placed in an empty Chapstick tube)

Sunglasses: Ott Full-Spectrum: Allergy Relief Shop, NEEDS

> > < <

Women's Personal Needs

YOU SHOULD AVOID
Bleaches, fragrances, pesticides and preservatives

LESS-TOXIC ALTERNATIVES

PADS & TAMPONS
Autumn Harp organic cotton tampons

Cotton Plus (organic cotton no-applicator tampons and sanitary pads)

Decent Exposures

Gladrags (cotton menstrual pads): Abundant Earth, Allergy Relief Shop, The Baby Lane, Earthwise Basics, Keepers

Gladrags Storage Bag: Abundant Earth, Allergy Relief Shop, The Baby Lane, Keepers

Granny Pads: B.Coole Designs

Grass Roots Natural Goods

Harmony Moon cotton pads & tampons: Natural Lifestyle

Heart of Vermont

Lotus Pad Co. (organic cotton sanitary pads)

Lunapads (100% cotton washable pads): Alternative Baby, Eco-Logique, Lunapads

Natracare (100% organic cotton, oxygen-bleached tampons): Allergy Relief Shop, GAIAM, Harmony, Natracare, Simmons Natural Body Care

Natracare Pads & Panty Shields (100% cotton – no additives): Allergy Relief Shop, GAIAM, Harmony, Natracare

Natural Choice (100% organic cotton menstrual pads): Simmons Natural Body Care

Organic cotton pads: Abundant Earth, Eco Baby, The Living Source, Pookie Doos

Organic cotton tampons: Abundant Earth, AEHF, Eco Baby, JAMS, The Living Source, Organic Essentials

Organic Essentials Tampons: Simmons Natural Body Care

Pandora Pads & Tampons

Plaid Pads: Plaid Pads, Pookie Doos

Sea sponges can be used instead of tampons

Tambrands (cotton tampons bleached with hydrogen peroxide – not organic)

NURSING SUPPLIES
Nursing Clothing: Eco Baby

Nursing & Maternity Wear: The Nurtured Baby

Organic Cotton Nursing Bra: The Nurtured Baby

Organic Cotton Nursing Bras and Breast Pads: Eco Baby, Pookie Doos

Organic Cotton Nursing Pads: Alternative Baby, B.Coole Designs, Ethical Shopper, Mama Moons, The Nurtured Baby

Pandora's Organic Nursing Pads: Pandora Pads

100% Natural Cotton Nursing Pads: Nursing Mothers Supplies

MISCELLANEOUS PRODUCTS

Autumn Harp Unpetroleum Jelly: Allergy Relief Shop, Environmentally Sound Products

Puritans Pride – V-Loe (70% Aloe Vera)

Soaking pots for cloth pads: The Baby Lane

Incontinence Resources: Earthwise Basics, Natural Baby

Note: www.borntolove.com gives a vast list of resources for women's special needs and incontinence products – some are organic, others are just 100% cotton

> > < <

Pesticides

YOU SHOULD AVOID

Pesticides are not tested for neurological damage, but these harmful chemicals are routinely used on crops and in our homes. Three types of pesticides of concern to the consumer are organophosphates, n-methyl carbamates, and organochlorines. *(See Pesticides on page 31, 41 and 230)*

All insecticides and herbicides containing organophosphates, organochlorines, herbicides, fungicides, synthetic pyrethrins and carbamates should be avoided. They contaminate air, water and food. High LD50 ratings afford less human toxicity, but this rating applies only to oral and skin absorption - not respiratory contamination or differing sensitivities due to size, age or health conditions.

Aerosol foggers are to be avoided because they dissipate slowly. They allow pesticides and carriers to deposit in the carpet and furniture. If there is unavoidable usage, choose less toxic alternatives, and ventilate with exhaust fans.

LESS-TOXIC ALTERNATIVES

Natural Pyrethrum

Natural Pyrethrum pesticides are derived from dried, powdered flowers of pyrethrums. However, pyrethrum can be synthetically created to resemble the natural substances in pyrethrum flowers. These are often mixed with a petroleum distillate or piperonyl butoxide. Synthetic pyrethroid pesticides include Resmethrin, Permethrin and Cypermethrin. Pyrethrum pesticides are neurologically active and appear to exacerbate allergy and asthma, as ragweed-sensitive people may cross-react to pyrethrum and pyrethroids. Still, pyrethrum pesticides offer a less-toxic alternative for selected indoor and outdoor pest control.

Negative Ion Field

A negative ion field repels insects: Silver Spur

> > < <

Ants, Carpenter Ants & Fire Ants

YOU SHOULD AVOID
All commercial insecticides

LESS-TOXIC ALTERNATIVES

FOR ANTS
Borax and sugar (50-50 mixture)
Boric acid and 1/3 cup of mint apple jelly
Castor oil on cracks
Caulk all entry points
Cayenne pepper
Chili oil (chili mixed with sesame oil)
Concern Citrus Home Pest Control: AEHF
Corn grits or corn meal (will cause them to explode)
Drax: Waterbury
Ginger barrier – ants don't like to cross it
Honey and boric acid mixture
Jalapeño pepper spray: grind several jalapeños, mix with 1 quart water and boil 15 minutes. Let stand overnight then strain. Mix with water, pour into a spray bottle and spray. Label "Ant Spray."
Jecta (injectable borate for painted, sealed or hard-to-reach wood): Nisus
The Lil Hummer (suction cracks and crevices): Miracle Marketing
Logic (growth regulator)[n]: Marshall Grain Co.
Mint planted near entryways discourage ants
Niban Granular Bait (boric acid) and a Snuffer (Nisus Corp.) for use inside and outside: Nisus Corp., Biocontrol Network
Nibor (fine borate powder): Nisus Corp.
Peppermint (plant in yard)
Red chili pepper
Remove food sources – place all food in sealed containers
Pharoah Ants (methoprene growth regulator)
Red chili pepper & dried peppermint (sprinkled in specific areas)
Safer Ant & Crawling insect Killer: AEHF
Soapy water
Stickem (barrier)
Sticky Stuff
Tanglefoot Pest Barrier: Tanglefood Co.
Terro Ant Killer (bait containing Boric Acid): Allergy Relief Shop

FOR CARPENTER ANTS
Abamectin sulfluramide insecticidal bait: Gardens Alive, MSD Agvet, Peaceful Valley
Bora-Care (inject into wall areas with bait gun): Nisus Corp., Allergy Relief Shop

Boric Acid (inject into wall areas with bait gun)

Diatomaceous Earth: AEHF, Allergy Relief Shop, Garden-Ville, Natural Animal

Drione[a] (silica gel and pyrethrin): Target Specialty Products, Roxide International, and The Natural Gardener

Electrogun: Michelin Service Co.

Etex

Isothermics heat treatment

Natural pyrethrums (contains pyrethrins and carriers)[a]: Allergy Relief Shop, Peaceful Valley, Roxide International

Py-Rin (without Piperonyl Butoxide)

Bug Buster-O[a]: Monterey Lawn & Garden (contains petroleum)

Nematode mite

Niban (Granular Boric Acid): Nisus Corp., Biocontrol Network

Nibor (fine borate powder): Nisus Corp.

Scalding water (pour into the nests)

Silica Aerogel (inject into wall areas with bait gun)

Tim-Bor (Disodium Octaborate Tetrahydrate) – inject into walls with bait gun): Nisus, U.S. Borax, Marshall Grain Co.

FOR FIRE ANTS

Amdro (growth regulator)[a]

Abamectin sulfluramide insecticidal bait: Gardens Alive, MSD Agvet, Peaceful Valley

Boric acid with drying agents: Orcon

Citrex[a]: Marshall Grain Co.

Fire Ant Hormone Bait: Natural Gardening Research Center

Logic - Fenoxycarb (growth regulator)[a]: Marshall Grain Co.

Neo-Life Green Soap: The Living Source

Parasite Fire Mite: Biofac, Inc.

Tansy (herb) plant around the house.

True Stop (contains .21% Rotenone – natural insecticide found in all plants)

Zap Herbal Powder

> > < <

Carpet Beetles

YOU SHOULD AVOID
Paradichlorobenzene and organophosphate insecticides

LESS-TOXIC ALTERNATIVES
Frequently vacuum upholstery and carpet
Steam clean carpet to remove lint, hair and dust

In Clothes:
Organic pyrethrum (to kill)[a]
Repeated freezing and thawing

186   *Less-Toxic Alternatives*

Store airtight with camphor[n]
Store in sealed bags

> > < <

Note: For Fleas & Ticks, See Pet Care Section

> > < <

Flies

YOU SHOULD AVOID
Insecticide strips and aerosols.

LESS-TOXIC ALTERNATIVES
Agro-BioTech Corp House Fly Trap: AEHF
Basil herb plants and crushed leaves
Beneficial Insects: Hydro Gardens
Fly swatter and/or flypaper
Fly traps, swatters and catchers: Marshall Grain Co.
Lavender (dried)
Neem Oil – Bioneem: Biocontrol Network, Peaceful Valley, Ringer, Safer
Orange Peel
Safer Fly Scoop, Indoor Fly Trap: AEHF
Sure Fire Fly Scoop: Allergy Relief Shop
Sudbury Bye Fly (trap with attractant): AEHF
Terro Fly Catchers & Fly Swatters: Allergy Relief Shop

> > < <

Lawn & Garden Care

YOU SHOULD AVOID
Commercial preparations that may contain chemical contaminants such as organophosphates and carbamates because they act as nerve toxins. Ninety-five percent of the commercial pesticides used on lawns are carcinogenic. Many have not been tested for long-term health affects only for a limited number of health effects.

LESS-TOXIC ALTERNATIVES
FOR LAWN & GARDEN PESTS
Azatin: Hydro Gardens
Beneficial insects and worms (earthworms, ladybugs, lacewings, and/or praying
     mantis – control undesirable pests): BioFac, Garden-Ville, Hydro Gardens,
     Marshall Grain Co., Natural Gardening Co.
BioSafe
Chrysanthemums (natural pyrethrums)
Gardens Alive
Garden-Ville

Insect Killing Soap[a]: Allergy Relief Shop
Insect Oil: Gardens Alive or Garden-Ville
Ivory Liquid: mix 2-4 Tbsps. with 1 gallon water, use as a spray.
Ladybug Lures – Safer (attracts beneficial ladybugs): AEHF
Marigolds
Natural Guard Insecticidal Soap
Nematodes: Garden-Ville, Hydro Gardens
Neem Oil – Bioneem: Biocontrol Network, Peaceful Valley, Ringer, Safer
        (Works on army worms, web worms, hornworms, gypsy moths, field crickets, grasshoppers, white flies, leafminers, aphids, weevils, mealy bugs, and mosquitoes.)
Onion, garlic and pepper: mix 1 onion and several cloves of garlic with 2 tsps. red pepper and 2 cups water. Let this mixture sit one day, then strain through an old nylon. Add 1 tsp. detergent and 5 to 6 cups of water. Use as a spray.
Organic insecticides[a]: Monterey Lawn & Garden, Marshall Grain Co.
Ringer Insecticidal Soap: Gardens Alive, Garden-Ville
Rotenone[a] (root of tropical plant): Gardens Alive, Marshall Grain Co.
Sabadilla[a] (seeds of South African lily): Garden-Ville
Safer Houseplant Insecticidal Soap: AEHF
Shaklee Basic H or Neo-Life Green: mix 3 Tbsps. to 4 gallons of water, and spray around the foundation of the home to decrease insects. Also you can use as plant spray.
Turplex (safer alternative for golf courses): Agri-Dyne

FOR APHIDS, SPIDER MITES & WHITEFLIES
Aphid/White Fly Trap: Natural Gardening Co.
Arbico: Arizona Biological Co.
Azatin: Hydro Gardens
Beneficial Insects: Hydro Gardens
Buttermilk and flour diluted with one gallon of water. Use as a spray.
Encarsia formosa (natural pest that kills whiteflies): Garden-Ville
Garlic Spray
Insect Killing Soap[a]: Allergy Relief Shop
Ivory Liquid: mix 3 drops to gallon of water and spray.
Jalapeños: grind several fresh jalapeños, add water, boil, let stand overnight, strain. Mix with quart of water and use as a spray.
Ladybug Lures (attracts them to your garden) – Safer: AEHF
Ladybugs and lacewings: BioFac, Garden-Ville, Marshall Grain Co., Natural Gardening Co.
Liquid Seaweed: Garden-Ville
Margosan-O: Ringer
Natural Guard Insecticidal Soap: Walmart stores
Neem Oil – Bioneem: Biocontrol Network, Peaceful Valley, Ringer, Safer
Organica K-Neem Oil: AEHF

Less-Toxic Alternatives

Ringer Insecticidal Soap: Gardens Alive, Garden-Ville

Safer Insecticidal Soap &Houseplant Insecticidal Soap: AEHF, Marshall Grain Co.

Safer Houseplant Sticky Stakes (controls fungus gnats, whiteflies, blackflies, thrips and other flying insects): AEHF

Safer Rose & Flower Insect Killer: AEHF

Safer Sticky White Fly Traps: AEHF

Soap flakes: mix 2 Tbsps. with one gallon of water for use as a spray. Use a strong spray of water to knock the insects off the plants. Repeat every third day for 9 days to break up the egg cycle.

Soybean Oil: Natural Gardening Co.

Tangle-Traps: Tanglefoot Co.

FOR BLACK SPOT & POWDERY MILDEW

Baking soda spray (4 Tbsp. baking soda, 1 drop detergent and 2.5 Tbsps. oil in 1 gallon water)

Copper & sulfur fungicides[a]

Fungicidal Soap

Oil with soap: Mix 3 drops Ivory or alternate liquid detergent with 2/3 Tbsp. vegetable oil, add 1 quart water (spray)

For powdery mildew on roses: mix 1 Tbsp. baking soda and 2.5 Tbsp. mineral oil in 1 gallon water

OR 3-5 Tbsp. mineral oil and 1 Tbsp. detergent in 1 gallon water

FOR CRICKETS

Inside - Boric Acid, Roach Proof

Inside - Silica Aerogel (100% pure): Cabot Corp

Neem Oil – Bioneem: Biocontrol Network, Peaceful Valley, Ringer, Safer

Outside - Neem Oil – Margosan-O: Ringer

Bioneem: Biocontrol Network, Peaceful Valley, Ringer, Safer

Outside or attic – Niban Granular Bait (boric acid) and a Snuffer (Nisus Corp.) for use: Nisus Corp., Biocontrol Network

Keep grass mowed and back from the house – restrict vegetation near the house - keep outside lights turned off (that attracts crickets)

FOR GRASSHOPPERS / LEAFHOPPERS

Insect Killing Soap[a]: Allergy Relief Shop

Insecticidal Soap with Citrus Oil: Gardens Alive, The Natural Gardener, Peaceful Valley

Ladybugs: BioFac, Garden-Ville, Marshall Grain Co.

Neem Oil – Bioneem: Biocontrol Network, Peaceful Valley, Ringer, Safer

Nolo Bait: Hydro Gardens

FOR GRUBS

Nematodes: Garden-Ville, Hydro Gardens

Ringer

Safer Insect Killer

FOR GYPSY MOTHS
Neem Oil – Bioneem: Biocontrol Network, Peaceful Valley, Ringer, Safer
Safer Gypsy Moth Trap: AEHF

FOR LEAFMINERS
Azatin: Hydro Gardens
Beneficial Insects: Hydro Gardens
Neem Oil – Bioneem: Biocontrol Network, Peaceful Valley, Ringer, Safer

FOR MEALY BUGS
Beneficial Insects: Hydro Gardens
Insect Killing Soap□: Allergy Relief Shop
Ladybugs: BioFac, Garden-Ville, Marshall Grain Co.
Margosan-O: Ringer
Neem Oil – Bioneem: Biocontrol Network, Peaceful Valley, Ringer, Safer
Safer Insecticidal Soap & Houseplant Insecticidal Soap: AEHF, Marshall Grain
     Co.

FOR SCALE
Beneficial Insects: Hydro Gardens
Dormant Oil
Insect Killing Soap□: Allergy Relief Shop
Natural Guard Insecticidal Soap: Walmart stores
Ringer Insecticidal Soap: Ringer
Safer Insecticidal Soap: AEHF, Marshall Grain Co.

FOR SNAILS & SLUGS
Beer traps
Decoliate snails (destroys garden snails and eggs): Garden-Ville, Natural
     Gardening Co.
Perform late evening search and destroy
Remove tall grass and debris from vicinity of garden
Safer Slug & Snail Copper Barrier Tape: AEHF
Sluggo (organic)□: Monterey Lawn and Garden
Snail Bar Barrier
The Pit, Snail & Slug Trap – Safer: AEHF

FOR WEB WORMS & ARMY WORMS
Neem Oil – Bioneem: Biocontrol Network, Peaceful Valley, Ringer, Safer
Worm-Ender□: Monterey Lawn and Garden

NATURAL FERTILIZERS
AFM
Auntie Fuego Soil Conditioner (citrus oil and molasses blend): Garden-Ville
BioSafe
Comfrey leaves make a nitrogen-rich fertilizer. Soak several large leaves in a
     bucket of water for 3 days. Use the solution to water plants. Compost the
     leaves.

Compost Bioactivator: Allergy Relief Shop
Corn Meal Gluten (contains 10% nitrogen content)
Compost and vermicompost
Gardens Alive
Garden-Ville (organic fertilizers and natural foliar feeding products)
Marshall Grain Co.
Medina: The Living Source
Natural fertilizers and organic gardening supplies are now locally available, check with garden shops
Nitron Nature Meal & Formula A-35: Allergy Relief Shop
Organic fertilizers[□]: Abundant Earth, Monterey Lawn and Garden
Vitalize Natural Plant Food: Allergy Relief Shop

NATURAL HERBICIDES (WEED CONTROL)

Amazing Lawn: Gardens Alive
Corn Meal Gluten (inhibits weed germination and root development): Marshall Grain Co.
Herbicidal Soap: Ringer, Peaceful Valley, Gardens Alive
Marshall Grain Co.
Quik Weed Killer (organic)[□]: Monterey Lawn & Garden

~ Feed Your Lawn & Garden Organic Food ~

> > < <

Mice

YOU SHOULD AVOID
Poisons that contain toxins

LESS-TOXIC ALTERNATIVES
Galvanized steel trap: Real Goods
Sure Fire Smart Mouse Trap: Allergy Relief Shop

> > < <

Mosquitos & Other Biting Insects

YOU SHOULD AVOID
Applying insecticides to skin or clothes. May contain DEET (a nerve toxin)

LESS-TOXIC ALTERNATIVES
Avena Bugoff
Basil and sage
Blocker Kid's Spray & Light Country Lotion (DEET free): AEHF
Citronella candles or Citronella in olive oil base[□]: Marshall Grain Co.
Citronella, chamomile tea and witch hazel
Green Ban

Jungle Juice: Nutri Biotics
Lavender Oil
Mosquito Net Canopy: Real Goods
Mosquito Torpedo: The Living Source
Natrapel spray and lotion (aloe vera and 10% citronella): Allergy Relief Shop,
    Environmentally Sound Products Gardeners Supply Co.
Neem Oil – Bioneem: Biocontrol Network, Peaceful Valley, Ringer, Safer
Pennyroyal with or without eucalyptus
Skeeter Off (natural)
Skeeter Skatter⁰: Simmons Natural Body Care
Skeeter Shooo: Allergy Relief Shop
Solar Sound Waves (mosquito guard): Real Goods
Summit Mosquito Dunks: AEHF

Homemade Mosquito Repellant:
    2 oz. vegetable oil
    1/4 tsp. citronella and eucalyptus
    1/8 tsp. each pennyroyal, cedar, and rose geranium oils
    Combine, label and apply to skin. Keep away from mouth and eyes

Vitamin note: Taking 50-100 mg. B per day repels mosquitos (include a B
    Complex to achieve B vitamin equality.

FOR MOSQUITOS IN LAKES & PONDS
Bacillus Thuringiensis Israelensis (Liquid or Mosquito Dunks): Biofac, Hydro
    Gardens, Marshall Grain Co., Real Goods Ringer
Altosid® – Methoprene growth regulator: Specialty Products
These two products are most effective if used together.
Mosquito Dunks: AEHF, Marshall Grain Co.

> > < <

Moths

YOU SHOULD AVOID
Moth balls, moth flakes, mothproof shelf paper, and products that contain
    paradichlorobenzene or naphthalene

LESS-TOXIC ALTERNATIVES
AFM Herbal Moth Mixture: The Living Source
Agro-BioTech Codling Moth Trap: AEHF
Bay leaves, dried lemon peels or whole peppercorns
Brush clothes often (eggs are fragile and are easily destroyed)
Cedar Chips enclosed in cotton sachet⁰ or Cedar Oil
Clothes moth trap: Natural Gardening Co.
Hang clothes on an outside line (air and sunlight eliminate moths)
Herbal sachet: Abundant Earth
Lavender (dried)
Neem Oil – Bioneem: Biocontrol Network, Peaceful Valley, Ringer, Safer

Pheromone Trap: Insects, Ltd.
Repeated freezing and thawing of articles (destroys moths and eggs)
Richards Moth-Away (herbal – mint-fresh scent): AEHF
Rosemary and mint
Safer Clothes Moth Alert: AEHF
Sure Fire Clothes Moth Alert: Allergy Relief Shop
Wash woolens before storing (if washable) or run through dryer on warm cycle
    before storing – repeat every 2 or 3 months to kill moth larvae

Natural Moth Recipe:
    ½ lb. Rosemary, ½ lb. Mint, ¼ lb. Thyme, 2 lbs. Cloves, ¼ lb. ginseng
    Make a sachet of these herbs and hang in the closet.
For Flour & Meal Moths:
Safer Pantry Pest Trap: AEHF
Sure Fire Pantry Pest Trap: Allergy Relief Shop, Vermont Country Store
Panty Moth Trap: Natural Gardening Co.

> > < <

Roaches & Silverfish

Roaches adversely affect those with allergies and can cause asthmatic reactions

YOU SHOULD AVOID

Organophosphate, organochlorine and carbamate insecticides. High LD50
    (applied worldwide) ratings afford less mammalian toxicity, but refers
    only to oral and skin absorption. Does not include absorption by the lungs
    or account for individual differences.
Foggers, aerosols and pest motels that contain the above.
Pest control agencies

LESS-TOXIC ALTERNATIVES

Abamectin sulfluramide insecticidal bait: Gardens Alive, MSD Agvet, Peaceful
    Valley
Agro-BioTech Roach Trap: AEHF
Azatin: Hydro Gardens
Bait Gun: Specialty Products
Baking soda mixed half and half with powdered sugar (roaches cannot belch,
    so they will explode)
Boric Acid Powder (put under cabinet drawers, refrigerators, and in cracks -
    keep away from children and pets)
Bois-d-arc apples (slice and place on ground under or around building)
Caulk or plug all cracks and crevices
Concern Citrus Home Pest Control: AEHF
Combat Roach Traps[a] (with hydramethylnon)
Cooper Brite Roach Prufe: AEHF, The Living Source
Fungal Roach Bait – BioPath: EcoScience

Gencore (roach growth regulator)[a]
Harris Roach Tablets (do not use around small children or animals)
Jecta (injectable borate for painted, sealed or hard-to-reach wood): Nisus
The Lil Hummer (suction for cracks and crevices): Miracle Marketing
Maxforce (hydramethylnon bait growth regulator)
Nematodes: Garden-Ville, Hydro Gardens
Niban Granular Bait (boric acid) and a Snuffer (Nisus Corp.) for inside and
    outside: Nisus Corp., Biocontrol Network
Nibor (fine borate powder): Nisus Corp.
Remove all food sources and store all food in closed containers
Roach Kil (orthoboric acid): Allergy Relief Shop
Roach Proof
Roach Trap: put Vaseline and food inside open jars. Roaches crawl inside and
    cannot escape
Sea Bright Roach traps and bait: NEEDS

Make your own roach balls
    2 cups Boric Acid
    1 cup flour
    ¼ cup margarine
    1 small onion (chopped)
    Add enough water to form stiff dough. Roll into small balls. Place in the
    cupboards, behind the appliances and in closets. Keep away from small
    children and animals.

Homemade roach trap
    Grease inner neck of milk bottle and put a little raw potato or stale beer in
    it as bait. Once they get inside, they cannot get out.

FOR SILVERFISH
Diatomaceous Earth: AEHF, Allergy Relief Shop, Garden-Ville, Marshall Grain
    Co., Natural Animal
Inside:
    Agro-Biotech Silverfish Trap: AEHF
    Nibor (fine borate powder): Nisus Corp.
    Silica Aerogel (100% pure): Cabot Corp
    Roach Proof
Outside or attic:
    Niban Granular Bait (boric acid) and Snuffer: Nisus Corp., Biocontrol
        Network
    Snuffer (for dispensing Niban): Nisus Corp

> > < <

Spiders

LESS-TOXIC ALTERNATIVES
Agro-Biotech Spider Trap: AEHF
Glue boards
Natural pyrethrums[a]:** Allergy Relief Shop, Peaceful Valley, Roxide
International, Py-Rin (without Piperonyl Butoxide)
Bug Buster-O[a]: Monterey Lawn & Garden (contains petroleum) Tallon
Termite & Pest Control (California)
Niban Granular Bait (boric acid) for use inside and outside: Nisus Corp.,
Biocontrol Network
Silica Aerogel[a] (inject into wall with bait gun) (100% pure): Cabot Corp

> > < <

Termites

NOTE TO BUILDERS: If you are constructing a building, please read this
section carefully and use the correct means for termite control such as
nematodes, diatomaceous earth, silica gel, sand-gravel barriers, borate
derivatives, pyrethrins, termite shields and termite baits. Pay close attention
to water and drain pipes. Consider metal studs, and avoid pine and eucalyptus
woods which termites prefer.

YOU SHOULD AVOID
Organophosphates, organochlorines and synthetic pyrethroids

LESS-TOXIC ALTERNATIVES
Baits:
Sentricon System: Dow AgroSciences
Sulfluramide (above ground): FMC Corp., Specialty Products
Subtrafuse & Sentricon (below ground): American Cyanimid
Hydramethylnon: American Cyanimid
Bio-Blast (fungal, biological termiticide): EcoScience, Paragon
Bora-Care (treat wood studs before building): Nisus Corp.
Borax treated wood
Copper-8 Quinolinolate (9.6 oz.) If wood is in contact with soil.[a]
Copper shields on wood
Diatomaceous Earth: AEHF, Allergy Relief Shop, Garden-Ville, Marshall Grain
Co., Natural Animal
"First Line" (for subterranean termites only): Sterling Pest Mgt.
Jecta (injectable borate for painted, sealed or hard-to-reach wood): Nisus
Natural Pyrethrums[a]:** Allergy Relief Shop, Peaceful Valley, Roxide
International, Py-Rin (without Piperonyl Butoxide),
Bug Buster-O[a]: Monterey Lawn & Garden (contains petroleum) Tallon
Termite & Pest Control (California)
Nematodes: Garden-Ville, Hydro Gardens

Paraffin Wax – melted

Premise 75 (Imidacloprid): Bayer Corp.

Sand & gravel barrier - Bore 4.75 mm to 1.18 mm, 8" deep & wide

Spear (Nematodes)

Synthetic Pyrethroids[a]: The following synthetic pyrethroids are not generally recommended because they may be toxic to some and should be used only after careful consideration of the risk. If used, they should be mixed only with water.

> Demon TC[a] (a cypermethrin)
>
> Dragnet FT[a] – similar to Torpedo (contains piperonyl butoxide – contains no xylene)
>
> Tempo[a]
>
> Torpedo[a] (contains 5% xylene)
>
> Tribute[a]

Tallon Termite & Pest Control (California)

Termidor (active ingredient Fipronil): Aventis Environmental Science

Termite Proof

Tim-bor® (Disodium Octaborate Tetrahydrate) – can be used in wall voids: Nisus, U.S. Borax, Marshall Grain Co.

Wood treatment recipe: Mix 1 ½ cup boiled linseed oil and 1 oz. paraffin wax. Add mineral spirits to make 1 gallon.[a] Dip ends and joints in solution for 1-3 minutes. Label clearly.

You should be out of the house for 2 weeks past pesticide usage.

> > < <

DRYWOOD TERMITES

YOU SHOULD AVOID

Methyl bromide and toxic fumigants

LESS-TOXIC ALTERNATIVES

Abamectin sulfluramide insecticidal bait: Gardens Alive, MSD Agvet, Peaceful, Sterling Pest Mgt.

Bio-Blast (fungal, biological termiticide): Paragon

Electrogun: Michelin Service Co.

Heat Treatment: Isothermics

Natural pyrethrums[a]:** Allergy Relief Shop, Peaceful Valley, Roxide International, Py-Rin (without Piperonyl Butoxide)

> Bug Buster-O[a]: Monterey Lawn & Garden (contains petroleum) Tallon Termite & Pest Control (California)

> > < <

Wood Beetles

YOU SHOULD AVOID

All commercial insecticides

196

LESS-TOXIC ALTERNATIVES
Bio-Blast: Paragon
Bora-Care: Nisus Corp, Allergy Relief Shop
Dri-Die (silica ammonium fluorosilicate)
Drione[°] (silica gel and pyrethrums): Roxide International, The Natural Gardener
Silica Aerogel (100% pure): Cabot Corp
Electrogun: Michelin Service Co.
Kiln dried wood
Less toxic wood sealant
Natural pyrethrums[°]:** Allergy Relief Shop, Peaceful Valley, Roxide
    International, Py-Rin (without Piperonyl Butoxide),
      Bug Buster-O[°]: Monterey Lawn & Garden (contains petroleum) Tallon
        Termite & Pest Control (California)
Natural varnish[°]
Paint wood with a safe paint
Torpedo[°] (synthetic permethrin)

> > < <

Yellow Jackets & Wasps

LESS-TOXIC ALTERNATIVES
Insect Killing Soap[°]: Allergy Relief Shop
Insecticidal Soap - citrus oil plus pyrethrin[°]: Ringer, Peaceful Valley
Yellow jacket/wasp traps & baits: AEHF, Allergy Relief Shop, Environmentally
    Sound Products, Marshall Grain Co., NEEDS
Wasp stopper - 20% boric acid

FOR APPLICATION OF BAITS & BORA-CARE
Bait Gun: Specialty Products
Chemtech Multi-Foamer: Chemtech Supply

> > < <

**Natural pyrethrums should not be used in living area. May be toxic to some.
Even some natural pyrethrums contain petroleum distillates.

> > < <

Pet Care

Weekly shampooing, conditioning and treatment of pets will not only reduce the risk of fleas and ticks, it will also remove allergy-causing dander and other irritants.

To check for fleas in the house, put a bowl of water on the floor in a dark room, and place a light over it. Check the water the next morning for fleas (they are drawn to the light at night). This is a good measure of the flea population in the house.

Use cider vinegar[°] to remove pet odor.

You should test your pet for allergy to a product before using it. Avoid using products on pet's faces. Do not use products containing d-limonene or linalool on cats. Avoid organophosphates. If you wouldn't use it on yourself, avoid using it on your pets.

> > < <

Pet Beds, Litter Boxes, & Pet Accessories

LESS-TOXIC ALTERNATIVES
Chemical-Free, 100% Organic Pet Beds: Chemically Sensitive Living, Lifekind Products
Hemp Collars & Leads: A Happy Planet
Herbal Pet Collars: The Living Source,
Zeolite Kitty Litter Freshener: Absolute Environmental's

> > < <

Pet Shampoo & Treatments

LESS-TOXIC ALTERNATIVES
Allerpet: Absolute Environmental's, Priorities
Ambio-Clean: Rainman Int.
Fleabusters Shampoo®: Fleabusters
Groom Master Pet Shampoo (boric acid): Natural Animal
Herbal products for pet care: The Living Source, Priorities
Natural Animal Herbal Shampoo and Powders: Allergy Relief Shop
Natural Chemistry Fur and Feather: Allergy Relief Shop
Pet Organics Herbal Shampoo and treatments: The Living Source
Safer Flea Soap: Peaceful Valley
Yeast and Garlic Bits: Allergy Relief Shop
VIP Citrus Based Shampoo & Spray: Vet Express
For Dogs: Citrus Peel Spray (contains d-limonene and linalool, which kills all stages of the flea's life cycle). Simmer 6-8 citrus peels in 1-2 quarts of water for 2-3 hours. Adding more water as needed. (Can also use grated orange peel for a shorter cooking time) Let the liquid stand until it cools. Then strain. Add more water and spritz on dog beds and dogs, working the solution into the coat (do not use on cats).
For Cats: make an herbal brew of rosemary, rue or wormwood; cool, strain and gently sponge the cat.

> > < <

Fleas & Ticks

YOU SHOULD AVOID
Petrochemicals and pesticides in flea and tick collars.

LESS-TOXIC ALTERNATIVES
FOR FLEAS ON ANIMALS
Cedar chips in bedding

Citronella oilᵒ: Marshall Grain Co.

Diatom Dust Insect Powder (diatomaceous earth powder): Allergy Relief Shop

Diatomaceous Earth: AEHF, Allergy Relief Shop, Garden-Ville, Marshall Grain
    Co., Natural Animal

Dri-Die

Natural Animal Herbal Flea Collar & Insect Shooo: Natural Animal, Allergy
    Relief Shop

Flea Stop by Farnam Corp.

Garlic and Brewer's Yeast (tablet or powder – feed your pet daily): The Living
    Source

Herbal collars for dogs and cats: The Living Source, Priorities

Herbs in the animal's bedding: wormwood, oil of eucalyptus, oil of lavender,
    winter savory or tansy

Insect Killing Soapᵒ: Allergy Relief Shop

Natural Animal

Pennyroyal Oil (soak a piece of rope in it and place around pet's neck)

Pennyroyal herbs – plant around house – also use dried herbs

Pet Organics Herbal Flea Products: The Living Source

Ringers Entire Flea & Tick Spray (insecticidal soap and pyrethrins)
    (Can also be used on inside pets, carpets, bedding, floors and other areas
    where eggs hide): The Living Source

Safers Insecticidal Flea Soap (fatty acid-based soap)

Silica Aerogel works on cats and some dogs (100% pure): Cabot Corp.

Wash pet bedding at least once a week – more often during infestations

Homemade herbal flea powder
2 ounces pennyroyal, 1 ounce norwood, 1 ounce rosemary and 1 tsp. cayenne
    pepper

FOR TICKS
A tick will loosen if touched with a drop of Tincture of Merthiolate or a hot
    match. You can then pick the tick off with tweezers.

Diatomaceous Earth (apply outside): AEHF, Allergy Relief Shop, Garden-
    Ville, Marshall Grain Co., Natural Animal

Citrus Oil D-limonene or linalool (not on cats): Hansens Pet Systems

Insect Killing Soapᵒ: Allergy Relief Shop

Insecticidal Soap with Citrus Oil: Natural Gardener, Gardens Alive, Peaceful
    Valley

Natural pyrethrumsᵒ:** Allergy Relief Shop, Peaceful Valley, Roxide
    International, Py-Rin (without Piperonyl Butoxide),
        Bug Buster-Oᵒ: Monterey Lawn & Garden (contains petroleum): Tallon
        Termite & Pest Control (California)

Permaguard (diatomaceous earth and pyrethrums): The Living Source, Pristine
    Products
Plant sage outside to keep ticks away

FOR INSIDE FLEAS/TICKS
(For floors, carpets and upholstery)
Steam clean or heat treat carpet and upholstery every week for three weeks to
    get adults and larvae, then use HEPA vacuum daily; then at least once a
    week for a month. Discard or freeze vacuum bags after each use. Can
    then spray with a growth regulator.
Agro-BioTech Flea Trap: AEHF
Bonide Fleas Beater For Carpets: AEHF
Boric Acid - Roach Prufe: The Living Source
Carpet Stuff
Citra-Solv[a] - use ¼ cup in 1 gallon of water (use on floors)
Concern Citrus Home Pest Control: AEHF
Demize (d-limonene): Paragon, Marshall Grain Co.
Diatomaceous Earth (apply carefully outside): AEHF, Allergy Relief Shop,
    Garden-Ville, Marshall Grain Co., Natural Animal
Ecology Works Fleanix Flea Control[a]: Allergy Relief Shop
Enforcer Over Nite Flea Trap: AEHF
Insect Killing Soap[a]: Allergy Relief Shop
Methoprene Insect Growth Regulator - Precor[a] : Marshall Grain Co.
    Must be away for a week when used – use only as last resort.
Natural Citrus Carpet Powder: The Living Source
Rock Salt - pour 2 ounces of lavender oil over 2-3 quarts of rock salt. Sprinkle
    over areas - do not walk on it.
Safer[a] Entire Flea & Tick Spray (insecticidal soap and pyrethrins)
Sodium Polyborate[a] – Rx for Fleas Plus powder: Fleabusters
    Must be absent when applied to carpet and first vacuumed (with HEPA or
    water vac). Shampoo carpet for removal. Sprinkle rock salt in the carpet,
    and leave it for a few days before vacuuming.
Torus Fenoxycarb[a] (IG regulator)
Herbs and baking soda blended together.

FOR OUTSIDE FLEAS & TICKS – IN YOUR YARD
BioBuster (beneficial nematode): Fleabusters
D-limonene[a] (Do not use on cats or inside your house)
Diatomaceous Earth: AEHF, Allergy Relief Shop, Garden-Ville, Marshall Grain
    Co., Natural Animal
Insecticidal Flea Soap: Ringers
Nematodes: Garden-Ville, Hydro Gardens
Permaguard (diatomaceous earth and pyrethrums): Pristine Products
Plant sage to keep them away

> > < <

Part IV: Resource Directory
Knowledge needs to be applied
Products need to be located.

> >< <

We have tried to make this as up-to-date as possible.
If you discover any incorrect information
or know of changes in information, please contact the publisher.

> >< <

MAIL ORDER &
INTERNET RESOURCES

A Happy Planet *(multiple products)* .... (888) 946-4277
    2261 Market St. PMB #71, San Francisco, CA 94114
    Retail outlet: 3242 16th St., San Francisco, CA .... Fax: (415) 821-2770
    www.ahappyplanet.com/ahpstore

AEHF *(multiple products)* .... (800) 428-2343 or (214) 361-9519
    American Environmental Health Foundation .... Fax: (214) 361-2534
    8345 Walnut Hill Ln., Ste. 225, Dallas, TX 75231
    www.aehf.com   e-mail: aehf@aehf.com

AFM Enterprises, Inc. *(personal care, cleaners, paints, etc)* .. (619) 239-0321
    350 W. Ash St., #700, San Diego, CA 92101

Abrams Royal Pharmacy .... (800) 458-0804 or (214) 349-8000
    8220 Abrams Rd., Dallas, TX 75231

Absolute Environmental's Allergy Store ... (800) 771-2246 or (954) 472-0128
    3504 S. University Dr., Davie, FL 33328 .... Fax: (954) 464-9133
    www.allergystore.com e-mail: allergy@allergystore.com

Abundant Earth .... (888) 51-EARTH (513-2784) or (360) 386-2186
    762 W. Park Ave., Port Townsend, WA 98368 .... Fax: (360) 386-2196
    www.abundantearth.com e-mail: goodstuff@abundantearth.com

Air Technology Systems, Inc. *(air handling)* .... (301) 620-2033
    1572 Tilco Dr., Frederick, MD 21704

Aireox Research Corp. *(air handling)* .... (909) 689-2781
    11004 Hole Ave., Riverside, CA 92505

Alexandra Avery Purely Natural Skin Care *(sunscreen)* .... (503) 236-5926
    4717 SE Belmont St., Portland, OR 97215

Allegro Natural Dyes, Boulder, CO 80302 *(fabric dyes)* .... (303) 247-0784
Allergy Alternative .... (800) 838-1514 or (707) 838-1514
    526 Shagbark St., Windsor, CA 95492 .... e-mail: allergy@ap.net
    (heaters, air purification systems)
Allergy-Asthma Technology .... (800) 621-5545 or (847) 966-2952
    8224 Lehigh Ave., Morton Grove, IL 60053
    www.allergyasthmatech.com *(bedding, cleaning products)*
Allergy Control Products, Inc. *(multiple products)* .. (800) 422-DUST (3878)
    www.allergycontrol.com .... Fax: (203) 431-8963
Allergy Relief Shop, Inc. *(multiple products)* .... (800) 626-2810
    3360 Andersonville Hwy., Andersonville, TN 37705
    www.allergyreliefshop.com e-mail: allergy@ix.netcom.com
    Consultation Phone: (423) 494-4100 .... ARS Lab Phone: (423) 494-4109
Allergy Relief Store *(multiple products)* .... (800) 866-7464
    250 Watson Glen, Franklin, TN 37064 .... (615) 866-7464
    www.allergyreliefstore.com
Allermed Inc. *(air purification systems)* .... (972) 442-4898
    31 Steel Rd., Wylie, TX 75098
Allerx (a division of Dust Free) .... (800) 447-1100 or (972) 635-2580
    P.O. Box 1119, Royce City, TX 75189 .... Fax: (800) 929-9712
    www.allerx.com *(air filtration/purification & misc. allergy products)*
Alpine Industries *(vapor barrier)* .... (916) 926-2460
    P.O. Box 277, Mt. Shasta, CA 96067
Alternative Baby *(baby products)* .... (800) 469-1126
    www.alternativebaby.com see also www.alternativebaby.org
Alternative Undies *(clothing)* .... (888) 471-1935
    PMB 225, 1537 Fourth St., San Rafael, CA 94901
    www.pantyparlour.com
American Biltrite *(Duravinyl flooring)* .... (905) 507-2401
    90 Matheson Blvd. W., Mississauga, Ontario, Canada L5R 353
American Environmental Products *(lighting)* .... (800) 339-9572
    625 Mathews St., Fort Collins, CO 80524 .... Fax: (970) 482-5816
    www.sunalux.com
American Porcelain Enamel Co. of Dallas .... (214) 637-4775
    3506 Singleton Blvd., Dallas, TX 75212 *(porcelain panels)*
Appel Co. *(Orange Glo floor cleaner)* .... (303) 740-7637
    8765 E. Orchard Rd., Englewood, CO 80111
Arizona Biological Co. *(pesticides)* .... (800) 767-2847 or (520) 826-9785
    18701 N. Lago Del Oro Pkwy., Tucson, AZ 85737
Arizona Health Foods .... (800) 333-4172
    13802 N. 32nd St. #14, Phoenix, AZ 85032
    www.arizonahealthfoods.com e-mail: goodhealth@azhf.com

Aroma Vera, Inc. *(aromatic oils)*............... (800) 669-9514 or (310) 280-0407
    5901 Rodeo Rd., Los Angeles, CA 90016 .... www.aromavera.com
Atlantic Recycled Paper Co. .... (800) 323-2811 or (410) 747-7314
    20 Winters Ln., Catonsville, MD 21228
Aubrey Organics *(cosmetics, personal care products)* .... (800) 282-7394
    4419 N. Manhattan Ave., Tampa, FL 33614 .... Fax: (813) 876-8166
    www.aubrey-organics.com   e-mail: marketing@aubrey-organics.com
Aura Cacia *(essential oils)* .... (800) 437-3301 or (707) 795-1312
    Weaverville, CA *(to locate a distributor)* .... www.auracacia.com
Auromere *(herbal toothpaste, soaps, herbs, oils)* .... (800) 735-4691
    2621 W. Hwy. 12, Lodi, CA 95242
    www.auromere.com   e-mail: sasp@lodinet.com
Aventis Environmental Science *(termaticide)*
    95 Chestnut Ridge Rd., Montvale, NJ 07645
B.Coole Designs *(clothing)* .... (800) 992-8924 or (707) 575-8924
    (Formerly Richman Cotton Co.) 2631 Piner Rd., Santa Rosa, CA 95401
    www.bcoole.com   e-mail: info@bcoole.com
The Baby Lane *(baby items)* .... (888) 387-0019 or (252) 634-9937
    4523 Rivershore Dr., New Bern, NC 28560 .... Fax: (509) 357-4529
    www.thebabylane.com   e-mail: lisa@thebabylane.com
Basic Coatings, Inc. *(wood treatment)* .... (800) 441-1934
    P.O. Box 677, Des Moines, IA 50303
    www.basiccoatings.com   e-mail: bcinfo@basiccoatings.com
Bauer Inc., Eddie *(clothing)* .... (800) 426-8020 / Fax: (800) 414-6110
    Redmond, WA 98052 .... www.eddiebauer.com
Biocontrol Network .... (800) 370-4301 or (615) 370-4301
    (Integrated pest management products) .... Fax: (615) 370-0662
    5116 Williamsburg Rd, Brentwood, TN 37027
    www.biconet.com   e-mail info@biconet.com
BioFac, Inc. *(beneficial insects)* .... (800) 223-4914
    P.O. Box 36, Mathis, TX 78368 .... Fax: (361) 547-9660
    www.Biofac.com   e-mail: info@biofac.com
BioShield Paint Company (See Eco Design)
Bison Specialties *(fabrics)* .... (406) 259-6342
    9230 Pryor Rd., Billings, MT 59101
Blue Canoe *(organic clothing)* .... (888) 923-1373 or (707) 923-1373
    P.O. Box 543, 390-A Lake Benbow Dr., Garberville, CA 95542
    www.bluecanoe.com e-mail: info@bluecanoe.com Fax: (707) 923-1374
Blue Star, Inc. *(tents)* .... (800) 752-8877
    6980 U.S. Hwy. 10E, Missoula, MI 59802
Born to Love *(baby's and women's special needs)* .... (905) 725-2559
    445 Centre St. S., Oshawa, ON, Canada L1H 4C1
    www.borntolove.com .... Fax: (905) 725-3297

Bossaire Inc. *(air handling)* .... (612) 378-0049
   2901 4th St. SE, Minneapolis, MN 55414 .... Fax: (612) 378-2604
   www.bossaire.com   e-mail: bossaire@mm.com
Cabot Corp. *(pesticides)* .... (800) 222-6145
   700 E. U.S. Hwy. 36, Tuscola, IL 61953-9643
Canary Fashion Inc. *(clothing)* .... (212) 274-8223
   161 Grand St., New York, NY 10013
Capitol City Mattress Co. Inc. *(bedding)* .... (615) 227-2751
   900 Main St., Nashville, TN 37206
Carousel Carpet Mills *(carpets)* .... (707) 485-0333
   1 Carousel Ln., Ukiah, CA 95482
C-Cure of California *(grouts, sealers)* ...... (800) 325-6851 or (909) 947-0028
   1420 S. Bon View Ave., Ontario, CA 91761 .... Fax: (909) 947-4095
   www.c-cure.com (Larry Wilson) .... Order fax: (800) 547-7557
Chambers *(carpets and bedding)* .... (800) 334-9790
   P.O. Box 7841, San Francisco, CA 94120-7841
Chemically Sensitive Living *(multiple products)* .... (888) 891-7293
   377 Wilburn Ave. #213, Swansea, MA 02777
   www.chemsenlvng.com   e-mail: business@chemsenlvng.com
Chemtech Supply Inc. *(pesticides)* .... (800) 848-7578 or (480) 833-7578
   1905 S. MacDonald, Mesa, AZ 85210
Childsake *(toys, crafts, etc.)* .... (650) 595-1765 / Fax: (650) 595-2895
   P.M.B. 88, 2033 Ralston Ave., Belmont, CA 94002-1737
   www.childsake.com e-mail: store@childsake.com
Clearly Natural Products *(soaps)* .... (707) 762-5815
   P.O. Box 750024, Petaluma, Ca 94975-0024 .... Fax: (707) 762-5816
   www.clearlynaturalsoaps.com e-mail: info@clearlynaturalsoaps.com
The Cloth Bag Company .... (770) 393-0058
   1249 Pitts Rd., Atlanta, GA 30350
   www.clothbag.com e-mail: sales@clothbag.com
Collins Aikman Floor Covering Division . (800) 241-4902 or (214) 749-0663
   1519 Hi Line Dr., Dallas, TX 75207 *(Sutherland Mill carpets)*
Cordwainers *(shoes)* .... (603) 463-7742
   67 Candia Rd., Deerfield, NH 03037
Corning/Revere Customer Information Center .... (800) 999-3436
   140 Washington Ave., P.O. Box 7369, Endicott, NY 13761
   www.corningware.com e-mail: ccpci@mmcweb.com
Costa Rica Natural *(recycled paper)* .... (305) 666-0034 or (800) 777-3378
   5000 SW 75th Ave., Miami, FL 33155 .... Fax: (800) 443-8977
   www.ecopaper.com
Cotton Plus, Inc. *(natural cotton fabrics)* .... (806) 428-3345
   822 Baldridge St., O'Donnell, TX 79351 .... Fax: (806) 439-6647
   www.cottonplus.com

Less-Toxic Alternatives

The Country Store *(multiple products)* ..... (888) 747-6764 or (804) 737-6764
   412 Acreview Dr., Highland Springs, VA 23075
   e-mail: revision@gte.net
Coyuchi Inc. *(bed linens)* .... (888) 418-8847 or (415) 663-8077
   P.O. Box 845, Point Reyes Station, CA 94956......... Fax: (415) 663-8104
   www.coyuchiorganic.com   e-mail: info@coyuchiorganic.com
Crown City Mattress .... (626) 452-8655 / Fax (626) 452-1590
   11134 Rush St, South El Monte, CA 91733
The Dasun Co. .... (800) 433-8929 or (760) 480-8929
   P.O. Box 668, Escondito, CA 92033 .... Fax: (760) 746-8865
   (air filtration, cleaning products)
Decent Exposures .... (800) 524-4949 or (206) 364-4540
   P.O. Box 27206, Seattle WA 98125-1606
   www.decentexposures.com *(baby needs, women's needs and clothing)*
Dellinger Inc. *(carpet)* .... (706) 291-4447
   75 Eden Valley Rd. SE, Rome, GA 30161
Denny Wholesale Services .... (800) 327-6616 or (954) 971-3100
   3500 Gateway Dr., Pompano Beach, FL 33069 .... Fax: (954) 972-0910
   www.dennywholesale.com e-mail: dennywholesale@aol.com
   (vapor barrier – for product information and area dealers)
Denver Tent Co. *(tents)* .... (303) 399-3232
   4004 Grape St., Denver, CO 80216
Dermalight Systems *(UV light – mold inhibitor)* .... (818) 995-4274
   13425 Ventura Blvd., Sherman Oaks, CA 91423
Desert Aire Co. *(industrial dehumidifiers)* .... (414) 357-7400
   8300 W. Sleske Court, Milwaukee, WI 53223 .... www.desert-aire.com
Desert Essence Cosmetics .... (800) 848-7331 or (817) 734-1735
   9700 Topanga Canyon Blvd., Chatsworth, CA 91311
   www.desertessence.com/products.htm *(Australian tea tree oil products)*
Designs by Droste *(metal cabinets for kitchen & bath)* .... (817) 763-5031
   4818 Camp Bowie, Fort Worth, TX 75107
Deva Lifewear Inc. *(clothing)* .... (800) 222-8024
   P.O. Box 266, Westhope, ND 58793 .... Fax: (800) 251-1746
   www.devalifewear.com   e-mail: deva@ndak.net
Diamond Brand Inc. *(wood toothpicks)* .... (800) 777-7942 or (207) 645-2574
   1800 Caloquet Ave., Caloquet, MN 55720 .... www.diamondbrand.com
Diamond Organics .... (888) ORGANIC (675-2642)
   P.O. Box 2159, Freedom, CA 95019 .... Fax: (888) 888-6777
   www.diamondorganics.com   e-mail: info@diamondorganics.com
Dickson Bros. Inc. *(water treatment)* .... (972) 288-7537
   204 N. Galloway Ave., Mesquite, TX 75149
Dixie Peterson *(masks & signs)* .... (417) 842-3279
   1095 SW 90th Rd, Oronogo, MO 64855

Dow Agrosciences Co. *(pesticides)* .... (800) 686-6200
    9330 Zionsville Rd., Indianapolis, IN 46268 .... www.dowelanco.com
Drugstore.com *(supplements, cosmetics - not all their products are less-toxic)*
    www.drugstore.com
Dust Free *(see also Allerx)* .... (800) 441-1107 or (972) 635-9564
    P.O. Box 519, 1112 Industrial, Royse City, TX 75189
    www.dustfree.com .... Fax: (800) 929-9712 or (972) 635-2713
Eagle Cabinets & Construction *(furniture)* .... (870) 453-3245
    Hwy. 62 E., Flippin, AR 72634
Earth Friendly Products *(multiple products)* .... (800) 335-ECOS (3267)
    44 Greenbay Rd., Winnetka, Illinois 60093
    www.ecos.com   e-mail: ecos@mcs.com
Earth Science *(hair & body care)* .... (800) 222-6720 or (909) 371-7565
    P.O. Box 1925, Corona, CA 91718 .... Fax: (909) 371-0509
Earth Speaks *(organic clothing)* .... (718) 694-8338
    69 Columbia St., Brooklyn, NY 11201
    www.earthspeaks.com   e-mail: info@earthspeaks.com
Earth Weave Carpets .... (706) 695-8800 / Fax: (706) 695-8885
    P.O. Box 6120, Dalton, GA 30722 .... www.earthweave.com
Earthlings *(children & infant wear)* ... (888) GO BABY O or (805) 643-2590
    592 E. Main St., Ventura, CA 93001
    www.earthlings.net   e-mail: orders@earthlings.net for catalog
Earth's Best *(baby food)* .... www.earthsbest.com
Earthwise Basics *(children's needs)* .... (800) 791-3957 or (802) 254-2235
    214 Elliot St., Ste. 2, Brattleboro, VT 05301 .... Fax: (802) 254-4254
    www.ediapers.com   e-mail: candc@ediapers.com or
    www.naturaltoys.com   e-mail: elves@naturaltoys.com
    (women's & baby's needs and incontinence supplies)
Ecco Bella *(sunscreen)* .... (877) 696-2220
    www.eccobella.com
Eco-Baby   www.ecobaby.com .... (888) ECOBABY or (619) 562-9606
    322 Coogan Way, El Cajon, CA 92020 .... Fax: (619) 562-0199
Eco-Bags Products Inc. .... (800) 720-2247 (914) 944-4556
    42 Stone Ave., Ossining, NY 10562 .... Fax: (914) 944-4609
    www.eco-bags.com   e-mail: Inquiries@ecobags.com
Eco Design – The Natural Choice .... (800) 621-2591 or (505) 438-3448
    (Also BioShield Paint Company and Livos Plant Chemistry)
    1365 Rufino Circle, Santa Fe, NM 87505
    www.bioshieldpaint.com   e-mail: edesignco@aol.com
EcoExpress *(gift baskets)* .... (800) 733-3495 / Fax: (415) 884-3036
    85 Galli Dr., Ste. E, Novato, CA 94949 .... www.ecoexpress.com
Eco-Logique *(women's needs)* .... (800) 680-9739 or (613) 596-6389
    P.O. Box 32073, 1386 Richmond Rd., Ottawa, ON, Canada K2B1A1
    www.eco-logique.com .... Fax: (613) 820-1626

Eco-Mall *(multiple resources for less-toxic products)*
   www.ecomall.com *(on-line environmental shopping center)*
Eco-Organics *(hemp & cotton clothing, body care)*.... (888) ECO-FASHION
   New Jersey 07304 .... www.eco-organics.com
EcoScience Corporation *(pesticides)* .... (800) 998-2467 or (732) 676-3000
   17 Christopher Way, Eatontown, NJ 07724-3325 ..... Fax: (732) 676-3031
   www.ecosci.com   e-mail: wsmith@ecoscience.com
Eco Smarte of Dallas / Ft. Worth Inc *(water treatment)* .... (817) 543-1681
   Arlington, TX 76002
Ecosport, Inc. *(clothing)*........................... (800) 486-4326 or (828) 687-7011
   3871 Sweeten Creek Rd., Arden, NC 28704 .... Fax: (828) 687-7077
   www.ecosport.net .... Fabric division (908) 272-7500
Edcor *(fruit and vegetable wash)* Dept. CG, 351-K Oak Place, Brea, CA 92621
ENutrition *(personal care products)* .... (800) 641-5558
   8550 Balboa Blvd. Ste. 140, Northridge, CA 91325
   www.enutrition.com
Environmental Health Center .... (214) 368-4132
   8345 Walnut Hill Ln, Ste. 220, Dallas, TX 75231 ... Fax: (214) 691-8432
   www.ehcd.com
Environmentally Sound Products *(multiple products)*............. (800) 886-5432
   P.O. Box 214, 167 Main St., Eldred, PA 16731
Ethical Shopper .... (877) 4-e-ethic (433-8442)
   www.ethicalshopper.com *(On-line source for multiple product lines)*
Euroclean *(vacuum—see Nilfisk)*
Euro Marble & Granite *(flooring)*.. (214) 741-9002
   161 Pittsburg St., Dallas, TX 75207
EuroSteam *(special cleanups)*... (817) 297-7745
   110 S. Hampton, Crowley, TX 76036 .... Fax: (817) 297-6675
   www.eurosteam.com
Everpure, Inc. *(water treatment)* .... (800) 942-1153 or (630) 654-4000
   660 Blackhawk Dr., Westmont, IL 60559 .... Fax: (630) 654-1115
   http://www.everpure.com/consumer/distributor.html *(for distributors)*
FMC Corp. *(pesticides)*........................... (800) 321-1FMC or (800) 321-3621
   P.O. Box 8, Princeton, NJ 08543 .... www.fmc.com
Fair Trade Naturals *(clothing)*.............. (888) NOCHEMS or (888) 662-4367
   www.algomaya.com
Feeling Goods *(furniture, household goods)* .... (877) 349-2102
   5511 Keybridge Dr., Boise, ID 83703 .... Fax: (877) 349-2103
   www.feeling-goods.com e-mail: info@feeling-goods.com
Filter Queen *(vacuums)*............................ (800) 344-1840 or (216) 986-8008
   www.filterqueen.com   e-mail: marketing@filterqueen.com
Flea Busters *(pet care)* .... (800) 666-3532
   6555 NW 9ᵗʰ Ave., Ste. 412, Fort Lauderdale, FL 33309
   www.fleabuster.com

Forbo Industries *(vinyl flooring, vapor barriers)* .... (800) 233-0475
   P.O. Box 667, Hazelton, Pa 18201 .... www.forbo.com
Foust, E.L. Co. .... (800) EL-FOUST (353-6878) or (630) 834-4952
   P.O. Box 105, Elmhurst, IL 60126 .... Fax: (630) 834-5341
   www.foustco.com   e-mail: sales@foustco.com
   (water filtration & air purification)
FoxFiber *(fabrics)* .... (520) 684-7199
   Natural Cotton Colours, Inc., P.O. Box 66, Wickenburg, AZ 85358
   www.foxfibre.com   e-mail: nodyes@foxfiber.com
Fred Nelson & Associates *(See The Safe Reading & Computer Box Co.)*
Friedrich AC Co. *(air purifiers)* .... (800) 541-6645 or (210) 357-4480
   4200 N. Pan Am Expwy., P.O. Box 1540, San Antonio, TX 78295-1540
   www.bestaircleaner.com or www.friedrich.com
Furnature *(organic upholstered furniture and bedding)* .... (617) 792-3169
   319 Washington St., Boston, MA 02135-3395 .... Fax: (617) 787-0350
   www.furnature.com   e-mail: furnature@tiac.net
GAIAM – See Harmony
Gardeners Supply Company .... (888) 833-1412 or (802) 660-3505
   128 Intervale Rd., Burlington, VT 05401 .... Fax: (800) 551-6712
   www.gardeners.com   e-mail: info@gardeners.com
Gardens Alive *(pesticides)* .... (812) 537-8650
   776 Rudolph Way, Lawrenceburg, IN 47025 .... Fax: (817) 537-5108
   www.gardensalive.com e-mail: gardenhelp@gardensalive.com
Gardenville, Inc. *(pesticides - several area stores)* .... (210) 651-6115
   Office: 7561 E. Evans Rd., San Antonio, TX .... www.garden-ville.com
Garnet Hill *(clothing, bedding)* .... (800) 622-6216 or (603) 823-5545
   231 Main St., Franconia, NH 03580 .... Fax: (888) 842-9696
   (bedding, home furnishings and clothing) .... www.garnethill.com
Gazoontite *(multiple products)* .... (415) 931-2230
   Main store: 2157 Union St., San Francisco, CA ..... www.gazoontite.com
   (Stores also in Costa Mesa, CA, & New York City) ....
Gemplers *(masks)* .... (800) 382-8473 / Fax: (800) 551-1128
   www.gemplers.com
Gloucester Co. Inc. .... (800) 343-4963 or (508) 528-2200
   235 Cottage St., Franklin, MA 02038 *(caulking and sealers)*
Golden Furniture Maker *(natural wood furniture)* .... (561) 586-5157
   3599 23rd Ave. S. #5, Lake Worth, FL 33461 .... Fax: (571) 586-5130
   www.woodever.com e-mail: woodever@earthlink.net
Goodkind Pen Company, Inc .... (800) 947-2250 or (207) 594-6207
   The Goodkind Bldg., 500 Main St., Rockland, ME 04841
   (wood writing pens) .... Fax: (207) 594-5840
Granny's Old Fashioned Products *(cleaning, laundry, hair care, personal care)*
   P.O. Box 256, Arcadia, CA 91006 *(for list of distributors)*

Grass Roots Natural Goods *(multiple products)* .... (800) 226-0924
   13 S. Linn St. #9, Iowa City, IA 52240 .... Fax: (319) 354-7853
   www.g-roots.com   e-mail: info@grng.com
Green Babies *(baby & infant clothing, dolls)*......................... (800) 603-7508
   www.greenbabies.com .... Fax: (914) 524-7906
Green Field Paper Co. *(organic paper)*..... (888) 402-9979 or (619) 338-9432
   1330 "G" St., San Diego, CA 92101 .... (619) 338-0308
   www.greenfieldpaper.com
Green iDeals *(On-line store for multiple product lines)*.......... (617) 864-0770
   1619 Massachusetts Ave., Cambridge, MA 02138-2753
   www.greenideals.com .... (617) 249-2067
GreenLine Paper Company *(non-chlorine paper)*................... (800) 641-1117
   631 S. Pine St., York PA 17403 .... Fax: (717) 846-3806
   www.greenlinepaper.com
GreenMarketplace.com .... (888) 59-EARTH
   5808 Forbes Ave., Pittsburgh, PA 15217 .... Fax: (412) 420-6404
   (On-line store for multiple product lines)
   www.greenmarketplace.com
Greenpeace *(clothing)* .... (415) 512-9025
   568 Howard St., 3rd Floor, San Francisco, CA 94105
Greenspan *(special cleaners)* .... Dept CG, Box 4656, Boulder, CO 80306
Hammons Products Co. *(organic nuts)* .... (417) 276-5121
   105 Hammons Dr., Stockton, MO 65785 .... www.black-walnuts.com
Harmony .... (800) 869-3446 or (800) 456-1177
   360 Interlocken Blvd. Ste 300, Broomfield, CO 80021
   www.gaiam.com .... Fax: (800) 456-1139
   (Catalog and online store for Whole Foods - multiple product lines)
Healthy Environments *(multiple products)* .... (800) 511-7732
   544 19th Ave, Seattle, WA 98122 .... www.healthye.com
Healthy Kleaner *(special cleanups)* .... (303) 444-3440
   Boulder, CO 80302
Heart of Vermont *(multiple products)* .... (800) 639-4123 or (802) 476-3098
   P.O. Box 612, Barre, VT 05641 .... www.heartofvermont.com
Heavenly Heat Saunas .... (800) MY SAUNA (697-2862)
   1106 Second St., #162, Encinitas, CA 92024 .... or (800) 533-0623
   e-mail: heavenly.heat@att.net .... or (760) 942-0478
Helios *(carpet)* .... (800) 843-5138 or (910) 627-7200
   335 Summit Rd., Eden, NC 27288
Hendricksen Naturlich .... (707) 824-0914
   (flooring, carpet, rugs, pads, and interiors)
   P.O. Box 1677, Sebastapol, CA 95473-1677
Hogil Pharmaceutical Corp. *(lice removal)*............................. (914) 696-7600
   2 Manhattanville Rd. Ste. 106, Purchase, NY 10577
   www.hogil.com   e-mail: hogil@aol.com

Honeysuckle Dreams *(children's toys)*.................................... (301) 217-0546
   1613 Auburn Ave., Rockville, MD 20850
   www.honeysuckledreams.com e-mail: honeysuckledreams@email.com
Humco Holding Group *(concrete sealer)*............................ (903) 831-7808
   7400 Alumax Rd., Texarkana, TX 75501 *(contact for distributors)*
   www.humco.com
Humidex (Air Tech Equip. Ltd.) .... (800) 416-9111 / Fax: (506) 532-6991
   1095 Ch Ohio Rd., Boudreau-Ouest, NB, Canada E4P 6N4
   www.humidex.ca e-mail: humidex@nbnet.nb.ca *(dehumidifiers)*
Hydro Gardens, Inc. *(beneficial insects)* .... (800) 634-6362
   P.O. Box 25845, Colorado Springs, Co 80936 .... or (719) 495-2266
   8765 Vollmer Rd., Colorado Springs, CO 80908
   www.hydro-gardens.com .... *(both numbers are phone or fax)*
   (Website has excellent explanation of use and value of beneficial insects)
Icynene, Inc. *(insulation system)*............... (888) 946-7325 or (905) 890-7325
   5805 Whittle Rd., Ste. 110, Mississaga, Ontario L4A2J1
   www.icynene.com
Ilami Furniture Gallery *(custom made furniture)* .... (972) 239-5278
   5909 Belt Line Rd, Ste. 110, Dallas, TX 75240 .... Fax: (972) 239-5290
   www.ilami.com
Insects, Ltd. *(pesticides)*............................ (800) 992-1991 or (317) 896-9300
   16950 Westfields Park Rd., Westfield, IN 46074
   www.insectslimited.com e-mail: insectsltd.@aol.com
International Light Inc. *(UV light – mold inhibitor)* .... (978) 465-5923
   17 Graf Rd., Newburyport, MA 01950
Island Hemp Wear *(clothing - also links to other hemp resources)*
   www.islandhemp.com e-mail: hemp@hawaiian.net
JAMS Natural Kids Products .... (877) 727-5267 or (609) 324-3938
   P.O. Box 8171, Trenton, NJ 08650 .... Fax: (609) 538-0091
   (children's needs) .... www.jamskids.com
James River Traders *(clothing)* .... (757) 827-6000
   James River Landing, Hampton, VA 23661
Janice's *(multiple products)*.. (800) JANICES (526-4237) or (973) 691-2979
   198 U.S. Hwy. 46, Budd Lake, NJ 07828-3001 .... Fax: (973) 691-5459
   www.janices.com e-mail: info@janices.com .... Fax: (973) 691-5459
K.B. Cotton Pillows, Inc. .... Fax: (888) 829-5292
   www.kbcottonpillows.com
Keepers! Inc. *(baby's & women's needs)* .. (800) 799-4523 or (503) 282-0436
   P.O. Box 12648, Portland, OR 97212 .... Fax: (503) 284-9883
   www.gladrags.com   e-mail: orders@gladrags.com
Kiss My Face *(personal care items available at retail stores and on web)*
   P.O. Box 224, Gardiner, NY 12525
   www.kissmyface.com

Kooltronic, Inc. / TherMax Division .... (800) 929-0682 or (609) 466-8800
    30 Pennington-Hopewell Rd. .... FAX: (609) 466-1114
    P.O. Box 240, Pennington, NJ 08534-0240 .... *(air purification)*
    www.kooltronic.com/thermax
Land's End *(clothing, furniture)* .... (800) 963-4816
    Land's End Ln., Dodgeville, WI 53595
    www.landsend.com
Leydet Arromatics *(essential oils)* .... (916) 965-7546
    P.O. Box 2354, Fair Oaks, CA 95628
    www.leydet.com   e-mail: leydet@leydet.com
Life Tree Products (A division of Sierra Dawn) .... (707) 588-0755
    Box # 513, Graton, CA 95444 *(cleaning products)*
Lifekind Products .... (800) 284-4983 or (530) 477-5395
    10141 Evening Star Dr. , Bldg. #8 .... Fax: (530) 477-5399
    P.O. Box 1774, Grass Valley, CA 95945 .... www.lifekind.com
    (On-line and mail-order source for multiple product lines)
The Living Source *(multiple products)* .... (254) 776-4878
    P.O. Box 20155, Waco, TX 75702-0155 ...... Voice Mail: (800) 662-8787
    Lake Air Mall, 5301 Bosque Blvd., Waco, TX 76710
    www.livingsource.com   e-mail: livingsource@earthlink.com
Livos Phytochemistry of America Inc. .... (508) 477-7955
    800 Falmouth Rd., P.O. Box 1740, Mashpee, MA 02649
    www.livos.com   e-mail: info@livos.com .... Fax: (508) 477-7988
    See also Eco-Design
    (all natural –chemical free oils, stains, waxes & cleaners)
Lotus Pad Co. *(women's personal needs)* .... (541) 758-4110
    131 NW 4th, Ste. 156, Corvallis, OR 97330
    www.lotuspad.com   e-mail: lotuspad@peak.org
Lunapads *(women's needs)* .... (888) 590-2299
    825 Granville St., Ste. 504, Vancouver, BC, Canada V6Z 1K9
    www.lunapads.com
Maggie's Organic Products *(clothing)* .... (800) 516-4100
    (Available from Ethical Shopper)
Magshield – Magnetic Shield Corp. .... (888) 766-7800 or (630) 766-7800
    Perfection Mica Company .... Fax: (630) 766-2813
    740 N. Thomas Dr., Bensenville, IL. 60106 U.S.A.
    www.magshield.com   e-mail: shields@magnetic-shield.com
Mama Moon .... (877) 4ABABYMOON / Fax: (831) 475-7291
    3912 Portola Dr., Ste. 13 #1005, Santa Cruz, CA 95062
    www.mamamoon.com   e-mail: info@mamamoon.com
    (baby and women's special items)

Mapes Industries Inc. .... (800) 228-2391 or (402) 466-1985
    2929 Cornhusker Hwy., Lincoln, NB 68504 .... Fax: (800) 737-6756
    P.O. Box 80069, Lincoln, NB 68501 .... or Fax: (402) 466-2790
    www.mapesind.com .... *(porcelain panels)*
Marquis Dental Mfg. .... *for distributor call* (303) 344-5222
    15370 Smith Rd. Unit H, Aurora, CO 80011 .... *(wood toothpicks)*
Marshall Grain Company .... (800) -658-5699
    2224 E. Lancaster, Ft. Worth, TX 76103 .... or (817) 536-5636
    www.marshallgrain.com   e-mail: mgc@marshallgrain.com
    (pesticides, beneficial insects)
Medic Alert *(medical identification bracelet)* .... (800) 432-5378
    P.O. Box 381009, Turlock, CA 95381 .... www.medicalert.com
Melaleuca Inc. *(for distributor info)* .... (208) 522-0870
    (concrete cleaner, Melaleuca oil - mold inhibitor)
Mia Rose Products *(cleaning products)* .... (800) 292-6339 or (714) 662-5891
    1374 Logan, Costa Mesa, CA 92626
    www.miarose.com   e-mail: info@miarose.com
Michelin Termite Service Co. .... (800) 327-1548 or (305) 594-7697
    7254 NW 34th St., Miami, FL 33122-1124 .... *(pesticides)*
    email: sales@michelincanvas.com
Micro Warehouse Inc. *(radiation filters)* .... (888) 498-8497
    55 United States Ave., P.O. Box 69, Gibbsboro, NJ 08026
    www.warehouse.com   e-mail: info2@warehouse.com
Miele, Inc. *(vacuums)* .... (800) 843-7231 or (609) 419-9898
    9 Independence Way, Princeton, NJ 08540 .... Fax: (609) 419-4298
    Product specialist call: (800) 463-0260 .... Dealer list: (888) 785-2828
    www.miele.com/usa
Miller Paint .... (503) 255-0190 or (206) 784-7878
    12812 N.E. Whitaker Way, Portland, OR 97230 ...... Fax: (503) 255-0192
    1500 N.W. Leary Way, Seattle, WA 98107 .... Fax: (206) 781-0441
    www.millerpaint.com
Miracle Marketing *(lil hummer)* .... (800) 634-6102
    P.O. 520125, Salt Lake City, UT 84152
    www.vac-miracles.com   e-mail: cs@vac-miracles.com
Mom's Aloe Store .... (800) 444-ALOE
    www.aloevera.com   *(Exclusive online retailer for AloeCeuticals, Carrington Lab., and Caraloe products)*
Monterey Lawn & Garden Products *(pesticides)* .... (800) 421-2680
    P.O. Box 35000, Fresno, CA 93745-5000 .... or (559) 499-2100
    www.montereylawngarden.com .... Fax: (559) 499-1015
    e-mail: info@montereylawngarden.com
Mother Harts Infant Sheets *(for distributor information)*
    P.O. Box 4229, Dept. GA-220, Boynton, FL 33424

Less-Toxic Alternatives

Mountain Energy & Resources Inc. *(air handling)* .... (303) 279-4971
   15854 W. 6th Ave., Golden, CO 80401
MSD Agvet *(pesticides)* .... (908) 855-4277
   P.O. Box 2000, Rahway, NY 07065
Multi-Pure Corp. *(water treatment)* .... (800) 622-9206
   7251 Cathedral Rock Dr., P.O. Box 34630, Las Vegas, NV 89128
   www.multipure.com
Murco Wall Products *(paint and joint compound)* .... (800) 446-7124
   300 NE 21st St., Ft. Worth, TX 76106 .... e-mail: murco2@flash.net
My Favorite Planet *(clothing)* .... (212) 645-4641
   1740 Broadway, New York, NY 10019
National Allergy Supply *(air purification and vacuums)* .... (800) 522-1448
   1620 Satellite Blvd., Ste. D, Duluth, GA 30097 ...... Fax: (770) 623-5588
   www.natlallergy.com
National Biological Corp. *(UV lights)* ...... (800) 338-5045 or (303) 425-3388
   1532 Enterprise Pkwy., Twinsburg, OH 44087
Natracare *(women's needs)* .... (303) 320-1510 / Fax: (303) 320-3901
   191 University Blvd., Ste. 294, Ste. 294, Denver, CO 80206
   www.indra.com/natracare
Natural Animal *(pesticides & pet care)*.................................. (800) 274-7387
   7000 US Hwy. 1 N., St. Augustine, FL 32095 .... Fax: (804) 824-5100
   www.naturalanimal.com   e-mail: info@naturalanimal.com
Natural Baby *(baby items)* ... (800) 388-BABY (2229) / Fax: (330) 492-8290
   7835 N. Freedom Ave. N.W., Ste 2, North Canton, OH 44720-6907
   www.naturalbaby.com   e-mail: nbaby@cannet.com
The Natural Bedroom (See Crown Mattress)
The Natural Choice (See Eco Design)
Natural Cork *(flooring)* .... (800) 404-2675 or (706) 733-6120
   1710 N. Leg Court, Augusta, GA 20909 .... Fax: (706) 733-8120
   www.naturalcork.com   e-mail: info@naturalcork.com
The Natural Gardener *(pesticides, beneficial insects)* .... (800) 320-0724
   8648 Old Bee Caves Rd., Austin, TX 78735
The Natural Gardening Company .... (707) 766-9303
   P.O. Box 750776, Petaluma, CA 94975-0776 .... Fax: (707) 766-9747
   www.naturalgardening.com .... *(pesticides, beneficial insects)*
Natural Gardening Research Center *(pesticides)* .... (812) 623-4201
   P.O. Box 149, Sunman, IN 47041
Natural Lifestyle *(lighting)* .... (800) 752-2775
   16 Lookout Dr., Asheville, NC 28804-3330 ... www.natural-lifestyle.com
Natural Solutions Environmental, Inc. ...... (847) 577-7000 or (847) 675-9200
   4238 N. Arlington Heights, Arlington Heights, IL 60004
   www.naturalsolutions1.com *(vacuums)*.................. Fax: (847) 577-7045
Natural Water Environments .... (800) 944-4WET or (817) 355-0417
   Euless, TX 76039

Naturally Pure Alternatives *(water filtration)* .... (800) 736-7877
   575 Live Oak Ave., Ukiah, CA 95482-3730
   www.purewater.com   e-mail: info@purewater.com
Natures Carpet .... (800) 667-5001 or (604) 734-2758
   Colin Campbell & Sons Ltd. .... Fax: (604) 734.1512
   1428 W. 7th Ave., Vancouver, British Columbia, Canada V6H 1C1
   www.naturescarpet.com   e-mail: sales@colcam.com
NEEDS *(multiple products)* .... (800) 634-1380
   National Ecological and Environmental Delivery System
   P.O. Box 580, E. Syracuse, NY 13057 .... Fax: (800) 295-NEED
   www.needs.com   e-mail: needs@needs.com
Nigra Enterprises (Jim Nigra) .... (818) 889-6877
   5699 Kanan Rd. SCP, Agoura, CA 91301
   (water treatment, wood treatment, vacuums)
Nilfisk -Advance America Inc *(vacuums)* .... (800) NILFISK (645-3475)
   300 Technology Dr., Malvern, PA 19355 .... or (610) 647 6420
   www.pa.nilfisk-advance.com .... Fax: (610) 647 6427
   e-mail: questions@nilfisk-advance.com
Nirvana Safe Haven *(multiple products)* ... (800) 968-9355 or (925) 472-8868
   (Formerly Non Toxic Hotline) .... Fax: (925) 938-9019
   3441 Golden Rain Rd., Ste. 3, Walnut Creek, CA 94595
   www.nontoxic.com   e-mail: daliya@nontoxic.com
Nisus Corp *(pesticides)* .... (800) 264-0870
   215 Dunavant Dr., Rockford, TN 37853
   www.nisuscorp.com   e-mail: info@nisuscorp.com
NOPE *(shower curtains)* .... (800) 323-2811
   21 Winters Ln., Baltimore, MD 21228
Nova Natural Toys & Crafts .... (877) 668-2111 or (845) 426-3757
   817 Chestnut Ridge Rd, Spring Valley, NY 10977
   www.novanatural.com .... Fax: (877) 668-2444 or (845) 356-2304
Nursing Mothers Supplies .... (800) 688-6545 or (610) 254-8300
   www.nursingmothersupplies.com .... *(baby & women's needs)*
The Nurtured Baby .... (888) 564-BABY or (7040 549-4922
   4004 Keble Dr., Charlotte, NC 28269
   www.nurturedbaby.com
Nutech Energy Systems Inc. .... (519) 457-1904 / Fax: (978) 448-2754
   511 McCormick Blvd., London, Ontario, Canada N5W 4C8
   www.lifebreath.com   e-mail: nutech@lifebreath.com
   (Lifebreath air purification)
The Old-Fashioned Milk Paint Co. ..... (978) 448-6336 / Fax: (978) 448-2754
   436 Main St., Groton, MA 01450 .... www.milkpaint.com
Orcon *(pesticides)* .... (323) 937-7444
   5132 Venice Blvd., Los Angeles, CA 90019

Organic Bebé *(baby's needs)* .... (877) 644-0554
    233 Harvard Blvd., Lynn Haven, FL 32444 .... Fax: (801) 382-6001
    www.organicbebe.com   e-mail: organicbebe@home.com
The Organic Connection .... (800) WELNES-9
    523 Main St., New Rochelle, NY 10801
Organic Cotton Alternatives .... (888) 645-4452 or (505) 232-9667
    3120 Central S.E., Albuquerque, NM 87106 .... Fax: (505) 268-1323
    www.organiccottonalts.com .... *(bedding)*
Organic Essentials, Inc. *(women's needs)* .. (806) 428-3486 or (800)765-6491
    822 Baldridge, O'Donnell, TX 79351 .... Fax: (806) 428-3475
    www.organicessentials.com   e-mail: oeamber@pics.net
Organic Threads *(clothing)* .... (408) 897-3018
    P.O. Box 1109, Livermore, CA 94551-1109
Original Swiss Aromatics *(aromatic oils)* .... (415) 459-3998
    San Rafael, CA 94901
Oskri Organics *(organic clothing, bedding, toys, food)* .... (800) 821-3125
    P.O. Box 125, Thiensville, WI 53092
    www.oskri.com e-mail: info@oskri.com
Ott-Light *(lighting)* .... (800) 842-8848 / Fax: (813) 626-8790
    www.ott-light.com   e-mail: catalog@ott-lite.com
Our Cleaner World *(dry cleaning)* .... (214) 348-0234
    6611 Abrams Rd., Dallas, TX 75231
Pace Chemical Industries, Inc. .... (805) 499-2911
    Newbury Park, CA 91320 *(Crystal Aire wood treatments)*
Palmer Industries, Inc. .... (800) 545-7383 or (301) 898-7848
    10611 Old Annapolis Rd., Frederick, MD 21701
    www.palmerindustriesinc.com .... *(Vapor barrier, sealants, insulation)*
    e-mail: dapalmer@palmerindustriesinc.com
Pandora Pads *(women's needs)* .... (888) 558-PADS
    955 Frances Harriet Dr., Baton Rouge, LA 70815
    www.pandorapads.com
Paragon *(pesticides and pet care)* .... (800) 238-9254 or (901) 363-1427
    3635 Knight Rd., Ste. 7, Memphis, TN 38118
Patagonia *(sportswear – clothing)* .... (800) 638-6464 or (775) 747-1992
    8550 White Fir St., P.O. Box 32050, Reno, NV 89533-2050
    www.patagonia.com
Paul Penders Co. *(personal care products)* .... (707) 763-5828
    Petaluma, CA 94952
Peaceful Valley *(pesticides)* .... (916) 272-4769
    P.O. Box 2209, 12 Springhill Blvd, Grass Valley, CA 95945
Pecard Chemical Co. *(shoe care)* .... (800) 467-5056 or (920) 468-5056
    1836 Industrial Dr., Green Bay, WI 54302 .... Fax: (920) 468-1399
    www.pecard.com   e-mail: info@pecard.com

Peerless Imported Rugs .... (800) 621-6573 or (773) 472-4848
   3033 N Lincoln Ave., Chicago, IL 60657 .... Fax: (773) 525-4055
   www.peerlessrugs.com   e-mail: customerservice@peerlessrugs.com
Planet Products *(cleaning products)*
   23352 Mariano St., Woodland Hills, CA 91367
Planet Solutions *(cleaning products)* .... (954) 968-6699
   2150 NW 33rd St. #A, Pompano Beach, FL 33069 .. Fax: (954) 968-3456
Pookie Doos *(womens and baby needs)*
   www.pookiedoos.com   e-mail: ramona@pookiedoos.com
Power Quest Inc. *(Powerline - Solar Chargers)* .... (800) 637-2867
   3400 Corporate Way, Ste. C, Duluth, GA 30096
   www.powerexperts.com   e-mail: solar@powerexperts.com
Prestige-Exceptional Fabricare *(dry cleaning)* .... (301) 587-9740
   9420 Georgia Ave., Silver Spring, MD 20910
Priorities *(multiple products)* .... (800) 553-5398
   1451 Concord St., Framingham, MA 01701
   www.store.yahoo.com/priorities-online
Pristine Products *(pet care)* .... (800) 266-4YOU or (602) 955-7031
   2311 E. Indian School Rd., Phoenix, AZ 85016
Pure n Natural ...... (800) 237-9199 or (847) 470-1652 / Fax: (847) 470-1686
   5836 Lincoln Ave., #100, Morton Grove, IL 60053
   www.purennatural.com   e-mail: welcome@purennatural.com
Pure Water Place, Inc. *(water treatment)* .... (303) 776-0056
   15781 N. 83rd St., P.O. Box 6715, Longmont, CO 80501
Quill *(recycled papers)* .... (800) 982-3400 or (708) 634-4800
   P.O. Box 94080, Palatine, IL 60094-4080 .... Fax: (800) 789-8955
   www.quillcorp.com   e-mail: info@quillcorp.com
RH of Texas *(water treatment)* .... (214) 358-3998
   10052 Monroe Dr., Dallas, TX 75229
Radiant Heater Corp. .... (800) 331-6408 or (516) 477-8531
   P.O. Box 60, 74100-2 W. Front St., Greenport, NY 11944
   (ceramic radiant heaters and saunas)
Rainman Int. *(cleaning products, pet products)* .... (800) 892-7246
Real Earth Environmental Co. .... (800) 987-3326 or (310) 457-6331
   P.O. Box 728, Malibu, CA 90265 .... Fax: (310) 457-6441
   www.treeco.com   e-mail: treeco@treeco.com
Real Goods .... (800) 347-0070 or (800) 762-7325 or (707) 468-92921
   Catalog Sales: 200 Clara St., Ukiah, CA 95482 .... Fax: (800) 508-2342
   www.realgoods.com   *Note: Merged with GAIAM & Harmony*
   Stores in Hopland, Berkley, Los Gatos, and West LA, CA
Real Purity *(personal care)* .... (800) 253-1694 or (313) 572-9066
   13323 Washington Blvd., #304, Los Angeles, CA 90066
   www.realpurity.com .... Fax: (313) 572-2580

Real Recycled *(paper and many recycled products)* .... (800) 233-5335
   1541 Adrian Rd., Burlingame, CA 94010
Research Products Corp. .... (800) 334-6011 or (608) 257-8801
   1015 E. Washington Ave., Madison, WI 53703-2999 .... *(air handling)*
   AprilAire: www.aprilaire.com   SpaceGard: www.spacegardfilters.com
Reviva Labs *(skin soap)* .... (800) 257-7774 or (856) 428-3885
   705 Hopkins Rd., Haddonfield, NJ 08033 .... (856) 429-0767
   www.revivalabs.com   e-mail: revivalabs@aol.com
Ross, Frank T. & Sons Ltd. *(cleaners)* .... (416) 282-1107
   6550 Lawrence Ave., Toronto, Ontario, Canada
Royal Silk *(clothing)* .... (800) 227-6925 or (201) 392-0100
   810 31st St., Union City, NJ 07087
Roxide International *(pesticides)* .... (800) 431-5500 or (914) 235-5300
   P.O. Box 249, New Rochelle, NY 10802
The Safe Reading & Computer Box Co. .... (517) 689-6369
   4407 Swinson Rd., Rhodes, MI 48657 .... (517) 689-6877
   www.mcsrelief.com   *(see also Fred Nelson & Associates)*
Safer Alternatives .... (606) 442-5007
   P.O. Box 491663, Redding, CA 96049 .... Fax: (530) 365-0611
San Miguel de Allende, Inc. – Paul Ilami *(furniture)* .... (214) 760-9117
   1418 Slocum St., Dallas, TX 75207
The Sauna Warehouse *(pre-built saunas & kits)* .... (800) 906-2242
   20988 Bake Pkwy., Ste. 102, Lake Forest, CA 92630
   www.saunas.com   e-mail: sales@saunas.com ...... Fax: (949) 609-0166
Scientific Glass Co. Ltd. *(water treatment)* .... (505) 345-7321
   113 Phoenix Ave. NW, Albuquerque, NM 87107
Seventh Generation .....*(Available from GAIAM, Harmony and Whole Foods)*
Shepherd's Dream .... (800) 966-5540
   P.O. Box 3641, Santa Rosa, CA 95402 .... www.shepherdsdream.com
SierraPine Ltd. *(formaldehyde-free fiberboard)* .... (800) 676-3339
   3010 Lava Ridge Ct., Ste 220, Rosebille, CA 95661
   Call or visit the web site for list of distributors in your area
   www.sierrapine.com .... Fax: (916) 772-3415
Silver Spur *(negative ion field)*
   14048 N. 57th St., Scottsdale, AZ 85454
Simmons Natural Body Care *(skin soap)* .... (707) 777-1920
   42295 State Hwy. 36, Bridgeville, CA 95526
   www.simmonsnaturals.com   e-mail: simmonsnaturals@pon.net
Simplex Products *(vapor barrier)* .... (800) 345-8881 or (517) 263-8881
   1801 U.S. Hwy. 223, P.O. Box 10, Adrian, MI 49221
Sinan Company Natural Building Materials .... (530) 753-3104
   Box # 857, Davis, CA 95617

SOS from Texas *(clothing)* .... (800) 245-2339 or (806) 256-2033
    FM 1548, Shamrock, TX 79079 .... Fax: (806) 256-3611
    www.sosfromtexas.com   e-mail: gosostex@sosfromtexas.com
Space-Gard Filters *(See Research Products)*
Specialty Products *(pesticides – bait gun)* .... (215) 299-6000
    1735 Market St., Philadelphia, PA 19103 .... Fax: (215) 299-5999
Sterling Pest Mgt. *(pesticides)* .... (888) 872-9357 or (214) 320-1020
    (Dr. Gene Richardson) .... Fax: (214) 320-2580
    1215 Centerville Rd., Dallas, TX 75218
The SunBox Co. *(lighting)* .... (800) 548-3968 or (301) 869-5980
    19217 Orbit Dr., Gaithersburg, MD 20879-4149 ..... Fax: (301) 977-2281
    www.sunbox.com   e-mail: sunbox@aol.com
Sun Frost *(refrigerators)* .... (707) 822-9095
    824 L St., Arcata, CA 95521
Superior Floor Covering *(flooring)* .... (800) 247-4705 or (715) 842-5358
    901 E. Thomas St., Wausau, WI 54403
    www.superiorfloor.com   e-mail hardwood@superiorfloor.com
Superior Mattress Co. .... (817) 834-2866
    3804 NE 28th St, Ft. Worth, TX 76111
Swedish Clogs, Inc. *(shoes)* .... (800) 443-8167 or (904) 824-8844
    320 State Rd. 16, St. Augustine, FL 32095-1943
Tallon Termite & Pest Control .... (800) 779-2653 or (310) 376-0249
    123 W. Torrance, Redondo Beach, CA 90277 .... Fax: (310) 379-7415
    www.tallonterminte.com
Tanglefoot Co. *(pesticides)* .... (616) 459-4139 / Fax: (616) 459-4140
    314 Straight Ave. SW, Grand Rapids, MI 495046485
    www.tanglefoot.com   e-mail: tnglfoot@aol.com
Target Specialty Products *(pesticides)* .... (408) 293-6032
    1155 Mabury Rd., San Jose, CA 95133
Terressentials *(personal care products)* .... (301) 371-7333
    2650 Old National Pike, Middletown, MD 21769-8817
    www.terressentials.com .... Fax: (301) 371-5577
Texas Power Vac Inc. .... (800) 525-9005 or (254) 754-7606
    1721 Franklin Ave., Waco, TX 76701 .... *(duct cleaning)*
Texrite – Texas Cement Products, Inc. .... (713) 682-8411
    4000 Pinemont Dr., Houston, TX 77018
    www.texrite.com and www.texascement.com .... *(grouts)*
Thai Silk *(clothing)* .... (800) 722-7455 (650) 948-8611
    252 State St., Los Altos, CA 94022 .... Fax: 650) 948-3426
    www.thaisilks.com   e-mail: thaisilk@pacbell.net
The Thermos Co. *(food storage)* .... (800) 831-9242 or (847) 240-3150
    Corporate: 300 N. Martingale Rd., Ste. 200, Schaumburg, IL 60173
    www.thermos.com .... Fax: (847) 240-3211

Thirteen Mile Lamb & Wool Co. .... (406) 388-4945
    13000 Springhill Rd., Belgrade, MN 59714
    www.lambandwool.com   e-mail: becky@lambandwool.com
Tomorrow's World .... (800) 229-7571 or (757) 480-8500
    9665 First St., Norfolk, VA 23503 .... www.tomorrowsworld.com
Trinity Coatings Co. *(wood treatment)* ..... (800) 777-5683 or (817) 926-6811
    1800 Park Place, P.O. Box 721, Fort Worth, TX 76101
    www.trinitycoatings.com .... Fax: (817) 926-9346
Trinity Floor Corp. *(flooring)* .... (214) 943-1157
    1902 N. Beckley Ave., Dallas, TX 75208-2313
Tsoralite *(UV light – mold inhibitor)* .... (800) 331-3534
Under the Canopy ....(888) CANOPY 9 (226-6799)
    www.underthecanopy.com .... *(clothing & accessories)*
U.S. Borax, Inc. *(pesticides)* .... www.borax.com
    Western Office .... (800) 729-2672 or (661) 287-5400
        26877 Tourney Rd., Valencia, CA 91355 .... Fax: (661) 287-5495
    Eastern Office .. (800) 366-2672 or (773) 380-6301/ Fax: (773) 380-6309
        8600 W. Bryn Mawr Ave., Ste. 710-N, Chicago, IL 60631
Vermont Country Store *(clothing)* .... (802) 362-8440
    P.O. Box 3000, Manchester Center, VT 05255 .... Fax: (802) 362-0285
    Stores in Weston (Rt. 100) & Rockingham (Rt. 103)
    www.vermontcountrystore.com   e-mail: vcs@sover.net
Verve, Inc., Providence, RI 02907 *(chewing gum kit)* .... (401) 272-1204
Vet Express *(pet products)* .... (800) 458-7656
    P.O. Box 1168, Rhinelander, WI 54501
Vita-Mix Corp .... (800) 848-2649 / Fax: (440) 235-3726
    Household Division, Usher Rd., Cleveland, OH 44138
    (vacuum, food processors, cookware)
    www.vitamix.com   e-mail: household@vitamix.com
Vita Wave *(hair care)* .... (818) 886-3808
    www.vitawave.com
Waterbury *(pesticides)*.. (800) 845-3495
Whimsicality *(children's needs)*................ (888) 387-0019 or (252) 634-9937
    4523 Rivershore Dr., New Bern, NC 28560
    www.whimisicality.com
White Lotus Futon *(bedding)* .... (877) HAND MADE
    191 Hamilton St., New Brunswick, NJ 08901 .... Fax: (732) 828-415
    or 202 Nassau St., Princeton, NJ 085409 .... www.whitelotus.net
Whole Foods Inc. .... (512) 477-4455 / Fax: (512) 477-1301
    National office: 601 N. Lamar, Ste. 300, Austin, TX 78703
    Store and product list available on-line at www.wholefoodsmarket.com
    Multiple products - Over 100 retail stores in over 20 states and DC
    For catalog see Harmony   *Shop for products on-line at* www.gaiam.com

WinterSilks *(clothing)* .... (800) 648-7455
    11711Marco Beach Dr., Jacksonville, FL 32224 ...... Fax: (800) 548-0411
    www.wintersilks.com   e-mail: mailbox@wintersilks.com
Zodiac Pool Care Inc. .... (800) 937-7873 or (954) 735-9700
    3420 NW 53rd St., Ft . Lauderdale, FL 33309
    www.baracuda.com or www.nature2.com *(swimming pool water filters)*

> > < <

ORGANIC FOOD SUPPLIERS

A Happy Planet *(see page 201)*
Annie's Homeground *(organic pastas)* .... (781) 224-9639
    P.O. Box 128, Hampton, CT 06247 .... www.annies.com
Arrowhead Mills Inc. .... (806) 364-0730
    110 S. Lawton Ave., Hereford, TX 79045
Blackstock Coffee Co. Inc. .... orders: (877) 212-8505 or (905) 986-1444
    14041 Old Scugog Rd. unit 2, Blackstock Ontario, Canada L0B-1B0
    (Organic coffee & organic flavoring extracts)
    www.blackstockorganics.com
Cascadian Farm Inc. *(organic foods wholesaler)* .... (800) 624-4123
    719 Metcalf St., Sedro Wooley, WA 98284 .... or (360) 855-0100
    www.cfarm.com (includes retail store locator)
Chucks Seafood .... (541) 888-5525
    5055 Boat Basin Dr., Coos Bay, OR 97420
Colorado Prime Corp. *(wholesale poultry)* .... (303) 322-8516
    5805 E. 42nd Ave., Denver, CO 80216
Core Values Northeast *(apples)* .... www.corevalues.org
    A project of Mothers & Others
Czimer Game & Sea Foods, Inc. .... (708) 301-0502
    13136 W. 159th St. Lockport, IL 60551
Dale's Exotic Game Meats .... (800) BUY-WILD
    P.O. Box 368, Brighton, CO 80601 .... Fax: (303) 659-0255
Diamond Organics *(see page 205)*
Eberly Poultry Inc. .... (717) 336-6440
    1095 Mt. Airy Rd., Stevens, PA 17578 .... Fax: (717) 336-6905
    www.eberlypoultry.com
EcoExpress – Organic Food Gift Baskets *(see page 206)*
Eco-Organics .... (888) ECO-ORGANICS or (201) 333-8840
    300 Communipaw Ave., Jersey City NJ 07304
    www.eco-organics.com
Ethical Shopper 1-877-4-e-ethic (433-8442)
    www.ethicalshopper.com

Frankferd Farms Foods .... (724) 352-9500
    717 Saxonburg Blvd., Saxonburg, PA 16056 .... Fax: (724) 352-9510
    www.frankferd.com *(wide range of dairy-free, wheat-free and gluten-free organic products – also baby food)*
Garden Spots Finest .... (800) 829-5100
    438 White Oak Rd., New Holland, PA 17557
    www.gardenspotsfinest.com
Good Earth Organic Farm .... (903) 496-2070
    8629 FM 272, Celeste, TX 75423
    www.goodearthorganicfarm.com   e-mail: mail@goodearthorganicfarm
GreenMarketplace.com *(multiple product lines)* .... (888) 59-EARTH
    5808 Forbes Ave., Pittsburgh, PA 15217 .... Fax: (412) 420-6404
    www.greenmarketplace.com
The Healthy Trader .... (800) 636-2584
    380 Camino de Estrella #130, San Clemente, CA 92572
    www.healthytrader.com .... Fax: (949) 369-0726
Horizon Organic Dairy .... (888) 494-3020 or (303) 530-2711
    P.O. Box 17577, Boulder, CO 80308-7577 .... Fax: 303-652-1371
    6311 Horizon Ln., Longmont, CO 80503
    www.horizonorganic.com *(includes retail locator)*
Jaffe Bros. .... (760) 749-1133
    28560 Lilac Rd., Valley Center, CA 92082
Jedlicka Farm *(chicken, beef, pork and grains)* .... (319) 624-2686
    2019 Vincent Ave. N.E., Solon, Iowa 52333
Kennedys Natural Foods .... (703) 533 8488
    1051 W. Broad St., Falls Church, VA 22046
Living Tree Community .... (800) 260-5534 or (510) 526-7106
    www.livingtreecommunity.com .... Fax: (510) 526-9516
    (organic nuts, nut butters, dried fruits)
Long Life Teas .... (800) 887-4096
    www.long-life.com/products.htm
Meat Shop .... (253) 537-4490
    13419 Vickery Ave. E., Tacoma, WA 98446
Morinaga Nutritional Foods, Inc. .... (800) NOW-TOFU (669-8638)
    2050 W. 190th St. #110, Torrance, CA 90504
    www.morinu.com *(tofu products)*
MotherNature.Com .... (800) 517-9020
    www.mothernature.com
Mothers' Milk List *(nationwide organic dairy product suppliers list)*
    From Mothers and Others *(See Section H)* .... (212) 242-0010
    and Rural Vermont .... (802) 223-7222
    www.mothers.org/fieldwork/mo_field_milklist.html
Muir Glen Organic Tomato Products .... (800) 832-6345
    424 N. 7th St., Sacramento, CA 95814 .... www.muirglen.com

Natural Lifestyle *(see page 213)*
New Image Grass Beef (Jon & Wendy Taggart) .... (817) 866-2028
    324 HCR4103, Grandview, TX 76050 .... Fax: (817) 866-2304
    www.grassfedbeef.net / e-mail: sales@grassfedbeef.net
The Organic Connection .... (800) WELNES-9
    523 Main St., New Rochelle, NY 10801 .... or (914) 636-3080
Organic Provisions .... (800) 490-0044 or (215) 674-2217
    P.O. Box 756, Richboro, PA 18954-0756 .... Fax: (215) 443-7087
    www.orgfood.com   e-mail: info@orgfood.com
    (organic and kosher)
Organic Valley Family of Farms .... (888) 444-6455
    CROOP (Coulee Region Organic Produce Pool) Cooperative
    507 W. Main St., LaFarge, WI 54639 .... Fax: (608) 625-2600
    www.organicvalley.com *(includes organic products locator)*
Organic Wholesaler's Directory & Yearbook
    Community Alliance with Family Farmers .... (800) 852-3832
    Box 464, Davis, CA 95617
Oskri Organics *(see page 215)*
Ozark Co-Operative Warehouse .... (501) 521-COOP (4920)
    Box 1428, Fayetteville, AR 72702
    www.ozarkcoop.com   e-mail: warehouse@ozarkcoop.com
Purity Foods .... (517) 351-9231
    2871 W. Jolly Rd., Okmos, MI 48864 .... Fax: (517) 351-9391
    www.purityfoods.com   e-mail: purityfoods@voyager.net
Read-Massey Organic Farm.. (940) 872-5437
    Products sold at several locations in the Grapevine, TX area
    www.freerangechick.com   e-mail freerangechick@morgan.net
Shelton Poultry .... (909) 623-4361
    204 N. Loranne, Pomona, CA 91767 *(web site includes a directory of*
    health food stores that carry their products)
    www.shelton.com   e-mail: turkbaron@sheltons.com
Shiloh Farms Bakery .... (800) 362-6832 or (501) 298-3297
    One Hibler St., Sulfur Springs, AR 72768
    www.users.nwark.com/~shilohf   e-mail: shilohf@nwark.com
Special Foods .... (703) 644-0991
    9207 Shotgun Court, Springfield, VA 22153
Southern Brown Rice .... (800) 421-7423
    P.O. Box 185, Weiner, AR 72479 .... Fax: (870) 684-2239
    www.southernbrownrice.com   e-mail: office@southernbrownrice.com
    (Wholesale only – no retail sales, but will furnish product information)
SunOrganic Farms .... (888) 269-9888
    Box 2429, Valley Center, CA 92082 .... Fax: (760) 751-1141
    www.sunorganic.com

Sunnyland Mills .... (800) 501-8017 or (559) 233-4983
    4439 E. Annadale Ave., Fresno, CA 93725 .... Fax: (559) 223-6431
    www.sunnylandmills.com   e-mail: info@sunnylandmills.com
Texas Grass-Fed Beef
    Ted Slanker, R.R. 2, Box 175, Powderly, TX 75473 .... (903) 732-4653
    Eugene Haydon, P.O. Box 494, Florence, TX 76507 .... (254) 793-2307
    www.texasgrassfedbeef.com
    e-mail: naturalway@texasgrassfedbeef.com
Tree of Life .... (800) 800-2155 or (817) 477-3181
    105 Bluebonnet Dr., Cleburne, TX 76031
Turkey Farm .... (207) 778-2889
    209 Mille Hill Rd., New Sharon, ME 04955
Walnut Acres (Acirca, Inc.) .... (800) 433-3998
    4350 Fairfax Dr., Ste. 350, Arlington, Virginia 22203
    www.walnutacres.com or www.acirca.com
Welsh Family Organic Farm .... (319) 535-7318
    1509 Dry Ridge Dr., Lansing, IA 52151
Whole Foods Markets .... (512) 477-4455 / Fax: (512) 477-1301
    National office: 601 N. Lamar, Ste. 300, Austin, TX 78703
    Store list available on-line at www.wholefoodsmarket.com
    Over 100 retail stores in over 20 states and DC - have fresh organic foods
Wild Oats .... (800) 494-WILD (9453) or (303) 440-5220
    3375 Mitchell Ln., Boulder, CO 80301
    www.wildoats.com   e-mail: info@wildoats.com
Wilde Temptings .... (800) 434-4846
    4760 Lucerne Lakes Blvd. W., Ste. 401, Lake Worth, FL 33467
    www.wildetemptings.com   e-mail: wildetempt@earthlink.net
Wood Prairie Farm .... (800) 829-9765
    RFD 1, Box 164, Bridgewater, ME 04735

> > < <

NUTRITIONAL SUPPLEMENTS

AEHF   .... (800) 428-2343 or (214) 361-9519
    American Environmental Health Foundation .... Fax: (214) 361-2534
    8345 Walnut Hill Ln., Ste. 225, Dallas, TX 75231
    www.aehf.com   e-mail: aehf@aehf.com
Allergy Research Group .... (800) 545-9960 or (510) 487-8526
    (A Division of Scottsdale Scientific) .... Fax: (800) 688-7426
    30806 Santana St., Hayward, CA 94544 .... or Fax: (510) 487-8682
    www.nutricology.com   e-mail: info@nutricology.com
Alvita Herbal Teas .... (801) 756-9700
    600 E. Quality Dr., American Fork, UT 84003 .... Fax: (801) 763-0789

BioChem (Country Life) .... (631) 231-1031
    101 Corporate Dr., Hauppauge, NY 11788
Bio-Tech Pharmacal, Inc. .... (800) 345-1199 or (501) 443-9184
    P.O. Box 1992, Fayetteville, AR 72702 .... Fax: (501) 443-5643
    www.bio-tech-pharm.com
Bluebonnet Nutrition Corp. .... (800) 580-8866 or (281) 240-3332
    12915 Dairy Ashford, Sugar Land, TX 77478
    www.bluebonnetnutrition.com   e-mail: info@bluebonnetnutrition.com
Boericke & Tafel (hometherapeutic) .... (800) 888-4066 or (608) 221-9412
    518 Tasman St., Ste. C, Madison, WI 53714 .... Fax: (608) 221-9533
    www.boericketafel.com
Drugstore.com .... www.drugstore.com
    (Note: not all their products are less-toxic, but they do handle Boericke &
    Tafel, Nature Made & Nature's Bounty, Twin Labs)
Ecological Formulas .... (925) 827-2636
    1061 Shary Circle, Concord, CA 94518
Herbs for Kids (ZAND) .... (800) 232-4005 or (360) 384-5656
    A Division of Botanical Laboratories, Inc. .... Fax: (360) 384-1140
    1441 W. Smith Rd., Ferndale, WA 98248
    or 151 Evergreen Dr. Ste. #D, Bozeman, MT 59715
    www.zand.com or www.herbsforkids.com
iHerb.com .... (888) 792-0028 or (626) 358-5678
    Online herb store and health information website
Klaire Labs Inc. (Vital Life) .... (800) 533-7255 or (858) 350-7880
    140 Marine View Ave., Solana Beach, CA 92075 .... www.iHerb.com
The Living Source *(see page 211)*
Natrol   .... (800) 326-1520
    21411 Prairie St., Chatsworth, CA 91311 .... www.natrol.com
Nature Made Vitamins (Pharmavite) .... (818) 837-3633
    15451 San Fernando Mission, Mission Hills, CA 91345
Nature's Bounty .... (631) 244-2055
    90 Orville Dr., Bohemia, NY 11716 .... Fax: (631) 563-1623
    www.naturesbounty.com
Nature's Herbs (A TwinLab division)
    600 E. Quality Dr., American Fork, UT 84003 .... Fax: (801) 763-0789
    www.naturesherbs.com e-mail: village@naturesherbs.com
Nature's Life .... (714) 379-6500
    7180 Lampson Ave., Garden Grove, CA 92841
Nature's Resource Herbs (Pharmavite) .... (818) 837-3633
    15451 San Fernando Mission, Mission Hills, CA 91345
    www.natureresource.com
Nature's Sunshine *(available from the Healthy Trader)* .... (800) 223-8225
NEEDS *(see page 214)*

NutriCology .... (800) 545-9960 or (510) 487-8526
    (A Division of Scottsdale Scientific) .... Fax: (800) 688-7426
    30806 Santana St., Hayward, CA 94544 .... or Fax: (510) 487-8682
    www.nutricology.com   e-mail: info@nutricology.com
TwinLab (Twin Laboratories Inc.) .... (631) 467-3140
    2120 Smithtown Ave., Ronkonkama, NY 11779 .... www.twinlab.com
Tyler, Inc. .... (800) 869-9705 or (503) 661-5401
    2204 NW Birdsdale - Gresham, OR 97030 .... www.tyler-inc.com
Vitaline Corp. .... (800) 648-4755 or (541) 482-9231
    385 Williamson Way, Ashland, OR 97520 .... Fax: (541) 482-9112
    www.vitaline.com   e-mail: info@vitaline.com
ZAND Herbal Formulas .... (800) 232-4005 or (800) 371-8420
    A Division of Botanical Laboratories, Inc.
    1441 W. Smith Rd., Ferndale, WA 98248 .... www.zand.com

> > < <

PHARMACEUTICAL COMPOUNDING

Abrams Royal Pharmacy .... (800) 458-0804 or (214) 349-8000
    Bob Scarbrough, RPh., Compounding Specialist
    8220 Abrams Rd., Dallas, TX 75231
Apothecure, Inc. .... (800) 969-6601 or (972) 960-6601
    13720 Midway Rd., Ste. 109, Dallas, TX 75244
    www.apothecure.com   e-mail: gosborn@apothecure.com
College Pharmacy (Cheryl Patterson) .... (800) 888-9358 or (719) 262-0022
    3505 Austin Bluff Pkwy., Ste. 101, Colorado Springs, CO 80918
International Academy of Compounding Pharmacists .... (800) 927-4227
    For referral to a compounding pharmacist in your area . www.iacprx.org
Robertson's North Heights Pharmacy .... (870) 774-3666
    1201 E. 35th, Texarkana, AR 71854
Women's International Pharmacy .... (800) 279-5708
    5708 Monona Dr., Madison, WI 53716 .... (608) 221-7800
    13925 W. Meeker Blvd. #13, Sun City West, AZ 85375 .. (623) 214-7700

> > < <

LESS-TOXIC TRAVEL & RETREATS

Safe Travel Directory .... (561) 388-9042
    Nancy Westrum, 1501 Schooner Ln., Sebaskin, FL 32958
    www.mcstravel.resourcez.com
Adobe Hacienda – St. George Plantation, St. George Island, FL
    For chemically sensitive
    Bookings: Collins Real Estate .... (800) 423-7418

Conejos Cabins – Platora, CO .... www.conejoscabins.com
   Relatively safe – for those recovering from chemical sensitivity
   Bookings: Summer (719) 376-2547 / Winter: (417) 842-3279

> > < <

ENVIRONMENTAL ALTERNATIVES CONSULTATION

AEHF *(multiple products)* .... (800) 428-2343 or (214) 361-9519
   American Environmental Health Foundation .... Fax: (214) 361-2534
   8345 Walnut Hill Ln., Ste. 225, Dallas, TX 75231
   www.aehf.com   e-mail: aehf@aehf.com
The E.I. Answer Line (Share, Care & Prayer) .... (972) 964-8333
Environmental Health Center .... (214) 368-4132
   8345 Walnut Hill Ln. No 220, Dallas, TX 75231 ..... Fax: (214) 691-8432
   www.ehcd.com
Healthy Building Assoc. (Dan Morris) .... (206) 448-9135
   1932 1st Ave., Ste. 515, Seattle, WA 98101
   Indoor air quality, building materials & heating systems
International Institute for Bau-Biologie .... (727) 461-4371
   P.O. Box 387, Clearwater, FL 33757 .... Fax: (727) 441-4373
   Courses, seminars and home study on how to detect sick buildings
   www.bau-biologieusa.com   e-mail: baubiologie@earthlink.net
The Living Source *(See Mail Order Resources)*
Mary Oetsel *(Indoor air quality)*... (512) 288-2369
   Environmental Education and Health Services
   P.O. Box 92004, Austin, TX 78709
RCI Environmental Inc. .... (972) 250-6608
   17754 Preston Rd., Dallas, TX 75252

> > < <

Building & Remodeling Consultation

AEHF .... (800) 428-2343 or (214) 361-9519
   American Environmental Health Foundation .... Fax: (214) 361-2534
   8345 Walnut Hill Ln., Ste. 225, Dallas, TX 75231
   www.aehf.com   e-mail: aehf@aehf.com
Allergy Relief Shop, Inc. *(See Mail Order Resources)*
   Tommy Lyle / Both new construction and remodeling
Delgado Ecological Services .... (303) 841-7741
   www.eclu.org .... Fax: (303) 841-8776
Environmental Health Center .... (214) 368-4132
   8345 Walnut Hill Ln, Ste. 220, Dallas, TX 75231 ... Fax: (214) 691-8432
   www.ehcd.com

Doug George Homes Inc. .... (603) 749-5995
    126 Mast Rd., Dover, NH 03820-4427
Healthy Homes (Cecil Smith) .... (503) 666-8746
    305 Palmblad Dr, Gresham, OR 97030
The Living Source .... (254) 776-4878
    P.O. Box 20155, Waco, TX 75702-0155
    Lake Air Mall, 5301 Bosque Blvd., Waco, TX 76710
    www.livingsource.com   e-mail: livingsource@earthlink.com
Fred Nelson & Associates .... (517) 689-6369
    4407 Swinson Rd., Rhodes, MI 48657 .... (517) 689-6877
    www.mcsrelief.com
    Federal mortgages for the chemically sensitive (both remodeling and new
    construction), and kit for a stainless steel & glass safe room
Mary Oetsel *(Indoor air quality)*.. (512) 288-2369
    Environmental Education and Health Services
    P.O. Box 92004, Austin, TX 78709
Real Goods Design & Consulting .... (707) 468-9292 (ext. 2128)
    200 Clara Ave., Ukiah, CA 95482 .... Fax: (707) 462-4807
    www.solardevelopment.com   email: consul@realgoods.com

> > < <

Environmentally Safe Building & Restoration

BUILDING MATERIALS
GreenSpec Product Directory and Guideline
    c/o *Environmental Building News* .... (802) 257-7300
    122 Birge St. Ste. 30, Brattleboro, VT 05301 .... Fax: (802) 257-7304
    www.buildinggreen.com
See also Building Materials on pages 113-123)

CARPET &/OR DUCT CLEANING
Absolute Environmental's Allergy Store ... (800) 771-2246 or (954) 472-0128
    3504 S. University Dr., Davie, FL 33328 .... Fax: (954) 464-9133
    www.allergystore.com e-mail: allergy@allergystore.com
Texas Power Vac Inc. .... (800) 525-9005 or (254) 754-7606
    1721 Franklin Ave., Waco, TX 76701
National Air Duct Cleaners Association .... (202) 737-2926
    1518 K St., Ste. 503, Washington, DC 20005
Some local heating/AC firms and renovation companies perform these services,
but carefully check their procedures and any chemicals they use. Plan to
be away from home during the process. If contaminated ductwork is flex-
duct instead of metal, it may have to be completely replaced.

> > < <

ENVIRONMENTAL TESTING & EVALUATION

Isolate the incitant - Protect your greatest treasures.

Air

AEHF *(various types of testing)*................ (800) 428-2343 or (214) 361-9519
    American Environmental Health Foundation .... Fax: (214) 361-2534
    8345 Walnut Hill Ln., Ste. 225, Dallas, TX 75231
    www.aehf.com   e-mail: aehf@aehf.com
Anachem Inc. .... (800) 966-1186 or (972) 727-9003
    8 Prestige Circle Ste. 104, Allen, TX 75002 .... www.anachem.com
Analytical Services Inc. .... (800) 723-4432 or (802) 878-5138
    Box 515, 50 Allen Brook Ln, Williston, VT 05495 .. Fax: (802) 878-6765
    www.analyticalservices.com   e-mail: info@analyticalservices.com
Anderson Labs .... (802) 295-7344
    30 River St., Dedham, MA 020026 .... www.andersonlaboratories.com
    Also offers brochures and information on indoor air pollution
Cetech, Inc. .... (972) 276-9407
    602 N. 1st St., Garland, TX 75040
Chemical Analysis Inc. .... (972) 255-4100
    Irving, TX 75038
Chem-Safe Environmental Inc .... (509) 968-3973
    400 S. Main St., Ellensburg, WA 98926
EASI (Environmental Analytical Solutions, Inc.) .... (504) 469-3685
    2501 Lexington Ave., Kenner, LA 70062
Electro-Analytical Laboratories .... (440) 951-3514
    7118 Industrial Park Blvd., Mentor, OH 44060 .... (440) 951-3774
Environmental & Toxicology International Inc .... (800) 296-7053
    P.O. Box 75477, Washington DC .... (202) 546-7053
    11244 Waples Mill Rd., Fairfax, VA 22030 .... (703) 273-9621
Environmental Process Inc. (EPI) .... (612) 377-8316
    1220 Glenwood Ave., Minneapolis, MN 55405
Environmental Testing & Technology .... (760) 436-5990
    1106 2nd St., Encinitas, CA 92024
Hauser Laboratories .... (800) 241-2322 or (303) 443-4662
    5555 Airport Blvd., Boulder, CO 80301 .... Fax: (303) 441-5803
    www.hauserlabs.com .... *(some types of air testing)*
Megaclean .... (972) 279-4300
    15330 Lyndon B Johnson Freeway, Mesquite, TX 75150
Myotech Biological Inc. .... (800) 272-3716(903) 626-4429
    Rt 1, Box 182, Jewett, TX 75846

RCI Environmental Inc. .... (972) 250-6608
    17754 Preston Rd., Dallas, TX 75252
Texas Power Vac Inc. .... (800) 525-9005 or (254) 754-7606
    1721 Franklin Ave., Waco, TX 76701
3-M Organic Vapor Monitor .... (800) 243-4630
    3-M Occupational Health & Environmental Safety Div. ... Fax: 542-9373
Call your area EPA office for a list of air quality testing firms in your area.
(See also page 163 for carbon monoxide meters.)

> > < <

ELF / EMF / Microwave / RF Radiation

AEHF   *(see page 228)*
Allergy Relief Shop, Inc. *(see page 202)*
ELF Magnetic Surveys .... (800) 749-9873
    Box 860-295, HCR-2, Tucson, AZ 85735 .... Fax: (602) 822-2355
Safe Environments - Berkeley, CA 94702 .... (510) 549-9693
Your local electric company may also be able to provide testing for EMF
(See also page 163 for EMF, ELF, RF and Microwave Meters)

> > < <

Formaldehyde

AEHF *(See page 228)*
Air Quality Research .... (800) 818-5894 or (919) 941-5509
    100 E. Main St., Ste. C, Carboro, NC 27510
    www.airqualityresearch.com

> > < <

Lead

AEHF *(see page 228)*
Allergy Relief Shop, Inc. *(see page 202)*
Environmentally Sound Products *(see page 207)*
Frandon Lead Check Kit .... (800) 359-9000
    Frandon Enterprises, 511 N. 48th St., Seattle, WA 98103
Leadcheck Swabs .... (800) 262-5323
    Hybrivet Systems, P.O. Box 1210, Farmington, MA 01701
Lifekind Products *(lead in water) (see page 111)*
Suburban Water Testing Labs *(lead in water)* .... (800) 433-6595
    4600 Kutztown Rd., Temple, PA 19560 .... www.h2otest.com

> > < <

Mold

AEHF *(see page 228)*
Allergy Relief Shop, Inc. *(see page 202)*
Allerx (a division of Dust Free) *(see page 202)*
Analytical Services Inc. *(see page 228)*
Biolyne (Todd Below) .... (716) 639-7420
    1576 Sweet Home Rd., Buffalo, NY 14228 .... www.biolyne.com
Environmental Health Center *(see page 228)*
Myotech Biological Inc. *(see page 229)*
Northeast Center for Environmental Medicine .... (315) 488-2856
    2800 W. Genesee St., Syracuse, NY 13219

> > < <

Pesticides (In Water)

AEHF *(see page 228)*
Suburban Water Testing Labs *(see page 229)*

> > < <

Pesticide Information

AEHF *(see page 228)*
Environmental Health Center *(see page 207)*
National Coalition Against Misuse of Pesticides .... (202) 543-5450
    701 E. St. SE, Washington, DC 20003
Pesticide Telecommunications Hotline .... (800) 858-7378
    NPTN, Oregon State University *(Toxicity rating for pesticides)*
    323 Weniger Hall, Corvallis, OR 97331-6502 .... nptn.orst.edu

> > < <

Radon

AEHF *(see page 228)*
Abundant Earth *(see page 201)*
AirChek (Radon Laboratory Arden) .... (828) 684-0893
    570 Butler Bridge Rd., Fletcher, NC 28732
Airtech Radon Testing and Laboratory Analysis .... (610) 857-0206
    Nevins Way, Coatesville, PA 19320
Allergy Relief Shop, Inc. *(see page 202)*
Environmental Health Center (A Division of NSC) .... (800) 557-2366
    National Safety Council, Radon Test Kit Offer
    P.O. Box 65731, Washington, DC 20036
    www.nsc.org/ehc/radon/coupon.htm
Environmentally Sound Products *(see page 207)*

Key Technology Inc. .... (800) 523-4964 or (712) 274-8310
    929 Mount Zion Rd., Lebanon, PA 17045
Mid America Radon Testing .... (913) 469-1997
    Shawnee Mission, KS 66202
Radon Environmental Testing Corporation .... (305) 255-8700
    11000 SW 71ˢᵗ Ln., Miami, FL 33173
Radon Hotline (EPA) .... (800) SOS-RADON
Radon Testing Corp. of America .... (800) 457-2366
    2 Hayes St., Elmsford, NY 10523
Radon Testing Laboratory Inc .... (919) 876-1876
    6851 Greystone Dr., Raleigh, NC 27615
Suburban Water Testing Labs *(air and water) (see page 229)*

> > < <

Toluene

AEHF *(see page 228)*

> > < <

Water

AEHF *(see page 228)*
Abundant Earth *(see page 207)*
Allergy Relief Shop, Inc. *(see page 208)*
Anachem Inc. .... (800) 966-1186 or (972) 727-9003
    8 Prestige Circle Ste. 104, Allen, TX 75002 .... www.anachem.com
Analytical Services Inc. *(see page 228)* .... (800) 723-4432
EPA Safe Drinking Water Hotline .... (800) 426-4791
    1200 Pensylvania Ave. NW, Mail Code: 4604, Washington, DC 20460
    www.epa.gov/safewater
Environmentally Sound Products *(see page 207)*
Lifekind Products *(see page 211)*
National Testing Labs .... (800) 458-3330
Real Goods *(see page 216)*
Suburban Water Testing Labs *(see page 229 - large range of tests)*
Water testing kits often available through County Extension Agents.

> > < <

Environmental Evaluations

AEHF *(see page 228)*
RCI Environmental Inc. *(see page 229)*

> > < <

ORGANIZATIONS

Their publications (on-line or periodically mailed) are also listed.

AEHF .... (800) 428-2343 or (214) 361-9519
   American Environmental Health Foundation .... Fax: (214) 361-2534
   8345 Walnut Hill Ln., Ste. 225, Dallas, TX 75231
   www.aehf.com   e-mail: aehf@aehf.com
Allergy & Asthma Network .... (800) 878-4403 or (703) 385-4403
   3554 Chain Bridge Rd., Ste. 200, Fairfax, VA 22030
The Allergy & Environmental Health Assoc.
   P.O. Box 871, Cambridge, Ontario, Canada N1R5X09
   Quarterly (Quarterly – $25)
Alliance for Bio-Integrity .... (515) 472-5554
   406 W. Depot Ave., Fairfield, IA 52556 .... www.bio-integrity.org
American Academy of Allergy & Immunology .... (800) 822-ASMA
   611 E. Wells St., Milwaukee, WI 53202 .... www.aaaai.org
   National Allergy Bureau Daily Pollen Counts .... (800) 9-POLLEN
   National Allergy Bureau's Indoor Allergy Hotline ..... (877) 9-ACHOOO
American Academy of Environmental Medicine (AAEM) .... (316) 684-5500
   7701 E. Kellogg, Ste. 625, Wichita, KS 67207 .... Fax: (316) 684-5709
   www.aaem.com
American College of Allergy, Asthma & Immunology .... (847) 427-1200
   85 W. Algonquin Rd., Ste. 550, Arlington Heights, IL 60005
   www.allergy.mcg.edu   (also search www.medem.com)
Asthma & Allergy Foundation of America ..... (800) 7-ASTHMA (727-8462)
   AAFA, 1233 20th St., NW, Ste. 402, Washington, DC 20036
   www.aafa.org   e-mail: info@aafa.org .... Fax: (202) 466-8940
The Campaign to Label Genetically Engineered Foods .... (425) 771-4049
   P.O. Box 55699, Seattle, WA 98155 .... Fax: (603) 825-5841
   www.thecampaign.org   e-mail: label@thecampaign.org
Candida & Dysbiosis Information Foundation .... (409) 694-8687
   P.O. Drawer JF, College Station, TX 77841-5146
   Annual Newsletter
Center for Health Environment & Justice .... (703) 237-2249
   150 S. Washington St., Falls Church, VA 22046
The CFIDS Assoc. of America .... (800) 442-3437 or (704) 365-2343
   P.O. Box 220398, Charlotte, NC 28222-0398 .... Fax: (704) 365-9755
   (Chronic Fatigue and Immune Dysfunction Syndrome)
   The CFIDS Chronicle (Quarterly – $30)
   www.cfids.org e-mail: info@cfids.org
   Also gives links to other CFIDS, FMS and ME webring sites
Chemical Injury Information Network (CIIN) .... (406) 547-2255
   505 Larime, P.O. Box 301, White Sulphur Springs, MT 59645

www.ciin.org .... Fax: (406) 547-2455
Our Toxic Times (contribution) John & Cynthia Wilson, Editors
Chronic Fatigue, Multiple Chemical Sensitivity & Gulf War Syndrome
The Chemical Sensitivity Disorders Assoc.
    122 Regina Dr., Potomac Falls, VA 20165
    Chemical Sensitivity Connection (Quarterly - $10)
DAMS (Dental Amalgam Mercury Syndrome) Inc. .... (800) 311-6265
    P.O. Box 7249, Minneapolis, MN 55407-0249 .... (612) 721-1144
    www.amalgam.org
    International DAMS Newsletter (Quarterly - $20)
Earth Share (National) .... (800) 875.3863 or (202) 537-7100
    3400 International Dr., NW, Ste. 2K, Washington, DC 20008
    www.earthshare.org .... Fax: (202) 537-7101
Earth Share of California   www.earthshareca.org .... (800) 368-1819
    49 Powell St., Ste. 510, Francisco, CA 94102
Earth Share of New York   www.earthshareny.org .... (800) 875-3863
    285 Broadway, Ste. 29, Saratoga Springs, NY 12866
Earth Share of Texas .... (800) GREENTX or (512) 472-5518
    814 W. 23rd St., Austin TX 78705 .... Fax: (512) 472-4930
    www.earthshare-texas.org   e-mail: ESTX@earthshare-texas.org
Earth Share of Washington .... (206) 622-9840
    1402 Third Ave., Ste. 825, Seattle, WA 98101 .... www.esw.org
Earth Share of Australia .... www.earthshare.org.au
    Phone: 02 66857904 (Int 61 2+)   Fax: 02 66857468 (Int 61 2+)
    P.O. Box 1655 Byron Bay, NSW 2481 Australia
ECHO (Ecological Health Organization) .... (860) 228-2693
    P.O. Box 0119, Hebron, CT 06248-0119
    hometown.aol.com/ECHOMCSCT/home.html
EMF Hotline .... (800) 858-7378 or (906) 743-3091
Endometriosis Association .... (800) 992-3636 or (414) 355-2200
    8585 N. 76th Place, Milwaukee, WI 53223 .... Fax: (414) 355-6065
    www.endometriosisassn.org
Environmental Health Center (NSC) .... (202) 293-2270
    A Division of the National Safety Council .... Fax: (202) 293-0032
    1025 Connecticut Ave., NW, Ste. 1200, Washington, DC 20036
    www.nsc.org/ehc/ehcdirec.htm
Environmental Health Coalition .... (619) 235-0281 / Fax: (619) 232-3670
    1717 Kettner Blvd., Ste. 100, San Diego, CA 92101
    www.environmentalhealth.org   e-mail: ehc@environmentalhealth.org
    Toxinformer .... Fax: (619) 232-3670
Environmental Health Network .... (415) 541-5075
    P.O. Box 1155, Larkspur, CA 94977
    The New Reactor (Bi-monthly – $25)

Environmental Research Foundation .... (410) 263-1584
    P.O. Box 5036, Annapolis, MD 21403-7036 .... Fax: (410) 263-8903
    Rachel's Environment & Health Weekly (free weekly e-newsletter)
    Archive index: www.monitor.net/rachel/rehw-index.html
    To subscribe e-mail: rachel-weekly-request@world.std.com
Environmental Working Group
    1718 Connecticut Ave., N.W., Ste. 600, Washington, DC 20009
    www.ewg.org.   e-mail: info@ewg.org
    For food news: www.foodnews.org
Fibromyalgia Coalition Intnl. / Getting Well Support Groups
    6101 Nall Ave., Mission, KS 66202 .... www.fibrocoaltion.org
    Conquering the Challenge ($16 year – bimonthly)
The Food Allergy Network .... (800) 929-4040
    10400 Eaton Place, Ste. 107, Fairfax, VA 22030-2208
    www.foodallergy.org .... Fax: (703) 691-2713
    (website includes food allergy product alerts and food recalls – you can
    even sign up for e-mails of all food alerts!)
Foundation for Toxic Free Dentistry
    P.O. Box 608010, Orlando, FL 32860-8010
HEAL – Human Ecology Action League, Inc. .... (404) 248-1898
    P.O. Box 29629, Atlanta, GA 30359-0629 .... Fax: (404) 248-0162
    www.hometown.aol.com/HEALNatnl/index.html
    e-mail: HEALNatnl@aol.com
    The Human Ecologist (Quarterly – $26)
Health & Environment Resource Center .... www.herc.org
Healthy House Institute .... (812) 332-5073
    430 N. Sewell Rd., Bloomington, IN 47408 .... www.hhinst.com
The Herb Research Foundation .... (800) 748-2617 or (303) 449-2265
    1007 Pearl St., #200, Boulder, CO 80302 .... Fax: (303) 449-7849
    www.herbs.org
IAQ INFO .... (800) 438-4318 or (202) 484-1307 or (301) 585-9020
    Indoor Air Quality Information Clearinghouse - an EPA service
    P.O. Box 37133, Washington, DC 20013-7133
    e-mail: iaqinfo@aol.com
Institute for Solar Living .... (707) 744-2017 / Fax: (707) 744-1682
    Real Goods Trading Corp. Solar Living Center
    P.O. Box 836, 13771 S. Hwy. 101, Hopland, CA 95449
    www.solarliving.org   e-mail: isl@rgisl.org
Invisible Gardener Organization .... (310) 457-4438
    P O Box 4311, Dept W3, Malibu, CA 90265 .... Fax: (310) 457-5003
    www.invisiblegardener.com
MCS (Multiple Chemical Sensitivity) Advocacy Fund
    www.mcsadvocacyfund.org

MCS Referral and Resources .... (410) 362-6400
    508 Westgate Rd, Baltimore, MD 21229-2343 .... Fax: (410) 362-6401
    www.mcsrr.org   email: donnaya@rtk.net
MCS Survivors .... www.mcsurvivors.com
    (A resource web site for MCS and EI – lots of links to other sites)
Mothers & Others .... (212) 242-0010
    40 W. 20th St., New York, NY 10011-4211
    www.mothers.org   e-mail: mothers@mothers.org
    The Green Guide for Everyday Life (17 yr / $25)......... (888) ECO-INFO
National Asthma Education and Prevention Program
    National Heart Lung & Blood Institute / National Institutes of Health
    P.O. Box 30105, Bethesda, MD 20824
    www.nhlbi.nih.gov/about/naepp/index.htm
National Center for Environmental Health Strategies .... (856) 429-5358
    1100 Rural Ave., Voorhees, NJ 78043
    The Delicate Balance
National Coalition Against the Misuse of Pesticides .... (202) 543-5450
    701 E. St., #200, Washington, DC 20003
    www.csn.net/ncamp or www.ncamp.org
    Pesticides and You (Quarterly – $25) *Technical Report* (Monthly – $20)
National Institute of Environmental Health Sciences .... (800) 643-4794
    P.O. Box 12233, Research Triangle Park, NC 27709 .... (919) 541-3345
    www.niehs.nih.gov
National Institute of Occupational, Safety & Health .... (800) 356-4674
    (NIOSH) - Director, Hubert H. Humphrey Bldg. ...... Fax: (513) 533-8573
    200 Independence Ave., SW, Rm. 715H, Washington, DC 20201
    www.cdc.gov/niosh/about.html
National Nutritional Foods Association (NNFA) .... (949) 622-6272
    3931 MacArthur Blvd., Ste. 101 Newport Beach, CA 92660
    www.nnfa.org .... Fax: (949) 622-6266
National Pesticide Telecommunications Network .... (800) 868-PEST
    EPA-sponsored service at Oregon State University
    333 Weniger Hall, Corvallis, Oregon 97331-6502 ... Fax: (541) 737-0761
    www.ace.orst.edu/info/nptn   e-mail: nptn@ace.orst.edu
Natural Resources Defense Council .... (212) 727-2700
    40 W. 20th St., New York, NY 10011 .... Fax: (212) 727-1773
    Regional offices in Washington, DC, San Francisco & Los Angeles
    www.nrdc.org
NSF International (National Sanitation Foundation .... (734) 769-8010
    3475 Plymouth Rd., Ann Arbor, MI 48105 (tests products)
Northwest Coalition for Alternatives to Pesticides .... (514) 344-5044
    (NCAP) P.O. Box 1393, Eugene, OR 97440 .... Fax: (541) 344-6923
    www.pesticide.org   e-mail: info@pesticide.org.

Occupational Safety & Health Assoc. (OSHA) .... (202) 693-1999
   U.S. Department of Labor, OSHA, Office of Public Affairs
   200 Constitution Ave., Room N3647, Washington, DC 20210
   www.osha.gov .... To report emergency: (800) 321-OSHA (6742)
Organic Consumers Association / BioDemocracy Campaign
   (Facts on the hazards of genetically engineered foods
   6114 Hwy 61, Little Marais, MN 55614,
   www.purefood.org   e-mail: staff@purefood.org
   Activist or Media Inquiries: (218) 226-4164 / Fax: (218) 226-4157
   BioDemocracy News (published every 6 weeks) *Organic View* (bi-weekly)
Organic Farming Research Foundation .... (831) 426-6606
   P.O. Box 440, Santa Cruz, CA 95061 .... Fax: (831) 426-6670
   www.ofrf.org   e-mail: research@ofrf.org
Organic Trade Association .... (413) 774 7511
   74 Fairview St., P.O. Box 547, Greenfield, MA 01302
   www.ota.com   e-mail: info@ota.com .... Fax: (413) 774-6432
Pesticide Action Network of North America (PANNA) .... (415) 981-1771
   49 Powell St., Ste. 500, San Francisco, CA 94102 .. Fax: (415) 981-1991
   www.panna.org   e-mail: panna@panna.org
Price-Pottenger Nutrition Foundation .... (800) 366-3748 or (619) 574-7763
   P.O. Box 2614, La Mesa, CA 91943-2614
   www.price-pottenger.org   e-mail: info@price-pottenger.org
Protect All Children's Environments (PACE) .... (704) 724-4221
   2261 Buck Creek Rd., Marion, NC 28752 .... Fax: (704) 724-4177
   www.main.nc.us/pace
Rachel Carson Council
   8940 Jones Mill Rd., Chevy Chase, MD 20815
   The Rachel Carson Council News (Quarterly – Contribution)
SAFE (Smokefree Air For Everyone) .... www.pacificnet.net/~safe
   P.O. Box 246 Newbury Park, CA 91320
Safe Schools - Irene Ruth Wilkenfield .... (318) 984-2766
   205 Paddington Ave., Lafayette, LA 70508
   www.head-gear.com/SafeSchools   e-mail: ndgb37b@prodigy.com
   (Resource center for environmental health strategies for the classroom)
Share, Care & Prayer, Inc. .... www.sharecareprayer.org
   P.O. Box 2080, Frazier Park, CA 93225
   Share, Care & Prayer Journal (3 per year – contribution)
   Also have a tape and book library and a pen pall directory
Texas Organic Grower's Association .... www.texasorganicgrowers.com
   P.O. Box 15211, Austin, TX 78761
   Charlie Townsend – e-mail: townsend@hillsboro.net ...... (254) 694-3067
   Sue Johnson .... (512) 282-0153
Texas Pesticide Information Network .... www.texascenter.org/txpin

Texans for Alternatives to Pesticides (TAP) .... (713) 523-2TAP (2827)
    3015 Richmond, Ste., Houston, TX 77098
    Contact: Rebeka Perrella, Executive Director
    www.nopesticides.org   e-mail: nopesticides@hotmail.com
U.S. Consumer Product Safety Commission .... (800) 638-2772
    4330 East-West Hwy., Bethesday, MD 20814-4408 .... www.cpsc.gov
    Product recall and safety information
The Vanguard (chemical injury educ. org.) .... (512) 338-1108
    P.O. Box 26152, Austin, TX 78755-0152 .... Fax: (512) 338-1190
    www.austin360.com/community/groups/vanguard

> > < <

EPA Regional Offices
(U.S. ENVIRONMENTAL PROTECTION AGENCY)

National Office: www.epa.gov
    1200 Pennsylvania Ave., NW, Washington, DC 20460
    Indoor air quality home page: www.epa.gov/iaq
EPA Region 1 .... (617) 223-4845
    JFK Federal Bldg. # 2203, Boston, MA 02203
    Connecticut, Maine, Massachusetts, New Hampshire, Rhode Island, and
    Vermont
EPA Region 2 .... (212) 264-2515
    26 Federal Plaza, New York, NY 10278
    New Jersey, New York, Puerto Rico, and U.S. Virgin Islands
EPA Region 3 .... (215) 597-8320
    841 Chestnut St., Philadelphia, PA 19107
    Delaware, Maryland, Pennsylvania, Virginia, West Virginia, and District
    of Columbia
EPA Region 4 .... (404) 881-3776
    345 Courtland St., NE., Atlanta, GA 30365
    Alabama, Florida, Georgia, Kentucky, Mississippi, North Carolina, South
    Carolina, and Tennessee
EPA Region 5 .... (312) 353-2205
    230 S. Dearborn St., Chicago, IL 60604
    Illinois, Indiana, Michigan, Minnesota, Ohio, and Wisconsin
EPA Region 6 .... (214) 655-7208
    1445 Ross Ave., Dallas, TX 75202-2733
    Arkansas, Louisiana, New Mexico, Oklahoma, and Texas
EPA Region 7 .... (913) 236-2803
    726 Minnesota Ave., Kansas City, KS 66101
    Iowa, Kansas, Missouri, and Nebraska
EPA Region 8 .... (303) 283-1710

One Denver Place, Ste. 1300, 999 18th St., Denver Co. 80202
Colorado, Montana, North Dakota, South Dakota, Utah, and Wyoming
EPA Region 9 .... (415) 974-8076
215 Fremont St., San Francisco, CA 94105
Arizona, California, Hawaii, Nevada, Pacific Islands, and Tribal Nations
subject to U.S. law
EPA Region 10 .... (206) 442-7660
1200 Sixth Ave., Seattle, WA 98101
Alaska, Idaho, Oregon, and Washington

> > < <

Support Groups

Please notify us if you know of a support group for the chemically sensitive or environmentally ill, and we will try to add it to future editions.
Chronic Fatigue Syndrome and Fibromyalgia Support Group of DFW
(Dallas/Fort Worth, TX) www.virtualhometown.com/dfwcfids
Getting Well Support Groups (Fibromyalgia Coalition Intnl.)
6101 Nall Ave., Mission, KS 66202 .... www.fibrocoaltion.org
HEAL – Human Ecology Action League, Inc. .... (404) 248-1898
P.O. Box 29629, Atlanta, GA 30359-0629 .... Fax: (404) 248-0162
www.hometown.aol.com/HEALNatnl/index.html
e-mail: HEALNatnl@aol.com
Internet MCS Support Groups
http://groups.yahoo.com/group/MCS-CI-exile
http://groups.yahoo.com/group/MCS-Christian-Support
Missouri Support Group (Dixie Peterson) .... (417) 842-3279
1095 SW 90th Rd, Oronogo, MO 64855 (southwest Missouri)
Share, Care & Prayer, Inc. .... www.sharecareprayer.org
P.O. Box 2080, Frazier Park, CA 93225

> > < <

PUBLICATIONS
Periodicals (Including E-Zines)

Acres U.S.A. (12 issues/year – $24) .... (800) 355-5313 or (512) 892-4400
P.O. Box 91299, Austin, TX 78709 .... Fax: (512) 892-4448
Organic gardening magazine   Book catalog – free
www.acresusa.com e-mail: info@acresusa.com
Allergy Hotline ($35 for 12 months) .... (407) 628-1377
Hotline Printing & Public Relations
P.O. Box 161132, Altamonte Springs, FL 32716

Alternative Medicine .... (415) 435-1779
    1650 Tiburon Blvd., Tiburon, CA 94920 .. www.alternativemedicine.com
And He Will Give You Rest ($15 year) .... (610) 237-1698
    Rest Ministries, P.O. Box 502886, San Diego, CA 92150
    Newsletter for those who live with chronic illness or pain
Better Nutrition .... (770) 988-9991
    Sabot Publishing Co., Inc.
    900 Circle 75 Pkwy NW, Ste. 205, Atlanta, GA 30339
    www.betternutrition.com
Building with Nature (6 issues/year – $35) .... (707) 579-2201
    Architect Carol Venolia, P.O. Box 4417, Santa Rosa, CA 95402
Canary News ($20 per year - monthly) - MCS
    Lynn Lawson, 1404 Judson Ave., Evanston IL 60201
    e-mail: Lynnword@aol.com
Delicious .... (303) 939-8440
    New Hope Natural Media, 1301 Spruce St., Boulder, CO 80302
    www.healthwell.com
E, The Environmental Magazine (6 issues/year - $20) .... (203) 854-5559
    28 Knight St., Norwalk, CT 06851 .... Fax: (203) 866-0602
    P.O. Box 5098, Westport, CT 06881 .... www.emagazine.com
Environmental Building News .... (802) 257-7300
    Newsletter for environmentally responsible design and construction
    122 Birge St. Ste. 30, Brattleboro, VT 05301 .... Fax: (802) 257-7304
    www.buildinggreen.com
First for Women .... e-mail: firstforwomen@aol.com
    270 Sylvan Ave., Englewood Cliffs, NJ 07632
Greenkeeping (bi-monthly) .... (914) 246-6948
    (Focus on alternatives to toxic products in everyday living.)
    Box 110, Annandale-on-Hudson, New York 12504
Green Pages (Co-op America) .... (800) 58-GREEN or (202) 872-5307
    1612 K St. NW, Ste. 600, Washington, DC 20006 ... Fax: (202) 331-8166
    Online: www.greenpages.org (Printed version $5.95 + $2.00 ship)
Green Shopping Magazine (*free e-zine*) .... www.ecomall.com
Herbs for Health .... (800) 350-0952
    P.O. Box 7708, Red Oak, IA 51591 .... www.discoverherbs.com
Homegrown (6 issues/year - $15) .... (512) 9320-5576
    P.O. Box 913, Georgetown, TX 78627 (Texas organic gardening)
    www.homegrowntexas.com e-mail: judy@homegrowntexas.com
Interior Concerns Newsletter (6 issues/year – $35) .... (415) 389-8049
    131 W. Blithedale Ave., P.O. Box 2386, Mill Valley, CA 94942
Latitudes (6 issues/year $24) .... (561) 798-0472
    Learning disabilities, AD, hyperactivity
    214 Trace Court, West Palm Beach, FL 33411

Nutrition .... www.healthwell.com
Organic Food Business News .... (407) 628-1377
    Hotline Printing & Public Relations
    P.O. Box 161132, Altamonte Springs, FL 32716
Organic Gardening (6 issues/year – $15.96)
    Rodale Inc. .... (610) 967-5171
    33 E. Minor St., Emmaus, PA 18098-0099 .... Fax: (610) 967-8963
    www.organicgardening.com
Organic Style - Rodale Inc. *(see above)* .... www.rodaleorganicstyle.com
National Organic Wholesaler's Directory & Yearbook .... (800) 852-3832
    CAFF (Community Alliance with Family Farmers .... (530) 756-8518
    P.O. Box 363, Davis, CA 95617 .... e-mail: Nod@caff.org
Recognition of Multiple Chemical Sensitivity .... (410) 362-6400
    MCS Referral & Resources, 508 Westgate Rd., Baltimore, MD 21229
Safe Home Digest (monthly newsletter) .... (203) 966-2099
    (Monthly reviews of safer consumer products.)
    24 East Ave., Ste. 1300, New Canaan, CT 06840

> > < <

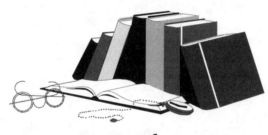

Books

Air Quality by Thad Godish. Chelsea, MI: Lewis Publ. 1985.

Allergies & the Hyperactive Child by D.J. Rapp. New York: Sovereign Books, 1982.

Allergy Self Help Book by Sharon Faelten. Emmaus, PA: Rodell Press, 1983.

The Bitter Truth About Artificial Sweeteners by Dennis W. Remington & Barbara W. High. Provo, UT: Vitality House International Inc., 1987.

Cassarett & Doull's Toxicology (The Basic Science of Poisons). Edited by Mary O. Amdur, John Doull, & Curtis Klaassen. New York: Pergamon Press.

Clean and Green by Annie Berthold-Bond. Woodstock, New York: Ceres Press, 1990.

Clinical Toxicology of Commercial Products by Robert E. Gosselin, Roger P. Smith, Harold C. Hodge with Jeannette E. Braddock. Baltimore: Williams & Wilkins.

Complete Book of Natural and Medicinal Cures by the editors of Prevention Magazine. Health Books, Rodale Press, 1994.

Coping with Your Allergies by N. Golos & F. G. Golbitz. New York: Simon and Schuester, 1986.

Diet for a Poisoned Planet by David Steinman. New York: Harmony Books, 1990.

Eating Clean – Overcoming Food Hazards. Center for Study of Responsive Law, P.O. Box 19367, Washington D.C.

The E.I. Syndrome by Sherry Rogers, M.D.

EPA Recognition & Management of Pesticide Poisonings (4th Edition) by Donald P. Morgan, M.D., Ph.D. Washington, DC: Health Effects Div., Office of Pesticide Programs, U.S. EPA, 1989.

Getting the Bugs Out: A Guide to Sensible Pest Management in the Home by W. Olkowski and H. Olkowski. New York: National Audubon Society, 1981.

The Healthy House (How to Buy One; How to Cure a Sick One; How to Build One) by John Bower. New York: Carol Publ. Group, 1997.

Healthy House Building by John Bower. Unionville, IN: Healthy House Institute, 1993.

Herbs for Health & Healing by Kathi Keville. Emmaus, PA: Rodale Press Inc., 1996.

If It's Tuesday it Must be Chicken by N. Golos & F. G. Golbitz. New Canaan, CT: Keats Publ, Inc., 1983.

Immunology by David Male. St Louis: C.V. Moseby Co., 1986.

The Impossible Child by Doris Rapp. Buffalo, NY, Practical Allergy Research Foundation, 1986.

Is This Your Child by Doris Rapp. New York: Morrow, 1991.

Is This Your Child's World by Doris Rapp.

Manual of Allergy & Immunology. Glenn Lawlor Jr., M.D.; Thomas J. Fisher, M.D. editors. Boston: Little, Brown & Co., 1981.

The Mother Earth Handbook edited by Judith S. Scheref. New York: Continuum Publ. Co., 1991.

No More Antibiotics by Mary Ann Block. Available from The Block Center, 1721 Cimarron Trail, Ste. 4, Hurst, TX 76054. 800-770-7039.

No More Ritalin - Treating ADHD Without Drugs, A Mother's Journey, A Physician's Approach by Mary Ann Block. Available from The Block Center, 1721 Cimarron Trail, Ste. 4, Hurst, TX 76054. 800-770-7039

Nontoxic and Natural by D. L. Dadd. Los Angeles: J. P. Tarcher, Inc. 1984.

The Non-Toxic Home by Debra L. Dadd. Los Angeles: J.P. Tarcher, Inc. 1986.

The Non-Toxic Home and Office (Protecting Yourself and Your Family from Everyday Toxics and Health Hazards) by Debra L. Dadd.

Nontoxic, Natural and Earthwise by Debra L. Dadd. Los Angeles: Jeremy P. Tarcher, Inc. 1990.

Nutritional Desk Reference by Robert H. Garrison Jr. and Elizabeth Somer. New Canaan CT: Keats Publishing, 1985.

Pesticides and Human Health by Wm. H. Hallenbeck and Kathleen M. Cunningham-Burns. New York: Springer-Verlog, 1985.

Rotational Bon Appetite by Stephanie Bauer and Barbara Maynard. Dallas: Environmental Health Center, 1986.

RX for Nutritional Healing (2nd Edition) by James F. Balch M.D. & Phyllis A. Balch CNC. Garden City Park, NY: Avery Publ. Group, 1997.

Save Your Money, Save Your Face by E. Brumberg. New York: Harper & Row, 1986.

Staying Healthy with Nutrition by Elson M. Haas, M.D. Berkley, CA: Celestial Arts, 1992

Toxicology - A Primer on Toxicology Principles & Application by Michael A. Kamrin. Chelsea, MI: Lewis Publ. 1988.

The Whole Way to Natural Detoxification by Jacqueline Krohn, M.D. Vancouver, BC: Hartley & Marks, Ltd., 1996.

Why Your House May Endanger Your Health by A. Zamm & R. Cannon. New York: Simon and Schuster, 1980.

Your Home, Your Health and Well-being by David Rousseau, W. J. Rea M.D. and Jean Enwright. Vancouver, BC: Hartley Marks, Ltd., 1988.

> > < <

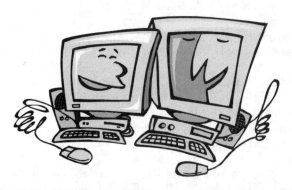

INFORMATION WEBSITES

Born to Love   www.borntolove.com ..... 905-725-2559 / Fax: 905-725-3297
445 Centre St. S., Oshawa, ON, Canada L1H 4C1
Website with links devoted to baby's and women's special needs
Camelia's Herbal Medicine Website
www.primenet.com/~camilla/herbs.htm
www.dirtdoctor.com (Howard Garrett's The Natural Way – Dallas, TX)
Saturdays 11-noon, Sunday 8-noon on News/Talk 820-WBAP
Website with great information and links about organic gardening

The Health Windows Corporation .... www.health.com
   Healthcare network that helps people become more knowledgeable
   and active in managing their personal health.
www.healthwell.com *(Natural health information source)*
Lassen Technologies .... www.snowcrest.net/lassen/mcsei.html
   Website for chemically sensitive & environmentally ill
Mother's Nature .... www.mothersnature.com/market
   620 Meadow Dr., McKinney, TX 75069
   Links to websites devoted to baby's and women's special needs.
Organic Hub *(Organic resource search engine)* .... www.organichub.com
Product Recall Websites:
   Consumer Reports Online .... www.consumerreports.org/Recalls
   eSafety.com (for parents) .... www.esafety.com/esafety_cfmfiles
   For Baby's Sake .... www.kohldesigns.com/safebaby
   KidSafe .... www.kidssafe.com/recalls
   KidSource .... www.kidsource.com/kidsource/content/recall.html
   Marketplace (Canada) .... http://cbc.ca/consumers/market
   National Highway Traffic Safety Administration .... www.nhtsa.dot.gov
   SafetyAlerts.com .... www.safetyalerts.com
   U.S. Consumer Product Safety Commission .... www.cpsc.gov
   U.S. Dept. of Agriculture - Food Safety & Inspection Service
   .... www.fsis.usda.gov/OA/recalls/rec_intr.htm
Ranchwest .... www.ranchwest.com
   P.O. Box 296, Cresson, TX 76035
   Website devoted to raising cattle without harmful chemicals
Simple Life .... www.simplelife.com
   Website devoted to organic cotton – organic cotton directory links to
   resources, organizations and other links.
Sustainable Cotton .... www.sustainablecotton.org
   Website devoted to making organic cotton a viable agricultural and
   economic alternative
Web Directory .... www.webdirectory.com
   An internet directory of environmental organizations.
Weil, Dr. Andres (M.D.) .... www.pathfinder.com/drweil
   A leader in integration of Western and alternative medicine. Teaches at
   and is founder of the Program in Integrative Medicine at the of Arizona
   Health Sciences Center in Tucson.

> > < <

NOTE: On some web browsers, you must add http:// to the front of all www addresses. Many of the web sites in Part IV have links to other sites that support less-toxic living.

Index

A

~ ~ ~

Notes

Use the space provided on the following three pages to list additional products that you have found to be less-toxic, and where they can be obtained. If you find products that you think will be beneficial to others, please let us know about these products so we can consider them for our next edition. Our mailing address is Optimum Publishing, P.O. Box 7435, Texarkana, TX 75505. Our e-mail address is gorman@optimumpublishing.com.

Updates

(Please note the following changes and additions as of May 1, 2002)

Information Changes

Canary Fashion Inc. - p. 204 (phone out of service)
Crown City Mattress - p. 204 (new phone) ... (800) 365-6563/(626) 452-8617
Diamond Organics - p. 204 (new phone) .... (888) 674-2642
Golden Furniture Maker - p. 208 (going out of business)
Nigra Enterprizes - p. 214 (out of business)
Superior Mattress Co. - p. 218 (phone out of service)
ThermoPly Storm Bracing - p. 116 (original only- must have foil on 2 sides
     - may not be tolerated by all)
Vita-Wave Perms – p. 177 (may not be tolerated by the chemically sensitive)

New Organizations, Web Resources & Resorts

CARES (p. 232) .... (719) 742-3310 or (866) 742-3310
     (Chemical Awareness, Research, Education & Solutions)
     PO Box 852, LaVita, CO 81055
     www.toxicfree.org e-mail: toxicfree@rmi.net
Linda Chae (MCS educational website) (p. 242) .... www.lindachae.com
"MCS" Beacon of Hope Foundation (p. 234) .... (843) 462-2681
     Peggy Trojano, Exec. Director
     56 Beidler Forest Rd., Dorchester, SC 29437
     e-mail: mcsbeaconofhope@yahoo.com
Pride and Joy Environmental Resort (add to p. 225) .... (321) 733-7804
     5685 S. A1A, Hwy. South Melbourne Beach, FL 32951
     www.pridejoyresort.com e-mail: info@pridejoyresort.com

New Products & Resources

A Beautiful Bed (p. 159) .... (800) 990-5519
     (silk and lambswool sheets and bedding) .... www.abeautifulbed.com
All Organic - links to organic foods and products .. www.allorganiclinks.com
Aluma-Foil (Vapor barrier – p.115) .... (800) 421-5947
     Advanced Foil Systems, Inc. .... www.afs-foil.com
     820 S. Rockefeller Ave. Ste. A, Ontario, CA 91761
Between the Sheets (pure silk sheets p. 159) ... 0044-1249-821517 (from US)
     18 Calne Business Centre, Harris Rd., Caine, Wiltshire, SN11 9PT, U.K.
     www.betweenthesheets.co.uk e-mail: info@betweenthesheets.co.uk
Duct Cleaning - power vac (consult your physician before anything is applied)
     Blackmon Mooring - www.blackmonmooring.com (for local dealers)
     Stanley Steemer - www.stanleysteemer.com (for local dealers)
ETEX Limited (Electrogun - p. 196) .... (702) 364-5911
     3200 Polaris Ave., Las Vegas, Nevada 89102 ... e-mail: etex1@aol.com
Healthguard Adhesive (p. 119) .... (706) 277-9767 or (800) 397-4583
     W.F. Taylor Co., 3601 South Hwy. 41 Dalton, GA 30720
     www.wftaylor.com

Leggett & Platt Inc. (Metal box springs p. 158) .... (972) 875-8401
    4100 South Interstate Highway 4, Ennis, TX 75119
Less EMF Inc. (p. 163, 165) .... (518) 392-1946 or (888) LESS EMF
    (Various EMF shield products including fabrics, garments, monitors, etc.)
    26 Valley View Ln., Ghent, NY 12075
    www.lessemf.com e-mail: lessemf@lessemf.com
Mosquito Guard (p. 191) & Tick Guard (p. 199) - for animals or humans
    Available at www.drugstore.com
        Or David Fingar .... (631) 725-6068 / fax (631) 725-8558
    www.tickcontrol.com e-mail: danjeta@optonline.net
Mosquito Repellant (p. 191) – rub catnip on your clothing
Rasco Bedding Co. - Makes & Bakes Mattresses (p. 158) ..... (903) 675-3145
    1515 W. Corsicana St., Athens, TX 75751
Sew Eco-Logical (Fabrics - p. 163) .... (541) 683-5828
    1280-B E. 28th Ave., Eugene OR 97403
    Fabrics and notions for clothing and home (including upholstery)
    www.seworganic.com e-mail: info@seworganic.com
Silicon Mask (HEPA or charcoal inserts - p. 112) Gempler
Steelcraft Mfg. Co. (metal kitchen cabinets - p. 113) .... (718) 277-2404
    352 Pine St., Brooklyn, NY 11208
Termi-Mesh Florida LLC (termites - p. 195) .... (407) 265-0665
    1660 N. County Rd. 427, Longwood FL 32750 ...... fax (407) 265-0982
    www.termi-mesh.com (termite-proofing mesh for new construction)
Termidor (p. 196) - certified providers by zip code - www.termidorhome.com
Thermal Life® Far Infrared Sauna – poplar wood saunas (p. 122)
    High Tech Health, Inc. .... (303) 413-8500 or (800) 794-5355
    2695 Linden Dr., Boulder, CO 80304 .... Fax: (303) 449-9640
    www.hightechhealth.com e-mail: billj@hightechhealth.com
WM Zinsser & Co. (Bin sheetrock & wood sealant - p. 121) . (732) 649-5000
    301 Cottontail Ln., Somerset, NJ 08873

New Organic Food & Seed Resources

Coleman Natural Beef & Coleman Lamb
    For a distributor near you – www.colemannatural.com
The Cook's Garden (organic seeds) .... (800) 457-9703 / Fax: (800) 457-9705
    PO Box 5010, Hodges, SC 29653-5010
    www.cooksgarden.com e-mail: info@cooksgarden.com
Petaluma Poultry .... (707) 763-1904 / (800) 556-6789
    For distributors in your area contact:
    P.O. Box 7368, 2700 Lakeville Hwy., Petaluma, CA 94955-7368
    www.healthychickenchoices.com or www.petalumapoultry.com
Sow Organic Seeds .... (888) 709-7333
    PO Box 527, Williams, OR 97544
    www.organicseed.com   e-mail: organic@organicseed.com

> > < <

Other Books by Carolyn Gorman

AT-CH-YOU!
(The Pollen and Dust Handbook)

This is an excellent resource for those who suffer
from pollen and mold allergies. It helps you determine
what plants and trees grow in your region during what seasons,
and can help you make decisions regarding where to live
based on the common regional pollens.

> > < <

FUNiGUS

FUNiGUS describes different types of mold, mildew and fungus;
where they are located; and the various types of reactions they produce.
This book includes treatment options and guidelines
for reducing mold exposure in your environment.

> > < <

OUR FRAGILE WORLD

This book is written for the family and
friends of people who suffer from Environmental Illness (EI)
and Multiple Chemical Sensitivities (MCS).
It helps them understand EI and MCS,
how these conditions originates,
the disease processes, and various treatment options.

> > < <

BOBBY & MARY LEARN ABOUT ALLERGIES
(A Children's Color & Learn Book)

This is a fun-filled learning experience that helps children
learn about allergies and how to deal with them.
It is full of coloring and activity pages;
plus it includes a story about an allergic child
written on a child's level, and a parent's resource section.
Illustrated by Brian Steward

(Limited quantity available - we will not be reprinting this book)

Order Form

Please make a copy of this form.
Print the following information.
Then send with a check or money order to:

OPTIMUM PUBLISHING

P.O. Box 7435, Texarkana, TX 75505-7435

(Please allow 2 to 3 weeks for delivery. Thank you.)

❏ Please send me the following:

___ copies *Less-Toxic Alternatives* .... @ $18.00 ea. . $ _____

___ copies *AT-CH-YOU!* .... @ $10.00 ea. . $ _____

___ copies *FUNiGUS* .... @ $ 6.00 ea. . $ _____

___ copies *Our Fragile World* .... @ $ 6.00 ea. . $ _____

___ copies *Bobby & Mary* (closeout) ...... @ $ 3.00 ea. . $ _____

TOTAL FOR BOOKS .... $ _____

Shipping & Handling (10% - $3.00 minimum) .... $_____

Sales Tax (in Texas add 8.25%) .... $_____

TOTAL ENCLOSED (Check or Money Order) ...... **$** _____

Name _____

Address _____

City _____ State ____ Zip _____

E-Mail Address _____

❏ Please put me on the mailing list for information about future offers.

Mrs. Gorman's books can be purchased from a number of book stores,
health food stores, and physicians.
They may be ordered direct from Optimum Publishing.
Or they can be ordered on the web at www.optimumpublishing.com.

Meet the Authors

Mrs. Carolyn Gorman is a health educator, widely recognized in the field of environmental medicine and allergies. She is a member of the *American Public Health Association* and the *New York Academy of Sciences*. Mrs. Gorman received a Master's Degree in Health Education from Texas Woman's University in Denton, Texas, and has been actively involved in clinical and environmental health education in the Dallas area for the past 20 years.

She has appeared on numerous local and national television and radio shows, and has served as a resource for many newspaper and magazine articles. Her speaking engagements include classroom appearances and regional panel discussions on environmental health, ecology, pollution, and corrective measures. She has also addressed medical conventions on the importance of patient education and healthy choices for everyday living.

Mrs. Gorman is the author of books and booklets for the chemically sensitive, allergic, environmentally ill, and those concerned about protecting our environment. Her books include *Less-Toxic Alternatives* (formerly titled *Less-Toxic Living*), *At-Ch-You*, *Our Fragile World*, *FUNiGUS,* and *Bobby & Mary Learn About Allergies (A Children's Color & Learn Book)*. She is also co-author *of The Mother Earth Handbook.*

Ms. Marie Hyde has a master's degree in Journalism from North Texas State University in Denton. She has written and edited many articles, newsletters and business publications; and has served as editor for books on a variety of subjects. She served as Mrs. Gorman's editor on the last four editions of *Less-Toxic Living*, as well as on most of her other publications.

They first met while Ms. Hyde was experiencing severe health problems due to environmental sensitivities. The two have tested many of the less-toxic alternatives in this book. They know that an environmentally sensitive individual can, indeed, live a healthier life while avoiding many of the toxins that plague our world today.

Mrs. Gorman and Ms. Hyde can be contacted through Optimum Publishing. P.O. Box 7435, Texarkana, TX 75505. You may send them e-mail messages at gorman@optimumpublishing.com.

> > < <